Advances in Exercise Adherence

ROD K. DISHMAN, PhD
University of Georgia
Editor

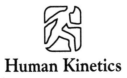

Human Kinetics

Library of Congress Cataloging-in-Publication Data

Dishman, Rod K.
    Advances in exercise adherence / Rod K. Dishman.
        p.   cm.
    Includes index.
    ISBN 0-87322-664-X
    1. Exercise. 2. Health behavior. 3. Patient compliance.
    I. Title.
    RA781.D548   1994
    613.7'1--dc20   93-47608
                                                                    CIP

ISBN: 0-87322-664-X

Developmental Editor: Larret Galasyn-Wright
Assistant Editors: Ed Giles, Julie Lancaster, Dawn Roselund, Anna Curry, Matt Scholz, and Dawn Barker
Copyeditor: Mary Weaver
Proofreader: Karin Leszczynski
Indexer: Joan K. Griffitts
Typesetter: Angela K. Snyder
Text Designer: Keith Blomberg
Cover Designer: Keith Blomberg
Printer: Edwards

Printed in the United States of America   10   9   8   7   6   5   4   3

Human Kinetics
Web site: http://www.humankinetics.com/

United States: Human Kinetics, P.O. Box 5076, Champaign, IL 61825-5076
1-800-747-4457
e-mail: humank@hkusa.com

Canada: Human Kinetics, 475 Devonshire Road, Unit 100, Windsor, ON N8Y 2L5
1-800-465-7301 (in Canada only)
e-mail: humank@hkcanada.com

Europe: Human Kinetics, P.O. Box IW14, Leeds LS16 6TR, United Kingdom
+44 (0)113-278 1708
e-mail: humank@hkeurope.com

Australia: Human Kinetics, 57A Price Avenue, Lower Mitcham, South Australia 5062
(08) 82771555
e-mail: humank@hkaustralia.com

New Zealand: Human Kinetics, P.O. Box 105-231, Auckland Central
09-523-3462
e-mail: humank@hknewz.com

Contents

Contributors

Tom Baranowski, PhD	Emory University Atlanta, Georgia
Steven N. Blair, PED	Cooper Institute for Aerobics Research Dallas, Texas
Kelly D. Brownell, PhD	Yale University New Haven, Connecticut
Karen J. Calfas, PhD	San Diego State University San Diego, California
Carl J. Caspersen, PhD, MPH	Centers for Disease Control Atlanta, Georgia
Guy Dirkin, PhD	United HealthCare Corporation Minnetonka, Minnesota
Rod K. Dishman, PhD	University of Georgia Athens, Georgia
Robert J. Donovan, PhD	University of Western Australia Nedlands, Western Australia
Gaston Godin, PhD	Laval University Quebec, Quebec
Han C.G. Kemper, PhD	Vrije Universiteit and Universiteit of Amsterdam Amsterdam, The Netherlands
Deborah Kendzierski, PhD	Villanova University Villanova, Pennsylvania
Abby C. King, PhD	Stanford University School of Medicine Stanford, California
Barbara J. Long, MD	San Diego State University San Diego, California
Bess H. Marcus, PhD	The Miriam Hospital and Brown University School of Medicine Providence, Rhode Island
Egil W. Martinsen, MD	Central Hospital of Sogn og Fjordane Forde, Norway
Robert K. Merritt, MS	Centers for Disease Control Atlanta, Georgia

Neville Owen, PhD

University of Adelaide
Adelaide, South Australia

Ralph S. Paffenbarger, Jr., MD, DrPH

Stanford University School of Medicine
Stanford, California

Nola J. Pender, PhD, RN

University of Michigan
Ann Arbor, Michigan

James O. Prochaska, PhD

University of Rhode Island
Kingston, Rhode Island

James F. Sallis, PhD

San Diego State University
San Diego, California

Roy J. Shephard, MD, PhD, DPE

University of Toronto
Toronto, Ontario
and Brock University
St. Catherine's, Ontario

Thomas Stephens, PhD

Thomas Stephens & Associates
Manotick, Ontario

Wendell C. Taylor, PhD, MPH

The University of Texas Health
    Science Center
Houston, Texas

Robert D. Weathers, EdD

Seattle Pacific University
Seattle, Washington

Christine L. Wells, PhD

Arizona State University
Tempe, Arizona

Denise E. Wilfley, PhD

Yale University
New Haven, Connecticut

Preface

Interest in exercise adherence has remained high since the 1988 publication of our initial book, *Exercise Adherence: Its Impact on Public Health. Healthy People 2000*, the national health promotion and disease prevention objectives in the United States for the year 2000, includes understanding the determinants of physical activity as an important area that needs more research. Since 1988, several scientific and professional consensus meetings sponsored by governments in Great Britain, Canada, and the United States have focused on the problem of understanding and increasing leisure-time physical activity. Interest in exercise adherence continues to grow in Europe and Australia. Theory has become more sophisticated, the research base continues to grow at an accelerating rate, and strategies for interventions to increase physical activity are now better studied and understood in ways that enhance their implementation and potential effectiveness.

In short, the problems and prospects outlined in our first book reflect many of the directions that have led research and practice during the past 6 years. About 30 doctoral dissertations and many more master's theses have addressed exercise adherence since 1988. Material from the first book is appearing in undergraduate textbooks, and the topic makes local and national news. But other things haven't changed. You still can't index exercise adherence: In my experience, the specificity and sensitivity of a computerized literature search on exercise adherence remain at about 10%.

There have indeed been advances in exercise adherence, both in the quantity and quality of theory and research and in interventions designed to increase and maintain physical activity. We now understand more fully that the exercise programs of the 1980s will not increase participation. We have learned that theories designed to increase interest in being active will not directly explain why well-intentioned people remain inactive or return to inactivity even after periods of successful exercise. We have seen that though many interventions can be accompanied by modest increases in physical activity, they may be short-lived without permanent changes in other circumstances that impede sustained activity.

Exercise as a behavior is best studied in the context of public health, we have discovered, but its determinants probably differ in a number of important ways from other health-related behaviors. Finally, though our theory and methods have become more sophisticated, no marked increase in leisure physical activity has occurred in industrialized nations during the past decade. Understanding and changing exercise adherence will require a mass action by scientists and professionals from many fields who have common interests in physical activity and public health.

Exercise adherence is not the domain of a single field. *Advances in Exercise Adherence* is dedicated to fueling efforts by scientists and practitioners in exercise science and sports medicine, preventive medicine, health psychology and behavioral medicine, epidemiology, nutrition, health promotion, rehabilitative medicine, communication and marketing sciences, and public policy—to name a few professional fields. But this diversity requires a single source to describe, integrate, and stimulate research and practice in exercise adherence, which is the undergirding purpose of this second book. Exercise adherence is not a North American problem alone. This book makes the first small step toward a more multicultural, multinational perspective. I wish more were known about ethnic, cultural, and gender aspects of exercise adherence to permit greater inclusiveness.

Because this book is intended as a sequel or companion to *Exercise Adherence*, the structure and topics are similar. Some original material and many new authors provide fresh perspectives of the knowledge that has accumulated. New topics, such as exercise adherence for older persons, weight loss, and international trends in physical activity patterns, reflect areas that were of great interest in 1988 but now have more mature knowledge. More attention has been devoted to children. We even include chapters on computers and marketing.

The trend toward studies of community- and population-based samples has increased generalizability beyond the largely clinical literature on North American caucasians that was surveyed for the 1988 book. Studies of African-Americans, Latino-Americans, and groups from countries other than the United States and Canada have appeared. Yet studies of children, older persons, women, ethnic minorities, and persons with physical disabilities are still relatively rare.

In many instances it is instructive to constrast the newer perspectives of this book with their counterparts from the 1988 volume. Methods used to measure physical activity and determinants in population studies of exercise adherence have not improved much. Some issues of theory remain unresolved or inadequately studied. And, despite some applications of new theory to exercise adherence, we need much more theory on maintenance of physical activity and relapse, rather than variations on old themes relating to the decision to start an exercise program. The debates over optimal and minimal types and amounts of physical activity for promoting health and adherence are more focused now than in 1988, but they are still unresolved by compelling evidence. The continuing need for a better blending of theory-driven research with the practical problems facing exercise professionals is painfully clear.

All in all, *Advances in Exercise Adherence*, combined with its predecessor, verifies a sustained but inadequate scholarly and professional interest in the fundamental questions still facing all who study and promote physical activity, exercise, and fitness for the benefit of the public's health: why people exercise and what good it does them.

Credits

Table I.1 is from "The Public Health Burden of a Sedentary Lifestyle" by J.M. McGinnis, 1992, *Medicine and Science in Sports and Exercise,* **24**, p. S197. Copyright 1992 by Williams & Wilkins Publishers. Reprinted by permission.

Table I.3 is from "Predicting and Changing Exercise and Physical Activity: What's Practical and What's Not" by R. Dishman. In *Toward Active Living: Proceedings of the International Conference on Physical Activity, Fitness, and Health* (pp. 97-106) by H.A. Quinney, L. Gauvin, and A.E.T. Wall (Eds.), 1994, Champaign, IL: Human Kinetics. Copyright 1994 by Human Kinetics Publishers, Inc. Reprinted by permission.

Table 1.2 is adapted from information appearing in *The New England Journal of Medicine,* "Physical Activity and Longevity of College Alumni" by R.S. Paffenbarger, Jr., R.T. Hyde, A.L. Wing, and C.C. Hseih, 1986, **315**, pp. 400-401 (letter). Adapted by permission.

Figure 3.12 is from "Leisure-Time Physical Activity in Scotland: Trends 1987-1991 and the Effect of Question Wording" by D.G. Uitenbroek and D.V. McQueen, 1992, *Sozial und Praventivmedizin,* **37**, pp. 113-117. Copyright 1992 by Birkhäuser Verlag AG. Adapted by permission.

Figure 4.1 is from "Sociobehavioral Determinants of Compliance With Health Care and Medical Care Recommendations" by M.H. Becker and L.A. Maiman, 1975, *Medical Care,* **13**, pp. 10-24. Copyright 1975 by J.B. Lippincott Co. Reprinted by permission.

Figure 4.2 is from *Understanding Attitudes and Predicting Social Behavior* (p. 8) by I. Ajzen and M. Fishbein, 1980, Englewood Cliffs, NJ: Prentice Hall. Copyright 1980 by Prentice Hall, Inc. Adapted by permission.

Figure 4.3 is from *Interpersonal Behavior*, p. 133, by H.C. Triandis. Copyright © 1977 by Wadsworth Publishing Company, Inc. Reprinted by permission of Brooks/Cole Publishing Company, Pacific Grove, CA 93950; and from "Use of Attitude-Behavior Models in Exercise Promotion" by G. Godin and R.J. Shephard, 1990, *Sports Medicine,* **10**, pp. 103-121. Copyright 1990 by Adis International Ltd. Adapted by permission.

Figure 4.4 is from *Understanding Attitudes and Predicting Social Behavior* (p. 100) by I. Ajzen and M. Fishbein, 1980, Englewood Cliffs, NJ: Prentice Hall; Copyright 1980 by Prentice Hall. Adapted by permission. "The Theory of Planned Behavior: Some Unresolved Issues" by I. Ajzen. In *Organizational Behavior and Human Decision Processes* (Vol. 50); a special issue on "Theories of Cognitive Self-Regulation" by E.A. Locke (Ed.), 1991. Copyright 1991 by the Academic Press. Adapted by permission; and "Prediction of Goal-Directed Behavior: Attitudes, Intentions, and Perceived Behavioral Control" by I. Ajzen and T.J. Madden, 1986, *Journal of Experimental Social Psychology,* **22**, pp. 453-474. Copyright 1986 by Academic Press. Adapted by permission.

Figure 5.1 and Table 5.2 are from "Exercise Self-Schemata: Cognitive and Behavioral Correlates" by D. Kendzierski, 1990, *Health Psychology,* **9**, pp. 69-82. Copyright 1990 by Lawrence Erlbaum Associates, Inc. Reprinted by permission.

Table 7.1 and 7.4 are from "Community Intervention for Promotion of Physical Activity and Fitness" by J.O. Holloszy, 1991, *Exercise and Sport Sciences Reviews,* **19**, pp. 247, 250. Copyright 1991 by Williams and Wilkins. Reprinted by permission.

Figure 8.1 is reprinted in part from the 1994 revised version of the Physical Activity Readiness Questionnaire (PAR-Q & YOU) by special permission from the Canadian Society for Exercise Physiology, Inc. Copyright © 1994, CSEP, Inc.

Figure 11.1 is from *Exercise and Children's Health* (p. 35) by T.W. Rowland, Champaign, IL: Human Kinetics. Copyright 1990 by Thomas W. Rowland. Reprinted by permission.

Introduction: Consensus, Problems, and Prospects

Rod K. Dishman

Understanding the knowledge, attitudes, and behavioral and social skills associated with adopting and maintaining regular exercise is a research need identified by *Healthy People 2000*, the U.S. national health promotion and disease prevention objectives for the year 2000 (U.S. Department of Health and Human Services, Public Health Service, 1991). Similar policies for understanding and increasing physical activity in other nations have appeared in the past few years (Fitness Canada, 1991; National Heart Foundation of Australia, 1985; Sports Council of Great Britain, 1990). An accelerated research agenda for understanding exercise adherence is timely because physical activity is a priority area for health promotion in *Healthy People 2000* (see Table I.1) and because the American Heart Association now recognizes physical inactivity as a major independent risk factor for coronary heart disease (Fletcher et al., 1992).

This introduction provides an overview of the knowledge and investigative methods that characterize the contemporary study of exercise adherence, with suggestions for future research and applications. First I summarize a recent review of literature on determinants and interventions that Jim Sallis and I conducted for a scientific consensus meeting held by the International Conference on Physical Activity, Fitness and Health (Bouchard, Shephard, & Stephens, 1994). The consensus reached at this meeting is generally consistent with that from a similar meeting, the U.S. National Heart, Lung, and Blood Institute (NHLBI) Workshop on Physical Activity and Cardiovascular Health (Sopko, Obarzanek, & Stone, 1992). Next I summarize a recent evaluation of the progress made since 1988 in understanding the determinants of physical activity when compared with earlier scientific consensus. This summary is supplemented with the key research recommendations from the International Conference on Physical Activity, Fitness and Health and the NHLBI workshop. Throughout, and at the conclusion of the chapter, I note how the chapters that follow address the theoretical and methodological issues raised in the current scientific consensus or how they are intended to bear on our recommendations for future research and application.

This book is limited to studies of exercise or physical activities consistent with definitions conventionally used in public health (Caspersen, Powell, & Christenson, 1985). Planning for participation, initial adoption of physical activity, continued

1

Table I.1   Physical Activity Objectives for the United States

Core objective	2000 target	Baseline
Health status		
Deaths from coronary heart disease	≤ 100 per 100,000	135 per 100,000
Overweight	≤ 20% of adults	26% age 20-74
Risk reduction		
Regular physical activity	≥ 30% age 6+	22% age 18+
Vigorous physical activity	≥ 20% age 18+	12% age 18+
Sedentary lifestyle	≤ 15% age 6+	24% age 18+
People ≥ age 65	22%	43%
People with disabilities	20%	35%
Strength/Flexibility activity	≥ 40% age 6+	Unknown
Overweight reduction	≥ 50% age 12+	< 30% age 18+
Services and protection		
Daily school physical education	≥ 50% grades 1-12	36% grades 1-12
Physical education time exercising	≥ 50% class time	27% class time
Worksite fitness programs	≥ 50% worksites 250-749 employees	32% worksites
Outdoor fitness trails	≥ 1 per 10,000 people	1 per 71,000 people
Routine counseling on exercise	≥ 50% primary care providers	30% providers

Reprinted from McGinnis (1992).

participation, or maintenance, and overall periodicity of participation (e.g., relapse, resumption, and seasonal variation) are characteristics of physical activity that require study. Relatively few direct comparisons of gender and studies of children, of people over age 65, of people with activity limitations, and of ethnic and minority groups, have been published. This fact makes it difficult to draw conclusions about how determinants in these cases may differ from general observations.

For the International Conference on Physical Activity, Fitness and Health, Jim Sallis and I (Dishman & Sallis, 1994) reviewed 33 studies on the determinants of physical activity and 20 intervention studies published since 1988, when *Exercise Adherence: Its Impact on Public Health* (Dishman, 1988a) was published. The studies sampled community and clinical groups, used various estimates of physical activities of differing intensities, and employed cross-sectional or prospective designs. Some studies reported multiple dependent measures or multiple subgroups of subjects. I will summarize here the tabular presentation of findings that can be obtained elsewhere (Dishman, 1994; Dishman & Sallis, 1994).

Determinants

We concluded that the studies generally had improved in concept and method compared with the literature before 1988 (Dishman, 1991; Dishman, Sallis, &

Orenstein, 1985). A limitation of earlier studies was their questionable generalizability to a population base because they were limited to clinical or other samples that were conveniently recruited. We found that 24 of 33 studies since 1988 used community samples, not samples from exercise programs, and 26 studies included men and women. The community-based studies included representative national samples from Australia (Bauman, Owen, & Rushworth, 1990; Owen & Bauman, 1992) and Canada (Stephens & Craig, 1990). Sample subjects ranged from high school students to people over age 65. People with low income and from minority groups were included in some studies. Nearly half of the studies (15 of 33) used a prospective, as opposed to a cross-sectional, design. Thus, whereas none of the studies permitted the causal inferences permitted by experimental research, the temporal sequence of assessing the independent variables (i.e., determinants) before the dependent variables (i.e., physical activity) provides more compelling directions for causal hypotheses than was true of earlier work. Prospective studies observed periods from several weeks to many years, permitting an estimate of the persistence of the relationships observed. The more persistent a relationship over time, the more likely it is to be causal. Also, much of the reduction in risk for chronic diseases in adulthood likely depends on frequent activity over many years. Thus, it is particularly important to understand what determines long-term physical activity. Although they have not been conducted, long-term prospective studies following children into adulthood, as well as retrospective studies of older adults retracing their activity histories, have particular promise for examining factors related to lifelong participation.

Another improvement in studies of determinants since 1988 has been an increase in the application of multidimensional theoretical models and assessment batteries. The study of multiple determinants recognizes the complexity of personal and cultural influences on physical activity and permits comparisons between determinants. This approach also provides directions to guide interventions that may need to be specialized for individuals or groups. It is necessary to understand the superiority of various determinants and theoretical models for predicting and explaining physical activity in order to increase the precision with which interventions can be applied.

Still, very few studies have empirically contrasted determinants or theories for predicting physical activity in the same sample of people. Most studies of determinants have ignored the well-known problem of measuring physical activity in a population base (Ainsworth, Montoye, & Leon, 1994; LaPorte, Montoye, & Caspersen, 1985). A continuing limitation of the determinants research is that virtually all studies focus on the maintenance versus dropout phase or do not discriminate between maintenance and adoption or the overall periodicity of activity patterns. Only a few studies since 1988 have addressed the problem of adoption (Kendzierski, 1990; Sallis, Hovell, & Hofstetter, 1992; Stephens & Craig, 1990). Because of the substantial number of sedentary adults in the population, it is essential to understand the determinants of physical-activity adoption. It may be that, as observed for long-term success in smoking cessation and weight loss, success in maintaining physical activity depends on repeated adoption or resumption of activity following periods of inactivity.

Theory for Physical Activity Determinants Research

In 1988 nine theoretical models were discussed that appeared relevant for understanding psychological influences on physical activity (Dishman, 1990). Some other relatively new models have been studied during the past 5 years. Studies of self-schemata (Kendzierski, 1988, 1990), social-cognitive theory (Dzewaltowski, 1989), and the transtheoretical, or stages of change, model (Marcus, Selby, Niaura, & Rossi, 1992), are discussed in this book. Bandura's (1986) social-cognitive theory assumes that personal factors, environmental events, and behavior function as interacting and reciprocal determinants. Bandura indicates that self-change operates via personal cognitive self-reactions stimulated by an internal process of comparing personal goals or standards and knowledge of personal attainment. Bandura and Cervone (1986) reported that individuals experiencing optimal motivation were dissatisfied with substandard performance, adopted challenging goals, and were confident (i.e., had high self-efficacy) in attaining those goals. Self-reactions to goals may interact with perceptions of self-efficacy to determine exercise motivation.

Another model, personal-investment theory (Tappe, Duda, & Menges-Ehrnwald, 1990), also has recently been applied to the study of exercise behavior. It is not yet clear how the key components of personal-investment theory differ from those of the other cognitive models that are all rooted in expectancy and goal-setting. The social-ecology framework (Stokols, 1992) can be applied to the study of social and physical environment influences on physical activity, but to my knowledge it has not been used.

An encouraging but rare sign for advancing more refined conceptualizations of physical activity is the publication of studies that directly contrast theoretical formulations. I know of three studies that involved comparisons with Ajzen and Fishbein's (1980) social psychological theory. In one comparison, a similar model that included past exercise was slightly more effective at predicting exercise than Ajzen and Fishbein's theory (Valois, Desharnais, & Godin, 1988). Two short-term studies indicated that social-cognitive theory, including self-efficacy ratings, was significantly more effective in predicting exercise than the Ajzen and Fishbein theory (Dzewaltowski, 1989; Dzewaltowski, Noble, & Shaw, 1990). More studies that compare theories are needed. Although it is interesting to contrast similar theories (see Figure I.1), from the standpoint of implementing interventions, it may be more useful to contrast very different theories.

Most social psychology models of the determinants of behavior recognize that ability moderates the impact of social and psychological variables on behavior (e.g., Ajzen, 1985), or such models posit the relationships among their variables on the assumption of equal ability among individuals. Because physical activity is a biologically based behavior, we must understand the role of genetic and biologic influences (e.g., maturation during childhood; Duncan & Duncan, 1991) on physical activity, as they may interact with or modify social and psychological determinants. Recent Canadian data suggest an important familial or heritable component of physical activity (Perusse, Leblanc, & Bouchard, 1988). In a study

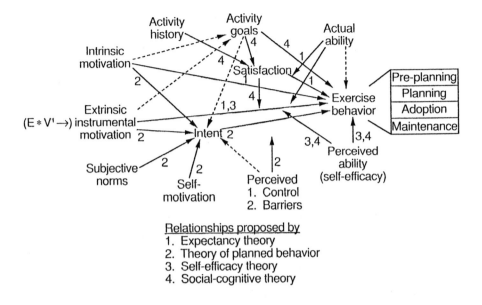

Figure I.1   Possible path relationships for competitive tests of components of popular decision theories applied to physical activity. Hypothesized causal connections between components are shown as solid lines leading from explanatory variables to endogenous, or dependent, variables (e.g., arrow connecting *Intrinsic motivation* and *Intent*). Hypothesized moderator effects are shown as solid lines connecting the moderator and the relationship that is hypothesized to be moderated (e.g., the line connecting *Satisfaction* and the line from *Extrinsic instrumental motivation* to *Exercise behavior*). E * V is the interaction of outcome-expectancy with outcome value or valence. Hypothesized mediator effects are shown as solid lines connecting the mediator and its hypothesized effect (e.g., Intent mediates the proposed influence of *Subjective norms* and *Exercise behavior*). Numbers adjacent to hypothesized effects refer to the theoretical model from which they stem. Broken lines represent other possible relationships not directly proposed by the theoretical models.

of family aggregation in a sample of more than 1,300 people, approximately 20% of the variation in daily physical activity was attributable to genetically transmissible factors (Perusse, Tremblay, Leblanc, & Bouchard, 1989).

Advances in the Measurement of Determinants

Most determinants of studies have used either unvalidated measures of potential determinants or general-purpose measures borrowed from the study of behaviors other than physical activity. Recently, investigators have begun to develop specific measures of potential determinants and to evaluate their reliability and validity. Measures of the following constructs have been reported:

- Physical self-perception (Fox & Corbin, 1989)
- Physical-activity enjoyment (Kendzierski & DeCarlo, 1991)
- Expected outcomes and barriers for physical activity (Marcus et al., 1992; Steinhardt & Dishman, 1989)
- Locus of control for physical-fitness behaviors (Whitehead & Corbin, 1988)
- Social support (Robbins & Slavin, 1988; Sallis, Grossman, Pinski, Patterson, & Nader, 1987)
- Self-efficacy (Sallis, Pinski, Grossman, Patterson, & Nader, 1988)

The proliferation of measures of psychological variables requires that researchers apply some degree of standardization. Better discriminant and convergent evidence for the validity of measures and their underlying constructs is needed to permit clear contrasts between social-cognitive variables such as outcome-expectancy values and self-perceptions. When different measures of the same purported construct are used, researchers may not be able to replicate the studies' findings. Also, there is a need to reconcile redundant measures before competing theoretical models of exercise behavior can be tested directly, for example, by structural models.

A number of potential environmental influences on exercise behavior have also been assessed, mainly by self-report. This can be a problem because the results of objective measures (e.g., distance from facilities) may differ from self-assessments (Sallis, Hovell, Hofstetter, Elder, Hackley, et al., 1990).

The Conundrum of Measuring Physical Activity

Despite advances in both theory and interventions in research on the determinants of physical activity and exercise during the past 5 years, concomitant advances have not occurred in the standardization of measurement technologies used in population-based surveys or intervention studies. The problem of measuring physical activity has received wide attention by researchers in public health (Ainsworth et al., 1994; LaPorte et al., 1985), but it has been ignored by those studying determinants of and interventions in physical activity. Nearly all the evidence supporting the theoretical models discussed in this book comes from self-reports of physical activity. The concurrent validity of the various self-reports has not been established (see Table I.2). We recently reported that the relationship between social-cognitive variables and self-reported free-living physical activity did not generalize to physical activity estimated by an electromechanical accelerometer (Dishman, Darracott, & Lambert, 1992). Because evidence for the validity of the activity self-reports used in past studies is weak or unreported, it is difficult to compare studies that do not agree or to conclude that our understanding of the determinants of free-living physical activity has advanced.

Determinants of Moderate Versus Vigorous Physical Activity

The growing evidence for the health benefits of moderate-intensity physical activity led the U.S. Public Health Service (U.S. Department of Health and

Table I.2 Free-Living Physical-Activity Assessment

Assessment procedure	Subject costs		Interference	Acceptability		Activity specifics
	Time	Effort		Personal	Social	
Calorimetry:						
Direct	VH	H-VH	H-VH	No	No	Yes
Indirect	VH	M-VH	H-VH	No	No	No
Surveys:						
Indirect calorimetry diary	M-H	M-H	VH	No	No	Yes
Task-specific diary	H-VH	VH	VH	?	Yes	Yes
Recall questionnaire	M-H	M-H	L	Yes	Yes	Yes
Quantitative history	L-M	L-M	L	Yes	Yes	Yes
Physiologic markers:						
Cardiorespiratory fitness	M-H	M-VH	L	?	?	No
Doubly-labeled water	M	M	L-H	Yes	Yes	No
Mechanical and electronic monitors:						
Heart rate	M-H	M-H	L-M	Yes	Yes	No
Pedometers	L	L	L-M	Yes	Yes	No
Electronic motion sensors	L	L	L-M	Yes	Yes	No
Accelerometers	L	L	L-M	Yes	Yes	No

Data from Ainsworth et al. (1994) and LaPorte et al. (1985).

Human Services, Public Health Service, 1991) and the American College of Sports Medicine (1990) to recommend that the public engage in regular moderate-intensity (as opposed to high-intensity) activity. The rationale for these recommendations and their potential impact is discussed in chapter 1 by Blair, Wells, Weathers, and Paffenbarger. However, few studies have directly examined differences between the patterns and determinants of moderate- and high-intensity physical activity (see chapter 3 by Caspersen, Merritt, & Stephens). Walking is the most commonly reported form of moderate-intensity activity (Stephens & Craig, 1990), but the absence of validated self-report measures of walking hinders research in this area.

Studies indicate that light, moderate, and vigorous leisure physical activities may be influenced by different factors. As noted in chapter 3, a decline in total leisure physical activity with advancing age is not seen for vigorous activities (e.g., ~60% of maximum METs) in people over age 65. Studies reporting separate analyses for moderate-intensity activities have noted increased levels of such activity with increasing age (Hovell et al., 1989; McPhillips, Pellettera, Barrett-Connor, Wingard, & Criqui, 1989; Stephens & Craig, 1990). Although men are found to have higher levels of total and vigorous activity, in at least two studies women reported more walking (Hovell et al., 1989; Stephens & Craig, 1990). In one community sample, psychological and social variables related to walking tended to have the same associations as those observed for vigorous exercise (Sallis et al., 1989), but they accounted for much less of the variance in walking. This might be explained by errors in measuring walking.

Studies are needed to determine the influence of injury and participants' subjective responses to it as determinants for adopting or maintaining physical activity. Injury is a reason commonly reported for stopping an exercise program (Sallis, Hovell, Hofstetter, Elder, Faucher, et al., 1990), but it is not known whether a person's history of injury or the expectation of future injury is a direct influence on adoption or resumption of an exercise program. Prospective studies are needed. Cross-sectional relationships between injury and physical activity can be misleading if people's exposures (i.e., total activity) are not equated, because the cross section of time will not determine whether or when a person resumes activity.

Determinants of Adoption Versus Maintenance of Physical Activity

Previous reviews (Dishman, 1990; Sallis & Hovell, 1990) have emphasized the need to distinguish between adoption, maintenance, and resumption of physical activity. I know of only one study that specifically assessed influences on resumption of exercise after dropout (Sallis, Hovell, Hofstetter, Elder, Faucher, et al., 1990), and it suggested that multiple episodes of dropout and resumption are common. Some progress has been made recently in research on adoption of physical activity. Factors that would motivate sedentary people to adopt have been reported (King, C.B. Taylor, Haskell, & DeBusk, 1990). Sedentary college students who perceived themselves as exercisers (self-schemata) stated they were likely to adopt exercise soon (Kendzierski, 1990) (see chapter 5 by Deborah Kendzierski). Adoption of vigorous exercise by a community sample of sedentary men during a 2-year period was predicted by self-efficacy, age (negative), and neighborhood environment. Adoption by women was predicted by level of education, self-efficacy, and friend and family support for exercise (Sallis et al., 1992).

Summary of Physical Activity Determinants Literature

Demographic variables continue to be associated with physical activity, but some could be considered selection biases rather than causal determinants. Education, income, male gender, and age (negative) are consistent correlates of physical-activity habits. Non-Hispanic whites appear to be more active than members of other ethnic groups, but it is difficult to separate the effects of ethnicity and socioeconomic status.

Nearly 20 cognitive variables have been studied since 1988. Among these, self-efficacy has received the most support as a determinant. The lack of prospective studies that control for physical activity habits before a cross-sectional observation, however, limits our confidence in the observed relationship between self-efficacy and activity and whether it is causal or reflects a selection effect. That is, active individuals report high self-efficacy because of past success due to factors other than self-efficacy. Self-schemata, self-motivation, outcome-expectancy values, perceived barriers, and intention to exercise have been reliably associated with physical activity in both community samples and supervised exercise programs. Knowledge about physical activity and health has not been reliably related to activity.

Physical activity during adulthood consistently predicts future activity, but no compelling evidence exists that activity patterns in childhood or early adulthood predict physical activity later in life. Likewise, other health-related behaviors, including smoking, are not usually related to overall leisure physical activity.

Social influences on physical activity have received little study. Social support from family and friends has consistently been related to physical activity in cross-sectional and prospective studies. Family influences on social-cognitive mediators of physical activity are discussed in chapter 12 by W.C. Taylor, Baranowski, and Sallis. Clinical anecdotes support the importance of group dynamics in reinforcing attendance at supervised programs, so more studies of group influences are needed.

Many environmental factors could influence physical activity, but few have been studied. The relationships reported between such factors and physical activity have been weak. The validity of assessing environmental factors by self-report is unknown. Objectively measured access to facilities, but not perceived access, has repeatedly been related to physical activity. Standardized measures are needed.

Despite earlier recommendations (Dishman, 1988b), little research has been conducted since 1988 on how characteristics of physical activity influence participation. Intensity of and perceived exertion during physical activity seem negatively related to participation, but there are not enough population-based studies on these topics to permit this conclusion. Assessing the intensity of physical activity is perhaps the most difficult of the many problems inherent in measuring physical activity in population samples (Ainsworth et al., 1994). Scales for perceived exertion have been validated as a substitute for measuring relative oxygen consumption for short-term incremental exercise but not for use in population studies (Dishman, in press).

Interventions

For the International Conference on Physical Activity, Fitness and Health, I conducted a quantitative meta-analysis of 20 studies done since 1988 of interventions to increase physical activity (Dishman, 1994; Dishman & Sallis, 1994). Results were transformed to a correlation coefficient (r) according to procedures outlined by Friedman (1968) and Rosenthal (1984). Consistent with Cohen's method (1977), population values of r approximating 0.01, 0.30, and 0.40 can be regarded as small, moderate, and large, respectively. Because it is useful to view the results of interventions in terms of success rates, r effects can be presented as binomial effect sizes (BES), report Rosenthal and Rubin (1982). BES can be interpreted as a measure of an intervention's success, that is, the change in the percentage of exercise adherents in the experimental group compared with that of a control group. A zero binomial effect size reflects a 50-50 chance of success. This approximates the median success rate, absent a behavior-change intervention, for supervised exercise programs involving both healthy adults and coronary heart disease patients.

The interventions, regardless of tradition or content, were usually associated with small to moderate effect sizes (i.e., r's ~ 0.15-0.20) for frequency of physical activity, with binomial effect sizes suggesting that exercise programs with success rates (based on attendance) approximating 40% might have increased success, to about 60%, with a behavioral intervention. The impact on changes in intensity and duration of physical activity is less clear. Since the size of these effects is comparable to those found for reduced intensity, duration, and frequency of exercise prescription in fitness-training studies for white males (Pollock, 1988), the superiority of behavior-change interventions over modifications in traditional fitness programming should be directly tested.

The following conclusions seem supported by the analysis summarized in Table I.3:

• Studies typically found that health education and behavior-modification or cognitive-behavior-modification principles could be implemented with exercise

Table I.3 Behavior-Change Interventions 1988-1992 (20 studies, 61 effects)

	Education counseling	Behavior modification	Behavior modification/ Cognitive-behavior modification	Exercise dose
Type	0.18 ± 0.25	0.23 ± 0.21	0.19 ± 0.28	0.14 ± 0.05
Activity measure	Self-report 0.14 ± 0.18	Heart rate 0.19 ± 0.20	Treadmill time 0.29 ± 0.20	$\dot{V}O_2$peak 0.02 ± 0.11
Study design	Randomized 0.17 ± 0.20	Non-equivalent control 0.17 ± 0.28	Uncontrolled cohort 0.41 ± 0.16	0.20 ± 0.24

Note. Summary of a meta-analysis of behavior-change interventions for exercise and physical activity from 1988 to early 1992. Effect sizes are presented as mean (unweighted by sample size) correlation coefficients ± standard deviations for different types of interventions, activity measures, and study designs. The value in the lower-right-hand corner represents the mean correlation for all 20 studies. Reprinted from Dishman (1994).

programs and were accompanied by increased frequency or time spent in the activity for limited periods.

• With the exception of studies closely linked with on-site programs or periodic supervision (e.g., worksites, clinics, schools), the studies did not demonstrate that exercise intensity or total activity was increased enough to increase physical fitness or reduce risk for morbidity or mortality.

• The quasi-experimental or uncontrolled designs used in about half of the literature limit conclusions about the causal nature of the increased physical activity that accompanied the interventions.

• Most studies have used indirect measures of physical activity (e.g., self-report) or indirect estimates of physical fitness based on heart rate or treadmill time. The validity of these methods for measuring physical activity was not established. Only a few studies attempted to verify self-reports of activity with expected increases in fitness (e.g., $\dot{V}O_2$peak, weight loss, heart rate). The effect size for increased fitness when $\dot{V}O_2$peak was measured was typically small, even when the effects for self-reported activity were large. Effects for self-reported physical activity appear larger (0.14 ± 0.18) than effects for changes in $\dot{V}O_2$peak (0.02 ± 0.11).

• The strength of scientific inference over the causal influence of an intervention depends on the research design used. The quality of designs used in exercise studies ranges from high (fully randomized) to moderate (matched or nonequivalent control group) to low (cohort study without a control group). Before 1988 most intervention studies used uncontrolled case and cohort designs (Dishman, 1991). Since 1988 most studies have used randomized or quasi-experimental designs with large samples of males and females of varying ages and thus offer more internal validity and generalizability. In general, the size of effects is inversely associated with the scientific quality of the study. The effect size for uncontrolled studies (0.41 ± 0.16) was twice that of randomized or quasi-experimental studies. The effect of the several interventions based on health education and fitness testing was comparable to that of behavior modification and cognitive-behavior modification. However, the scientific quality of most studies that have reported an effect of health education and fitness testing on exercise behavior has been weak.

Uncontrolled case and quasi-experimental multiple baseline studies published before 1988 commonly reported increases of 50% to 200% (Dishman, 1991). Because the baseline physical activity levels were low, however, the increased activity typically fell short of the frequency, duration, and intensity required to increase physical fitness (American College of Sports Medicine, 1990) and may not have reached the level of fitness (Blair et al., 1989) or the amount of increase in leisure physical activity (Paffenbarger et al., 1993) required to optimally decrease risk for disease morbidity or all-cause mortality. (See chapter 1 by Blair, Wells, Weathers, & Paffenbarger.) Only about half the studies reported a follow-up to the intervention, and they typically showed that increases in physical activity or fitness associated with the interventions diminished over time.

Before 1988 most interventions with physical activity and exercise lacked a compelling conceptual basis beyond simple behavior-modification principles. The relapse prevention model described by Dorothy Knapp (1988) in the first version of this book has received additional support since 1988 (King, Carl, Birkel, & Haskell, 1988; King, Frey-Hewitt, Dreon, & Wood, 1989; King, Haskell, C.B. Taylor, Kraemer, & DeBusk, 1991). Since then, however, it has become clearer that behavior change appears dependent upon the individual's readiness for change. The transtheoretical model (Prochaska & DiClemente, 1985) has recently been applied to physical activity. Prochaska and Marcus discuss this application in chapter 6. The transtheoretical model has been widely used to clarify the stages individuals progress through and the cognitive and behavioral processes they use while changing smoking behavior. The model proposes that individuals engaging in new behavior move through the stages of precontemplation, contemplation, preparation, action, and maintenance. Movement through these stages does not always occur in a linear manner and may be cyclical, as many individuals make several attempts at behavior change before reaching their goals. The processes of change are the cognitive, affective, and behavioral strategies people use as they progress through the stages of change, and those strategies are presumably unique to each stage of change. Process-oriented interventions targeted to individuals' specific stage of change may accelerate the adoption and maintenance of physical activity.

Since 1988 most studies have employed intervention packages, not single techniques, that have incorporated the following:

- Goal-setting based on initial fitness and desired outcomes
- Identifying personal costs and expected barriers to adoption and maintenance of an activity
- Developing strategies for eliminating or minimizing the impact of barriers to participation and for increasing support and reinforcement from friends, family, and housemates
- Planning a gradual progression of difficulty to optimize success and facilitate self-efficacy so clients have growing confidence in their physical ability to be active and to maintain the new pattern of activity
- Offering feedback from fitness testing and clients' self-monitoring of activity and progress
- Developing clients' personal strategies for returning to activity after inactivity due to flagging motivation, injury, vacation, and so forth.

It is not clear which components of the interventions are essential or are the most influential. Also, because of the research designs used, most of the studies have not provided compelling evidence that the components of the interventions were independently effective beyond social support and reinforcement.

Until 5 years ago most intervention studies used one-dimensional approaches with small numbers of people who were homogeneous in gender, race, ethnicity, health status, and economic and educational status. Recently, community-based interventions have applied psychological and behavioral theories for behavior change (King et al., 1992). These approaches go beyond the traditional practice of individual counseling and may include changes at organizational levels (community recreation centers, churches, diffusion strategies through schools), environmental levels (e.g., facility planning), and social (e.g., family interventions) levels. On the other hand, they may use cost-effective or convenient methods (e.g., mailings, telephone calls) for reaching large numbers of individuals who might not be reached by or amenable to traditional clinically based interventions. Examples of such interventions are discussed in chapter 7 by Abby King, and their application within the context of social marketing is described in chapter 10 by Donovan and Owen. Chapter 9 by Guy Dirkin illustrates how computers and telecommunication systems can be used to augment mediated interventions targeted toward increasing and maintaining leisure physical activity.

Future Directions

In 1988 (Dishman, 1988b) I evaluated the progress and priorities of the recommendations made by the 1984 Workshop on Epidemiologic and Public Health Aspects of Physical Activity and Exercise, sponsored by the U.S. Department of Health and Human Services (Powell & Paffenbarger, 1985). Jim Sallis and I recently provided our view of the progress made toward these recommendations, based on research and events since 1988 (Dishman & Sallis, 1994), for the International Conference on Physical Activity, Fitness and Health:

• The conceptualization and ranking of determinants according to their priority has not been achieved. Progress has been made, however, in identifying some strong and consistent correlates of physical activity. The demographic variables of age, education, gender, and socioeconomic status continue to be supported as determinants. Cognitive variables have been extensively studied, but only perceived barriers (negative), intention to exercise, mood disturbance (negative), perceived health or fitness, and self-efficacy have consistently been related to physical activity. The only behavioral variable predictive of current physical activity is activity level in the recent past. Social support from family and peers is also predictive of physical activity. Too few data on physical environmental influences (e.g., climate, access to facilities or parks) have been reported to allow the priority of these variables to be reliably estimated. Perceived exertion, or exercise intensity, is usually inversely related to physical activity participation.

Little or no progress has been made in identifying and ranking the interactions of personal attributes and environments as they influence physical activity. This remains a priority for the advancement of theory and the selection of effective interventions for different population segments and physical-activity settings, but it cannot occur until available theories are directly compared or remodeled based on analyses of data from large population-based studies or large-sample clinical studies.

Progress has been made in identifying cognitive factors and interventions that influence the planning and adoption of physical activity (Godin & Shephard, 1990; see chapter 4 by Gaston Godin) and in clarifying the effectiveness of behavioral and cognitive-behavioral interventions designed to increase and maintain physical activity (Dishman, 1991). The most effective components of these interventions, however, have yet to be identified. The relative importance, additivity, or interaction of population-based promotions of physical activity (based on social-cognitive and educational models) versus clinical interventions (based on principles of behavior modification or cognitive-behavior modification) requires study.

• Little or no progress has been made in understanding how determinants differ according to age, race, gender, ethnicity, socioeconomic level, health status, and fitness level or in identifying who is most likely to benefit from various intervention approaches. Research has increased in these areas, however, and they remain priorities.

Progress has been made in clarifying differences and similarities between determinants of moderate leisure physical activity and vigorous exercise related to fitness in supervised and free-living settings (Hovell et al., 1989; Sallis et al., 1986). Progress has also been made toward establishing that sport history (Dishman, 1988c) and age (Powell & Paffenbarger, 1985) are probably selection-bias effects, not true causes of contemporary inactivity. Family and peer influences, socioeconomic status, and education level may be selection-bias effects, but they have potential as true determinants. Their study remains a high priority.

Physical activity has not consistently been associated with other health behaviors. Although correlations may exist between physical activity and other health behaviors when variability within an individual is considered, variations between individuals for most health behaviors do not appear to be explained by variation in physical activity (Norman, 1986). This suggests that generalized health-behavior theories or interventions will not be useful for exercise applications when they focus on a population over a short time. Experimental or prospective studies are a high priority for deciding whether general or physical activity-specific theories and interventions are most effective for studying and increasing physical activity.

• Little or no progress has been made in understanding how perceptions and preferences for types and intensities are formed and whether they influence participation. This remains a high priority for free-living physical activity and for adoption in supervised leisure settings. Activity preferences may be less important for supervised exercise adherence, when activities vary and intensity is based on initial fitness level, but absolute intensity is still likely to be important.

Little or no progress has been made in understanding whether determinants and dispositions for physical activity differ at definable life stages. It does appear, however, that inactivity associated with age can be reversed with appropriate interventions (King et al., 1991; Powell & Paffenbarger, 1985). This priority has grown in importance because of the increase in elderly populations and a lack of evidence that schools have increased children's leisure physical activity (Iverson, Fielding, Crow, & Christenson, 1985).

Progress has been made in showing that stages in physical activity include planning, adoption, maintenance, and periodicity and that determinants may differ for each stage. (See chapter 6 by Prochaska & Marcus.) Decision-based theories and interventions appear helpful for increasing planning and adoption. Integrating decision theories with social-marketing strategies offers an important direction for future research and applications. (See chapter 10 by Donovan & Owen.) In addition, social support, self-motivation, self-regulatory skills, and interventions such as relapse prevention seem necessary for individuals to maintain or resume a physical-activity pattern. The origin and time course for intrinsic reinforcement of physical activity remains unknown, but understanding the process of personal motivation for physical activity remains a high priority for facilitating the success of public-health promotion. More studies using qualitative methods are encouraged in this area (e.g., Gauvin, 1989). Interaction among the fields of education, medicine, exercise science, behavioral science, public health, and public policy must be accelerated. Biologically oriented theories of reinforcement should receive more research attention, and more must be known about genetically transmissible dispositions toward physical activity and inactivity.

In addition, future studies must consider the unique cultural, economic, and political differences between nations. Theoretical models, evolving from ideologies that place responsibility on the self to effect behavior change (e.g., most of the decision theories studied in exercise settings), have less potential to explain or predict physical activity when social and environmental factors do not facilitate personal decision-making or direct personal control of behaviors such as exercise as a result of cultural or economic restraints. These concerns also apply to disadvantaged segments of the population in affluent societies.

The preceding recommendations were summarized and submitted for peer consensus by a subcommittee of the International Conference on Physical Activity, Fitness and Health (Bouchard et al., 1994). The subcommittee agreed upon the following research needs.

Research Needs for Determinants

- Determinants research should focus on personal and environmental variables that can be manipulated and applied in interventions. When feasible, findings from observational studies should be verified in experimental research. Genetic and biological influences on physical activity also need to be understood.

- Determinants and their relative importance are likely to vary for different populations, population subgroups, and cultures. Such differences should be investigated. Which determinants of physical activity do people of different sexes, ages, ethnic groups, education levels, and geographic locations share, and which determinants differ?

• More and better studies are needed of the determinants of various dimensions of physical activity—particularly activity of different intensities and types—and of sedentary behaviors.

• More studies are needed of the determinants for adoption of regular physical activity. Continued study of adherence, long-term maintenance, and relapse is also recommended.

• Determinants studies should use valid measures of physical activity and of potential determinants that are comparable across studies. Objective measures of environmental determinants should be developed.

Research Needs for Interventions

• The primary need is for the development and evaluation of effective approaches that encourage the adoption and long-term maintenance of physical activity. Personal, environmental, and physical activity characteristics found to be important in observational studies should be targeted in intervention research. Although interventions should be tailored to specific populations, subpopulations, and cultures, the means of tailoring are not well developed. Face-to-face interventions, suited for clinically based applications, should be compared with mediated interventions (e.g., through television, telephone, and mail) suited for population-based applications, to determine their relative effectiveness. Methods for documenting and improving the quality of intervention implementation (e.g., program leadership) should be studied.

• Interventions have disproportionately emphasized change in personal attributes (e.g., attitudes, intentions, self-efficacy) among exercise participants, but the interventions' effectiveness at changing such attributes is not established. Interventions that target variables in the social and physical environments should be evaluated.

• Valid measures should be developed for assessing the experiences and outcomes of physical activity that can reinforce participation and minimize relapse.

• There is a need to determine the types, intensities, durations, locations, social settings, and times of physical activity that may encourage its adoption and maintenance.

• Different measures of physical activity used in intervention studies should be standardized or reconciled.

A similar consensus was reached by working groups studying the determinants of physical activity and interventions in adults (King et al., 1992) and youth (Sallis, Simons-Morton, et al., 1992) at the National Heart, Lung, and Blood Institute's national meeting titled Physical Activity and Cardiovascular Health: Special Emphasis on Women and Youth. The groups' key recommendations called for

- better assessment tools that can provide detailed information on physical activity and its determinants;
- identification of appropriate interventions for various subgroups, including women, older people, minorities, and groups of varying states of health through the systematic exploration of cognitive, behavioral, psychological, developmental, social, and environmental determinants of physical activity;
- identification of effective intervention techniques to increase physical activity in children; and
- strategies for increasing the likelihood of active lifestyle behaviors that begin during childhood and can be carried into adulthood. The two key periods of interest are those when physical-activity levels typically decline: early adolescence and the transition between late adolescence and young adulthood (Sopko et al., 1992).

We hope that the chapters that follow accurately present the major contemporary approaches that address some of the consensus groups' key recommendations. This book has four parts:

- Exercise Adherence and Public Health
- Theory and Determinants of Physical Activity
- Interventions for Adoption and Maintenance
- Special Applications

The first section, Exercise Adherence and Public Health, provides an update of the expanding knowledge base from exercise epidemiology and clinical science. It focuses on the persistent debate over the dose-response requirements of physical activity and fitness adaptations for decreasing premature mortality (Blair, Wells, Weathers, & Paffenbarger, chapter 1, Chronic Disease: The Dose-Response Controversy) and depression and anxiety (Martinsen & Stephens, chapter 2, Exercise and Mental Health in Clinical and Free-Living Populations). These chapters integrate the authors' pioneering research with analyses and overviews of the extant empirical evidence. Collectively, their conclusions justify the public-health importance of understanding and increasing participation in leisure physical activity. The issue of a therapeutic dose of physical activity is also fundamental for studies of the determinants of participation, as such determinants may differ across levels of participation. Caspersen, Merritt, and Stephens describe current activity trends in Australia, Canada, Finland, and the United States in chapter 3, International Physical Activity Patterns: A Methodological Perspective. Physical activity trends provide a backdrop for targeting population segments for interventions to increase physical activity and for evaluating the effectiveness of such interventions. The tutorial provided on exercise epidemiology and the interpretation of surveillance data have broad implications for study of the determinants of leisure physical activity and for evaluation of the impact of the approaches described in several of the chapters that follow.

The second section, Theory and Determinants of Physical Activity, substantially expands previous coverage of the theoretically driven research on exercise adherence. Original investigators provide summaries of sustained research programs carried out since 1988 on the predictive validity of various decision theories for understanding exercise behavior. In chapter 4, Social-Cognitive Models, Gaston Godin describes his important research, which has spurred advances in the application of established theories of attitude, self-perception, and intention to our understanding of physical activity and exercise. Deborah Kendzierski describes her innovative work in chapter 5, Schema Theory: An Information Processing Focus. Her recent findings suggest that perception of oneself as an active or inactive person affects the way one perceives and appraises information about exercise and physical activity. These observations seem relevant to social-cognitive influences (discussed in chapters 4 and 12) and interventions (discussed in chapters 7, 8, & 10) designed to educate and persuade people about the benefits of being physically activity. Chapter 6, The Transtheoretical Model: Applications to Exercise, by Prochaska and Marcus, provides an overview of a benchmark approach that has proven effective for understanding relapse and the stages of successful behavior change in smoking cessation, weight loss, and psychotherapy. Instruments have been developed to measure the processes and stages of exercise adoption and maintenance and the related constructs of exercise-specific self-efficacy and decision-making. Studies applying the transtheoretical model with employees in the United States and Australia are discussed, along with observational and intervention studies designed to help researchers understand and increase the adoption of physical activity in community settings.

Part III, Interventions for Adoption and Maintenance, provides a broad but detailed view of current interventions designed for implementation in clinical and community settings (chapter 7, Clinical and Community Interventions to Promote and Support Physical Activity Participation, by Abby King) and the health-care environment (chapter 8, Health-Care Provider Counseling to Promote Physical Activity, by Pender, Sallis, Long, & Calfas). In chapter 7 King discusses her successful applied-research program at the Stanford Center for Research in Disease Prevention within a comprehensive review of behavior interventions. In chapter 8 Nola Pender and colleagues build a strong argument for the importance of health-care providers in initiating and supporting exercise behavior change. They describe project PACE as an example for practical implementation by health-care and exercise professionals of many of the ideas described in chapters 4, 6, and 7. Guy Dirkin provides a practically oriented and forward-looking discussion of using computers and telecommunication systems to monitor and support behavioral interventions for increasing and maintaining physical activity in chapter 9, Technological Supports for Sustaining Exercise. These chapters are followed by an insightful and comprehensive tutorial on social-marketing approaches to health-behavior change that focuses on community or population campaigns for exercise (chapter 10, Social Marketing and Population Interventions, by Donovan & Owen). Each chapter in this section offers many examples of how the theory discussed in Part II can be used to design, implement, and evaluate interventions for research and practical application.

In Part IV, Special Applications, physical activity and its determinants are discussed for population segments that are of growing interest to preventive medicine and public health. Han Kemper presents original findings from community-based research on youth in the Netherlands in chapter 11, The Natural History of Physical Activity and Aerobic Fitness in Teenagers. The approach described illustrates the importance of biocultural aspects of maturation in studies of physical activity determinants in youth. Taylor, Baranowski, and Sallis discuss family influences on physical activity in chapter 12, Family Determinants of Childhood Physical Activity: A Social-Cognitive Model. Their chapter provides a clear example of the application of general theory within a critical and understudied social context. Roy Shephard extends the social-psychology perspective to older people in chapter 13, Determinants of Exercise in People Aged 65 Years and Older. Recent findings from Canada (Stephens & Craig, 1990) indicate that, compared with young adults, older people have a similarly positive attitude about physical activity but feel they have less control over being active and are concerned about injury; older men feel less at ease than older women about beginning an exercise program. Strikingly, about 50% of older Canadians who are not physically active have no intention of becoming active. Despite their view of physical activity as beneficial, it is not a high priority for their leisure time. These findings emphasize the potential usefulness for older people of the applications of social-cognitive theory discussed in chapter 13, as well as other decision theories and interventions discussed in the preceding chapters. The book is appropriately concluded by chapter 14, Physical Activity and Diet in Weight Loss, by Wilfley and Brownell. Their chapter addresses the fundamental link between exercise and weight-loss programs for both effective outcomes and behavior change. Special reference is made to obese people and those with eating disorders. The authors describe results from clinical, worksite, and community interventions and provide a unique integration of psychological and physiological perspectives. Like chapters 12 and 13, this chapter comprehensively applies theory and practice to a crucial but poorly understood aspect of physical activity and public health. The chapter's message strongly reinforces a theme of several preceding chapters: that achieving an understanding of the ways physical activity complements—and is like and unlike—other health-related behaviors is both the underlying goal and the challenge of the contemporary study of exercise adherence.

Since 1988 advances have been made in understanding healthful outcomes associated with physical activity and exercise (chapters 1, 2, and 14), that physical activity can be increased (chapters 3 and 7), and how cognitive variables may influence the adoption and maintenance of physical activity. Much of the original research on these topics has been conducted by several contributors to this book (see chapters 4, 5, and 6). The theoretical models that encompass the major cognitive variables are readily applicable with such special groups as youth (chapters 11 and 12) and older people (chapter 13), but applications must consider biocultural factors that differ according to age and maturation. Applications of existing theories are also easily extended to special contexts such as health-care settings (chapter 8); the family (chapter 12) and the home; worksites, schools, and the community and population (chapters 7, 9, 10, and 14).

Well controlled experimental studies of the effectiveness of interventions applied in these settings are few, however. Also, few experimental manipulations of environmental factors (e.g., facility access) and social-cognitive variables (e.g., intentions, self-efficacy) show that changes in these factors directly influence exercise behavior. Correlational studies of these variables usually have not discounted that their relationships with contemporary physical activity might be due wholly or in part to past physical activity habits. The lack of experimental evidence limits our conclusions about how much of the observed association of physical activity with environmental and cognitive determinants is causal and how much reflects a selection effect. Active individuals may report strong attitudes, self-efficacy, and intentions because of past success, but such success may have been the result of factors other than attitudes, self-efficacy, and intentions.

Personal counseling, education, and persuasion campaigns can increase knowledge of and change attitudes about physical activity and can use peer models to build self-efficacy among the inactive. The effectiveness of interventions at accomplishing these outcomes has not usually been demonstrated (Ewart, C.K. Taylor, Reese, & DeBusk, 1983). It is unlikely that population interventions will be perfectly effective in increasing cognitive variables, so the behavioral impact (i.e., effect sizes) estimates from correlational data will overestimate causal effects. As Donovan and Owen illustrate in chapter 10, it is more likely that the behavioral impact of interventions designed to influence knowledge and attitudes will markedly diminish at each successive step—from initial public awareness to changes in intention to volitional attempts to be active to successful maintenance.

Correlations between self-reports of physical activity and such social-cognitive variables as self-efficacy, attitudes, and intentions commonly approximate 0.40 to 0.50 (Duncan & McAuley, 1993; Dzewaltowski et al., 1990; Godin & Shephard, 1990). Expressed as a binomial effect size, a correlation of 0.50 suggests that a success rate of 25% in adopting or maintaining exercise under control conditions would increase to 75% following an intervention whereby attitudes, self-efficacy, or intentions were increased. But Donovan and Owen demonstrate in chapter 10 that the use of a media campaign to accomplish an increase in intentions typically produces a much smaller behavioral effect. If, as they illustrate, only 3% of a sedentary audience intended to become active as the result of a media campaign, the effect would nonetheless be important for the 3 in 100 people helped by the intervention. Their example indicates, however, that effect sizes estimated from correlational studies far overestimate the true causal effect implied by the predictive relationship.

Direct behavioral change may not be a reasonable standard for evaluating the practical effectiveness of population interventions. The effectiveness of education campaigns applied in a community or population may be more appropriately evaluated by the extent to which they change awareness of the importance of physical activity and increase attention to advice on beginning a safe and effective exercise program rather than by direct changes in physical activity. Support systems by professionals (discussed in chapters 7, 9, & 14) can augment education and persuasion approaches and can also provide direct prompts, feedback and strategies, and reinforcers.

Many recent interventions have recommended more diverse and lower intensity activities than were recommended by exercise professionals 5 years ago (Dishman, in press). It seems likely that this practice could increase participation among many population segments, and it is consistent with the body of evidence on physical activity's apparent protective effects against early death due to coronary heart disease and other causes (see chapter 1) and for mental health (see chapter 3). However, it remains to be demonstrated whether the prevalence of physical activity, energy expenditure, and healthy outcomes will be increased by recommendations of low-intensity physical activity.

Although important gains have been made in the development of interventions to promote increased physical activity, most of the research has focused on one-dimensional interventions involving small numbers of highly selected subjects. A potentially more powerful strategy involves applying a community approach to intervention that spans multiple levels of analysis (personal, interpersonal, organizational/environmental, institutional/legislative) and aims to reach diverse population segments. In chapter 7 Abby King describes the application of psychological and behavioral theory to levels of intervention that extend beyond face-to-face counseling by a health or exercise professional to include organizational, environmental, and population-based settings. Several of these applications, as well as those Prochaska and Marcus discuss in chapter 6, promote the use of more economical or convenient avenues for reaching large numbers of inactive people. Specific examples are presented of community-based interventions for physical activity promotion in which strategies derived from social-cognitive theory and relapse prevention have been implemented, using convenient mediated delivery of the intervention (e.g., by telephone and mail). Several extensions of these ideas are proposed—using computers and telecommunication systems (see chapter 9) and marketing principles (see chapter 10). All these approaches are ripe for practical application and scientific evaluation.

Finally, much more must be learned about combining physical activity interventions with interventions designed to alter other health-related behaviors. Although correlational data have shown little association between physical activity and most other health behaviors (Norman, 1986), the clinical and community-based evidence Wilfley and Brownell discuss in chapter 14 suggests that pairing physical activity with diet not only enhances the outcome of weight loss and maintenance but may also increase adherence to both the diet and the physical activity plan. Because physical activity and the complex biological and psychological components underlying weight loss and maintenance may share several behavioral mechanisms, this chapter serves as a fitting conclusion for the book as well as a possible springboard for new approaches to understanding and changing physical activity.

References

Ainsworth, B.E., Montoye, H.J., & Leon, A.S. (1994). Methods of assessing physical activity during leisure and work. In C. Bouchard, R. Shephard, & T. Stephens (Eds.), *Physical activity, fitness, and health: International proceedings and consensus statement*. Champaign, IL: Human Kinetics.

Ajzen, I. (1985). From intention to actions: A theory of planned behavior. In J. Kuhl & J. Beckmann (Eds.), *Action-control: From cognition to behavior* (pp. 11-39). Heidelberg: Springer.

Ajzen, I., & Fishbein, M. (1980). Understanding attitudes and predicting social behavior. Englewood Cliffs, NJ: Prentice Hall.

American College of Sports Medicine. (1990). Position statement on the recommended quality and quantity of exercise for developing and maintaining fitness in healthy adults. *Medicine and Science in Sports and Exercise*, **22**, 265-274.

Bandura, A. (1986). *Social foundations of thought and action*. Englewood Cliffs, NJ: Prentice Hall.

Bandura, A., & Cervone, D. (1986). Differential engagement of self-reactive influences in cognitive motivation. *Organizational Behaviors and Human Decision Processes*, **38**, 92-113.

Baranowski, T., Bouchard, C., Bar-Or, O., Bricker, T., Heath, G., Kimm, S.Y.S., Malina, R., Obarzanek, E., Pate, R., Strong, W.B., Truman, B., & Washington, R. (1992). Assessment, prevalence, and cardiovascular benefits of physical activity and fitness in youth. *Medicine and Science in Sports and Exercise*, S240.

Bauman, A., Owen, N., & Rushworth, R.L. (1990). Recent trends and sociodemographic determinants of exercise participation in Australia. *Community Health Studies*, **14**, 19-26.

Blair, S.M., Kohl, H.W., Paffenbarger, R.S., Clark, D.G., Cooper, K.H., & Gibbons, L.W. (1989). Physical fitness and all-cause mortality: A prospective study of healthy men and women. *Journal of the American Medical Association*, **262**, 2395-2401.

Bouchard, C., Shephard, R., & Stephens, T. (Eds.) (1994). *Physical activity, fitness, and health: International proceedings and consensus statement*. Champaign, IL: Human Kinetics.

Caspersen, C.J., Powell, K.E., & Christenson, G.M. (1985). Physical activity, exercise, and physical fitness: Definitions, and distinctions for health-related research. *Public Health Reports*, **101**, 126-146.

Cohen, J. (1977). *Statistical power analysis for the behavioral sciences*. New York: Academic Press.

Dishman, R.K. (Ed.) (1988a). *Exercise adherence: Its impact on public health*. Champaign, IL: Human Kinetics.

Dishman, R.K. (1988b). Exercise adherence research: Future directions. *American Journal of Health Promotion*, **3**, 52-56.

Dishman, R.K. (1988c). Supervised and free-living physical activity: No differences in former athletes and non-athletes. *American Journal of Preventive Medicine*, **4**, 153-160.

Dishman, R.K. (1990). Determinants of participation in physical activity. In C. Bouchard, R.J. Shephard, T. Stephens, J.R. Sutton, & B.D. McPherson (Eds.), *Exercise, fitness, and health: A consensus of current knowledge* (pp. 75-101). Champaign, IL: Human Kinetics.

Dishman, R.K. (1991). Increasing and maintaining exercise and physical activity. *Behavior Therapy*, **22**, 345-378.

Dishman, R.K. (1994). Predicting and changing exercise and physical activity: What's practical and what's not. In H.A. Quinney, L. Gauvin, and A.E.T. Wall (Eds.), *Toward active living*. Champaign, IL: Human Kinetics.

Dishman, R.K. (in press). Prescribing exercise intensity for healthy adults using perceived exertion and exertional symptoms. *Medicine and Science in Sports and Exercise*.

Dishman, R.K., Darracott, C.R., & Lambert, L.T. (1992). Failure to generalize determinants of self-reported physical activity to a motion sensor. *Medicine and Science in Sports and Exercise*, **24**, 904-910.

Dishman, R.K., & Sallis, J.F. (1994). Determinants and interventions for physical activity and exercise. In C. Bouchard, R. Shephard, and T. Stephens (Eds.), *Physical activity, fitness, and health: International proceedings and consensus statement* (pp. 214-256). Champaign, IL: Human Kinetics.

Dishman, R.K., Sallis, J.F., & Orenstein, D. (1985). The determinants of physical activity and exercise. *Public Health Reports*, **100**, 158-171.

Duncan, T.E., & Duncan, S.C. (1991). A latent growth curve approach to investigating developmental dynamics and correlates of change in children's perceptions of physical competence. *Research Quarterly for Exercise and Sport*, **62**, 390-398.

Duncan, T.E., & McAuley, E. (1993). Social support and efficacy cognitions in exercise adherence: A latent growth curve analysis. *Journal of Behavioral Medicine*, **16**, 199-218.

Dzewaltowski, D.A. (1989). Toward a model of exercise motivation. *Journal of Sport and Exercise Psychology*, **11**, 251-269.

Dzewaltowski, D.A., Noble, J.M., & Shaw, J.M. (1990). Physical activity participation: Social cognitive theory versus the theories of reasoned action and planned behavior. *Journal of Sport and Exercise Psychology*, **12**, 388-405.

Ewart, C.K., Taylor, C.B., Reese, C.B., & DeBusk, R.F. (1983). Effects of early postmyocardial infarction exercise testing on self-perception and subsequent physical activity. *American Journal of Cardiology*, **51**, 1076-1080.

Fitness Canada. (1991). *Active living: A conceptual overview*. Ottawa, ON: Author.

Fletcher, G.F., Blair, S.N., Blumenthal, J., Caspersen, C., Chaitman, B., Epstein, S., Falls, H., Sivarajan Froelicher, E.S., Froelicher, V.F., & Pina, I.E. (1992). Statement on exercise: Benefits and recommendations for physical activity programs for all Americans. *Circulation*, **86**, 2726-2730.

Fox, K.R., & Corbin, C.B. (1989). The physical self-perception profile: Development and preliminary validation. *Journal of Sport and Exercise Psychology*, **11**, 408-430.

Friedman, H. (1968). Magnitude of experimental effect and a test for its rapid estimation. *Psychological Bulletin*, **70**, 245-251.

Gauvin, L. (1989). An experiential perspective on the motivational features of exercise and lifestyle. *Canadian Journal of Sport Sciences*, **15**(1), 51-58.

Godin, G., & Shephard, R.J. (1990). Use of attitude-behavior models in exercise promotion. *Sport Medicine*, **10**(2), 103-121.

Hovell, M.F., Sallis, J.F., Hofstetter, C.R., Spry, V.M., Elder, J.P., Faucher, P., & Caspersen, C.J. (1989). Identifying correlates of walking for exercise: An epidemiologic prerequisite for physical activity promotion. *Preventive Medicine*, **18**, 856-866.

Iverson, D.C., Fielding, J.E., Crow, R.S., & Christenson, G.M. (1985). The promotion of physical activity in the United States population: The status of programs in medical, worksite, community, and school settings. *Public Health Reports*, **100**, 212-224.

Kendzierski, D. (1988). Self-schemata and exercise. *Basic and Applied Social Psychology*, **9**, 45-61.

Kendzierski, D. (1990). Exercise self-schemata: Cognitive and behavioral correlates. *Health Psychology*, **9**, 69-82.

Kendzierski, D., & DeCarlo, K.J. (1991). Physical activity enjoyment scale: Two validation studies. *Journal of Sport and Exercise Psychology*, **13**, 50-64.

King, A.C., Blair, S.N., Bild, D., Dishman, R.K., Dubbert, P.M., Marcus, B.H., Oldridge, M., Paffenbarger, R.S., Powell, K.E., & Yaeger, K. (1992). Determinants of physical activity and interventions in adults. *Medicine and Science in Sports and Exercise*, **24**, S221-S236.

King, A.C., Carl, F., Birkel, L., & Haskell, W.L. (1988). Increasing exercise among blue-collar employees: The tailoring of worksite programs to meet specific needs. *Preventive Medicine*, **17**, 357-365.

King, A.C., Frey-Hewitt, B., Dreon, D.M., & Wood, P.D. (1989). Diet versus exercise in weight maintenance. *Archives of Internal Medicine*, **149**, 2741-2746.

King, A.C., Haskell, W.L., Taylor, C.B., Kraemer, H.C., & DeBusk, R.F. (1991). Group- versus home-based exercise training in healthy older men and women. *Journal of the American Medical Association*, **266**, 1535-1542.

King, A.C., Taylor, C.B., Haskell, W.L., & DeBusk, R.F. (1990). Identifying strategies for increasing employee physical activity levels: Findings from the Stanford/ Lockheed exercise survey. *Health Education Quarterly*, **17**, 269-285.

Knapp, D.N. (1988). Behavioral management techniques and exercise promotion. In R.K. Dishman (Ed.), *Exercise adherence: Its impact on public health* (pp. 203-235). Champaign, IL: Human Kinetics.

LaPorte, R., Montoye, H., & Caspersen, C. (1985). Assessment of physical activity in epidemiologic research: Problems and prospects. *Public Health Reports*, **100**(2), 131-146.

Marcus, B.H., Selby, V.C., Niaura, R.S., & Rossi, J.S. (1992). Self-efficacy and the stages of exercise behavior change. *Research Quarterly for Exercise and Sport*, **63**(1), 60-66.

McGinnis, J.M. (1992). The public health burden of a sedentary lifestyle. *Medicine and Science in Sports and Exercise*, **24**, S197.

McPhillips, J.B., Pellettera, K.M., Barrett-Connor, E., Wingard, D.L., & Criqui, M.H. (1989). Exercise patterns in a population of older adults. *American Journal of Preventive Medicine*, **5**, 65-72.

National Heart Foundation of Australia (1985). *Risk factor prevalence study* (No. 2-1983). Canberra, Australia: Author.

Norman, R.M.G. (1986). The nature and correlates of health behavior. *Health Promotion Studies Series* (No. 2). Ottawa, ON: Health and Welfare, Canada.

Owen, N., & Bauman, A. (1992). The descriptive epidemiology of physical inactivity in adult Australians. *International Journal of Epidemiology*, **21**, 305-310.

Paffenbarger, R.S., Hyde, R.T., Wing, A.L., Lee, I-Min, Jung, D.L., & Kampert, J.B. (1993). The association of changes in physical activity level and other lifestyle characteristics with mortality among men. *The New England Journal of Medicine*, **328**, 538-545.

Perusse, L., Leblanc, C., & Bouchard, C. (1988). Familial resemblance in lifestyle components: Results from the Canada Fitness Survey. *Canadian Journal of Public Health*, **79**, 201-205.

Perusse, L., Tremblay, A., Leblanc, C., & Bouchard, C. (1989). Genetic and familial environmental influences on level of habitual physical activity. *American Journal of Epidemiology*, **129**, 1012-1022.

Pollock, M.L. (1988). Prescribing exercise for fitness and adherence. In R.K. Dishman (Ed.), *Exercise adherence: Its impact on public health* (pp. 259-277). Champaign, IL: Human Kinetics.

Powell, K.E., & Paffenbarger, R.S., Jr. (1985). Workshop on epidemiologic and public health aspects of physical activity and exercise: A summary. *Public Health Reports*, **100**, 118-126.

Prochaska, J.O., & DiClemente, C.C. (1985). Common processes of self-change in smoking, weight control, and psychological distress. In S. Shiffman & T. Wills (Eds.), *Coping and substance use* (pp. 345-363). New York: Academic Press.

Robbins, S.R., & Slavin, L.A. (1988). A measure of social support for health-related behavior change. *Health Education*, **19**, 36-39.

Rosenthal, R. (1991). *Meta-analytic procedures for social research* (2nd ed.). Beverly Hills, CA: Sage.

Rosenthal, R., & Rubin, D.B. (1982). A simple, general purpose display of magnitude of experimental effect. *Journal of Educational Psychology*, **74**, 166-169.

Sallis, J.F., Grossman, R.M., Pinski, R.B., Patterson, T.L., & Nader, P.R. (1987). The development of scales to measure social support for diet and exercise behaviors. *Preventive Medicine*, **16**, 825-836.

Sallis, J.F., Haskell, W.L., Fortmann, S.P., Vranizan, K.M., Taylor, C.B., & Solomon, D.S. (1986). Predictors of adoption and maintenance of physical activity in a community sample. *Preventive Medicine*, **15**, 331-346.

Sallis, J.F., & Hovell, M.F. (1990). Determinants of exercise behavior. *Exercise and Sport Sciences Reviews*, **18**, 307-330.

Sallis, J.F., Hovell, M.F., & Hofstetter, C.R. (1992). Predictors of adoption and maintenance of vigorous physical activity in men and women. *Preventive Medicine*, **21**, 237-251.

Sallis, J.F., Hovell, M.F., Hofstetter, C.R., Elder, J.P., Faucher, P., Spry, V.M., Barrington, E., & Hackley, M. (1990). Lifetime history of relapse from exercise. *Addictive Behaviors*, **15**, 573-579.

Sallis, J.F., Hovell, M.F., Hofstetter, C.R., Elder, J.P., Hackley, M., Caspersen, C.J., & Powell, K.E. (1990). Distance between homes and exercise facilities related to frequency of exercise among San Diego residents. *Public Health Reports*, **105**, 179-185.

Sallis, J.F., Hovell, M.F., Hofstetter, C.R., Faucher, P., Elder, J.P., Blanchard, J., Caspersen, C.J., Powell, K.E., & Christenson, G.M. (1989). A multivariate study of determinants of vigorous exercise in a community sample. *Preventive Medicine*, **18**, 20-34.

Sallis, J.F., Pinski, R.B., Grossman, R.M., Patterson, T.L., & Nader, P.R. (1988). The development of self-efficacy scales for health-related diet and exercise behaviors. *Health Education Research*, **3**, 283-292.

Sallis, J.F., Simons-Morton, B.G., Stone, E.J., Corbin, C.B., Epstein, L.H., Faucette, N., Iannotti, R.J., Killen, J.D., Klesges, R.C., Petray, C.K., Rowland, T.W., & Taylor, W.C. (1992). Determinants of physical activity and interventions in youth. *Medicine and Science in Sports and Exercise*, **24**, S248-S257.

Sopko, G., Obarzanek, E., & Stone, E. (1992). Overview of the National Heart, Lung, and Blood Institute Workshop on physical activity and cardiovascular health. *Medicine and Science in Sports and Exercise*, **24**, S192-S195.

Sports Council of Great Britain (1990). *Sport, health, psychology, and exercise symposium*. London: Author.

Steinhardt, M.A., & Dishman, R.K. (1989). Reliability and validity of expected outcomes and barriers for habitual physical activity. *Journal of Occupational Medicine*, **31**, 536-546.

Stephens, T., & Craig, C.L. (1990). *The well-being of Canadians: Highlights of the 1988 Campbell's Survey*. Ottawa, ON: Canadian Fitness and Lifestyle Research Institute.

Stokols, D. (1992). Establishing and maintaining healthy environments: Toward a social ecology of health promotion. *American Psychologist*, **47**, 6-22.

Tappe, M.K., Duda, J.A., & Menges-Ehrnwald, P. (1990). Personal investment predictors of adolescent motivational orientation toward exercise. *Canadian Journal of Sport Sciences*, **15**, 185-192.

U.S. Department of Health and Human Services, Public Health Service. (1991). *Healthy people 2000: National health promotion and disease prevention objectives*. (DHHS Publication No. [PHS] 91-50212). Washington, DC: Government Printing Office.

Valois, P., Desharnais, R., & Godin, G. (1988). A comparison of the Fishbein and Ajzen and the Triandis attitudinal models for the prediction of exercise intention and behavior. *Journal of Behavioral Medicine*, **11**, 459-472.

Whitehead, J.R., & Corbin, C.B. (1988). Multidimensional scales for the measurement of locus of control of reinforcements for physical fitness behaviors. *Research Quarterly for Exercise and Sport*, **59**, 103-117.

Thanks to Jim Sallis for his collaboration on the reviews summarized here, to Charles Lance for his help in conceptualizing Figure 1, and to Donna Smith and Marlee Stewart for their help in preparing this manuscript.

PART *I*

Exercise Adherence and Public Health

CHAPTER *1*

Chronic Disease: The Physical Activity Dose-Response Controversy

Steven N. Blair
Christine L. Wells
Robert D. Weathers
Ralph S. Paffenbarger, Jr.

Does a lifetime of regular exercise decrease the incidence of chronic disease and increase longevity? Since antiquity the question has been debated by philosophers and physicians without resolution. Yet nearly everyone, scientists and laypeople alike, believes that regular exercise is important for optimal health. The literature on exercise and health has grown substantially over the past 20 years. Many randomized clinical trials now show that appropriate exercise programs may be expected to yield improvements not only in physical fitness but also in blood lipid levels, blood pressure, body composition, bone density, insulin sensitivity, and glucose tolerance. It seems reasonable to conclude that improvement in these clinical variables will lead to lower morbidity and mortality rates. Data supporting this conclusion are available but are primarily circumstantial. We do not have and probably will never have a randomized clinical trial of exercise as the primary factor for the prevention of chronic disease and premature mortality simply because of the complex logistics and enormous cost of such an undertaking. For the study to be truly definitive, researchers would need to randomly assign a large group of young people to a physically active lifestyle and a comparable group to a sedentary lifestyle. Potentially confounding variables, such as diet, stress, and smoking, would have to be strictly controlled. After several decades such a study probably would conclusively answer the exercise-health-longevity question, but only for the dose(s) of activity studied. Although such a study seems desirable, it is highly unlikely to occur and would probably be unethical. Of course, no randomized clinical trials have examined a lifetime of smoking and early death. But only fools (and perhaps the Tobacco Institute) suggest that the circumstantial evidence on smoking, disease, and mortality is too weak to draw causal conclusions from or to serve as a basis for action. Therefore, although the evidence linking exercise to chronic disease and premature death is less than perfect, it is reasonable to conclude that both are favorably affected by a lifetime of regular exercise.

Although it is widely accepted that appropriate activity exerts a positive influence on health and longevity, much less certainty exists about the quantification of appropriate exercise. Many who think regular exercise has health benefits probably define exercise as vigorous activity requiring a relatively high expenditure of energy. Aerobics classes, jogging, and cycling are prime examples of the types of activities that are popular and thought to be healthful. It now seems clear that important benefits can be obtained from moderate-intensity physical activity as well.

The principle of progressive overload is the guide for enhancing physical fitness, and Karvonen, Kentala, and Mustala (1957) made important early contributions to our understanding of training dose and fitness improvement. Cooper (1968) responded to requests for health-enhancing exercise prescriptions by presenting a point system based on intensity and duration of activity. The American College of Sports Medicine (ACSM) (1975) originally recommended average exercise intensities of at least 70% (60% to 70% initially) of maximal aerobic power for 20 to 40 minutes. Current ACSM guidelines (1991) recommend intensities as low as 40% of maximal aerobic power for 20 to 60 minutes—acknowledging that important health benefits and improvements in fitness may occur in some individuals with exercise of lower intensity. This chapter reviews selected classic and recent literature representing the growing body of evidence and the arguments supporting the relationships between physical activity and chronic disease, with special reference to the dose necessary for the desired effects.

All-Cause Mortality and Longevity

Table 1.1 shows the primary causes of death in the United States, with sex-specific, age-adjusted mortality rates. In 1980 the estimated life expectancies at birth were 71.8 years for men and 78.8 years for women. The age-adjusted death rates from all causes expressed per 100,000 people were 680 for men and 391 for women, yielding a sex ratio of 1.74. This means that men had a death rate almost 74% higher than women (Verbrugge & Wingard, 1987).

Excluding accidents (which rank third as a cause of death for males in the United States), the three leading causes of death for both men and women are diseases of the heart (primarily coronary heart disease), malignant neoplasms (cancer), and cerebrovascular diseases (primarily stroke). The sex ratios for these

Table 1.1   1980 Mortality Rates for the Leading Causes of Death in the United States

Cause of death	Age-adjusted mortality rate (per 100,000 population)			
	Males	Rank	Females	Rank
Diseases of the heart	206.7	1	108.9	1
Malignant neoplasms	166.3	2	112.7	2
Accidents	47.7	3	17.9	4
Cerebrovascular diseases	30.2	4	25.7	3
All causes	680.2	—	390.6	—

Data from Verbrugge and Wingard (1987).

chronic diseases range from 1.99 to 1.19, indicating that considerably more men than women die from all three.

Most investigations of physical activity and mortality have compared death rates of sedentary and active groups, and these findings are relevant to the relationship between physical activity and longevity. If sedentary individuals are more likely to die from diseases known to be the most common causes of death, longevity in that group will be decreased. Conversely, if active individuals are less likely to die from the primary causes of death, they will have increased longevity.

Physical Activity

Salonen, Puska, and Tuomilehto (1982) followed 3,978 men aged 30 to 59 years and 3,688 women aged 35 to 59 years from two counties in eastern Finland for seven years. Age-adjusted relative risks of death due to any disease in men were 1.9 for those with low physical activity at work and 1.5 for those with low physical activity at leisure. Corresponding values for women were 2.2 and 1.6, respectively.

Paffenbarger, Hyde, Wing, and Hsieh (1986a) followed 16,936 Harvard alumni for 16 years after they completed a mail survey on their exercise habits, including their usual walking, stair climbing, and sports participation. The exercise self-reports were converted to estimates of caloric expenditure and reported as kcal $\cdot$ week^{-1}. There was a steady decline in all-cause death rates across weekly caloric expenditure categories, from 94 per 10,000 man-years of follow-up in men who participated in less than 500 kcal $\cdot$ week^{-1} to 43 per 10,000 man-years in men in the 3,000 to 3,499 kcal $\cdot$ week^{-1} category. Men aged 35 to 79 years at baseline with less than 2,000 kcal $\cdot$ week^{-1} in exercise were compared with men with greater than or equal to 2,000 kcal $\cdot$ week^{-1}. The more active men gained 1.25 years of life up to age 80, compared with the sedentary men. Estimates

Table 1.2   Increased Longevity to Age 80 From Exercise Estimates From Harvard Alumni[a]

Baseline age (years)	Days exercising[b]	Days gained[c]	Hr gained/ hr of exercise[c]
40	260	507	1.95
50	195	438	2.25
60	130	339	2.61
70	65	161	2.47

[a]Exercise is defined as at least 2,000 kcal · week^{-1} obtained in 3 hr.
[b]Number of total days spent exercising from baseline age to age 80, if a person exercises 3 hr a week.
[c]Adjusted for blood pressure status, cigarette smoking, net gain in body mass index since college, and age of parental death.
Adapted from Paffenbarger et al. (1986b).

of gain in life compared to time the Harvard men spent exercising are shown in Table 1.2 (Paffenbarger, Hyde, Wing, & Hsieh, 1986b). For each hour spent exercising, Harvard alumni gain two hours in added life.

Physical Fitness

There are several problems inherent in the assessment of exercise habits. Present methods are imprecise and probably underestimate the true effect of exercise on mortality. Another way to address the exercise-mortality question is to use an assessment of physical fitness as a marker for exercise habits. Many mistakenly believe that physical fitness is primarily determined by genetic factors. This concept is not supported by recent work on the inheritance of fitness in monozygotic twins. This definitive study estimated that the genetic contribution to maximal aerobic power is approximately 40% or less (Bouchard et al., 1986).

Published reports on the relationship of fitness to exercise show correlations of 0.3 to 0.5 between responses to exercise questionnaires and fitness tests. This does not mean, however, that exercise habits are weakly related to fitness. More likely the low relationships are due to imprecise assessments of physical activity. At the Aerobics Activity Center in Dallas a record of exercise participation is obtained by having members enter reports on what they have done via remote computer terminals each day after their exercise session. This aggregate record is a more accurate summary of a person's exercise habits than can be obtained by questionnaire, and in this data base, correlations between the exercise record and performance on a maximal treadmill test are 0.7 to 0.8 (unpublished observations). Well-controlled randomized clinical trials also clearly show that increases in exercise are accompanied by increases in fitness. Thus, it seems logical that objective measures of fitness would be useful in studying the exercise-longevity question.

We (Blair et al., 1989) studied the relationship between maximal treadmill time and death rates in 10,224 men and 3,120 women who were followed for an average of slightly more than 8 years after a preventive medical examination at the Cooper Clinic. Age-adjusted all-cause mortality rates for the least fit (1st quintile) men were 3.44 times greater than for the most fit (5th quintile), and the death rate for the least-fit women was 4.65 times greater than that of their most-fit counterparts. Death rates per 10,000 person-years were 64.0, 26.3, and 20.3 for men of low (1st quintile), moderate (2nd and 3rd quintiles), and high (4th and 5th quintiles) fitness, respectively. For women in the same fitness categories they were 39.5, 16.4, and 7.4, respectively.

In the following sections we review the evidence that regular physical activity reduces risk of chronic suffering and premature death from cardiovascular diseases, diabetes, some cancers, obesity, and osteoporosis.

Hypertension

Using the Aerobics Center Longitudinal Study (ACLS) database, we (Blair, Goodyear, Gibbons, & Cooper, 1984) found that people with low physical fitness (as determined by a maximal treadmill test) had a relative risk (RR) of 1.52 for development of hypertension relative to fit people, after adjustment for sex, age, follow-up interval, baseline blood pressure, and body mass index (BMI). (These data were obtained for 4,820 men and 1,219 women 20 to 65 years of age who were normotensive at baseline.) More recently, we examined all-cause mortality in 10,224 healthy normotensive and 1,832 hypertensive but otherwise healthy men from the ACLS (Blair, Kohl, Barlow, & Gibbons, 1991). There were 240 deaths in the normotensive men and 78 deaths in the hypertensive men. For the normotensive men age-adjusted mortality rates per 10,000 man-years of follow-up ranged from 64.0 in the least-fit quintile to 18.6 in the most-fit quintile, for a RR of 3.4. For the hypertensive men the corresponding mortality rates were 110.5 to 24.8, for a RR of 4.5. The men were further classified into two baseline systolic blood pressure groups, those with pressure lower than 140 mmHg and those with pressure greater than or equal to 140 mmHg. Regardless of the blood pressure classification, the more fit men had lower mortality rates than the less fit men, and the relationship held after adjustment for age, serum cholesterol, resting systolic blood pressure, BMI, current smoking habits, and length of follow-up. We conclude that low physical fitness results in an increased risk for all-cause mortality in both normotensive and hypertensive men.

Coronary Heart Disease

Morris is generally credited with initiating the modern study of exercise and heart disease with his research on London transport workers and other occupational groups in the 1950s (Morris, Heady, Raffle, Roberts, & Parks, 1953). His more recent studies focus on mortality follow-up of middle-aged men in the British Civil Service.

Physical Activity

In 1980 Morris, Everitt, Pollard, Chave, and Semmence reported on men who had been asked to complete a detailed record of their physical activity during a Friday and Saturday. The activity records were used to classify the men as vigorous exercisers (VE) or nonvigorous exercisers (NVE). Vigorous exercise was defined as exercise at an intensity of at least 7.5 kcal · min^{-1}, a level equal to heavy industrial work. To be classified as VE, men had to report at least 5 min of sports or recreational activities at or above the intensity criterion, or at least 30 min of heavy work such as digging in the garden. Approximately 20% of the study participants were classified as VE, based on their exercise habits at baseline. The men were followed for mortality an average of 8.5 years, providing 150,000 man-years of follow-up. There were 475 deaths from coronary heart disease during follow-up. The coronary heart disease death rate was more than twice as high in NVE (2.9%) as in VE (1.1%). These results were not due to confounding by family history or other coronary heart disease risk factors, which were statistically controlled for in the analysis.

In 1990 Morris, Clayton, Everitt, Semmence, and Burgess reported the results of a 9.3-year follow-up of 9,376 male British civil servants who were age 45 to 64 at entry. There were 272 fatal cases of coronary heart disease and 202 nonfatal cases in 87,563 man-years of observation. Each man gave a detailed account of his physical activity for the previous 4 weeks. Using a variety of analyses, the researchers clearly showed that vigorous aerobic activity provided protection against coronary heart disease. Activities other than vigorous aerobic exercise were not associated with lower rates of coronary attack or mortality. The older cohort (55-64 years) showed a benefit associated with a lesser degree of aerobic exercise (i.e., a dose response) but not with other forms of exercise. This indicates that in older men less intense aerobic exercise may be adequate to reduce risk of coronary heart disease. Morris's work indicates that "it is the activity itself that protects" (p. 331), not self-selection, and further, that the exercise must be "continuing and current" (p. 332) and of the sort that contributes to cardiorespiratory fitness.

Leon, Connett, Jacobs, and Rauramaa (1987) reported mortality during follow-up of 12,138 men, aged 35 to 57 years at baseline, enrolled in the Multiple Risk Factor Intervention Trial. These men were in the upper 10% to 15% of risk, based on cigarette smoking, blood pressure, and serum cholesterol. Mortality surveillance was maintained at least 6 to 8 years, and 488 deaths were recorded. Exercise was assessed at baseline by an extensive leisure-time physical-activity (LTPA) questionnaire and interview. The men were asked about their participation in 62 individual activities over the previous 12 months. Frequency and duration of participation, along with the activity's energy cost, were used to calculate total energy expenditure in LTPA. All-cause and coronary heart disease death rates were higher in the 1st (most sedentary) tertile. Death rates were similar in the 2nd and 3rd tertiles. Results were unchanged after adjustment for age and other risk factors.

The study of Finnish men and women by Salonen et al. (1982) has particular relevance because Finnish people have the highest rate of coronary heart disease in the world. In addition to conducting the analysis of all-cause mortality discussed earlier, the researchers examined risk factors for cardiovascular disease (serum cholesterol, diastolic blood pressure, BMI, and smoking behavior). Age-adjusted and risk-factor-adjusted RR for acute myocardial infarction and fatal ischemic heart disease are shown in Table 1.3 (the two lower data panels will be referred to later). Age-adjusted RR values for low physical activity at work, at leisure, and at both work and leisure were highly significant for acute myocardial infarction for both men and women when compared with values associated with high levels of physical activity in the respective categories. However, risk-factor-adjusted RR values achieved statistical significance for acute myocardial infarction only for low physical activity at work. There was insufficient incidence of fatal ischemic heart disease in women for data analysis, but the pattern in men for fatal disease was similar to the findings for acute myocardial infarction.

Most of the studies reviewed by Powell, Thompson, Caspersen, and Kendrick (1987) on physical activity and coronary heart disease in women suggest no benefit for more active women. Is it likely that sedentary living habits are a coronary heart disease risk factor in men but not in women? We think not. The failure of several studies to find an inverse relationship between activity and coronary heart disease is probably due to methodological faults, such as inaccurate measurement of physical activity in women. Many of the studies' questionnaires, for example, do not assess activities such as child care and household chores. Several studies suggest that women respond to exercise in ways similar to men and that exercise improves women's risk status. The incidence of heart disease in women increases after menopause (Wenger, 1985), making the relationship in postmenopausal women between physical activity and known risk factors associated with coronary heart disease a topic of special interest. Cauley et al. (1986) examined the relationship between physical activity and high-density-lipoprotein cholesterol (HDL-C) subfractions in 255 white postmenopausal women with a mean age of 57.6 years. Using multiple regression analyses to control possible confounding factors, the researchers found that physical activity was independently and significantly related to total HDL-C and HDL-2. In fact, there was a "near linear relationship between frequency of sport activity and HDL-2" (p. 692).

A study of Finnish women aged 25 to 64 years reported similar but somewhat weaker results (Marti, Tuomilehto, Salonen, Puska, & Nissinen, 1987). High leisure-time physical activity showed an inverse association with a combined coronary heart disease risk estimate (smoking, serum cholesterol, and blood

Table 1.3 Age- and Risk Factor-Adjusted Relative Risks (RR) Associated with Low Physical Activity at Work and in Leisure Time in Finnish Men and Women

	Age-adjusted RR (90% CI)	Risk factor–adjusted RR (90% CI)
Acute myocardial infarction		
Men		
Low physical activity at work	1.6** (1.2, 2.0)	1.5** (1.2, 2.0)
Low physical activity at leisure	1.4** (1.1, 1.7)	1.2 (0.9, 1.5)
Low physical activity at both work and leisure	2.5*** (1.8, 3.7)	—
Women		
Low physical activity at work	2.7*** (1.8, 4.1)	2.4*** (1.5, 3.7)
Low physical activity at leisure	1.7** (1.1, 2.6)	1.5 (0.9, 2.5)
Low physical activity at both work and leisure	4.0*** (2.1, 7.9)	—
Fatal ischemic heart disease		
Men		
Low physical activity at work	1.6** (1.1, 2.3)	1.6* (1.1, 2.3)
Low physical activity at leisure	1.7** (1.2, 2.5)	1.4 (0.9, 2.5)
Women		
Insufficient incidence		

Cerebral stroke		
Men		
Low physical activity at work	2.0** (1.4, 2.9)	1.6* (1.1, 2.5)
Low physical activity at leisure	1.2 (0.8, 1.8)	1.0 (0.7, 1.5)
Women		
Low physical activity at work	1.8** (1.2, 2.8)	1.7* (1.1, 2.7)
Low physical activity at leisure	1.3 (0.8, 2.0)	1.3 (0.8, 2.0)
Death, all diseases		
Men		
Low physical activity at work	1.9*** (1.5, 2.5)	1.9*** (1.5, 2.5)
Low physical activity at leisure	1.9*** (1.5, 2.4)	1.5** (1.2, 2.0)
Low physical activity at both work and leisure	3.9*** (2.7, 5.5)	—
Women		
Low physical activity at work	2.4*** (1.6, 3.5)	2.2*** (1.5, 3.3)
Low physical activity at leisure	1.6** (1.1, 2.3)	1.6** (1.0, 2.3)
Low physical activity at both work and leisure	3.5*** (1.9, 6.3)	—

Note. CI = confidence interval.
$* = p < 0.05$. $** = p < 0.01$. $*** = p < 0.001$.
Data from Salonen et al., (1982).

pressure) and a positive association with HDL-C. In our opinion, the weaker results were at least partly due to the inclusion of young women and possible confounding by menopausal factors.

At least two studies have shown that regular aerobic exercise alters the lipoprotein profile in postmenopausal women. Seals, Hagberg, Hurley, Ehsani, and Holloszy (1984) reported that 6 months of high-intensity endurance training resulted in increased HDL-C and decreased triglyceride levels in elderly women. Whitehurst and Menendez (1991) recently reported that an 8-week walking program at 70% to 80% of predicted maximum heart rate also resulted in increased HDL-C and reduced triglyceride levels in 31 women with an average age of 69 years.

Duncan, Gordon, and Scott (1991) studied 102 sedentary premenopausal women to determine the effects of 24 weeks of walking. Three groups of subjects walked the same distance 5 days per week, but their speeds were varied such that the groups walked 3 mi in 36, 45, and 60 min, respectively, by week 14 and thereafter. Aerobic fitness increased in a dose-response manner in walkers as compared with sedentary controls; however, increases in HDL-C were similar among the three groups.

Although this evidence is indirect and circumstantial, it offers support to the hypothesis put forth in this paper—that regular exercise offers protection from coronary heart disease in both women and men and that women with low physical-activity levels are at increased risk for coronary heart disease.

The studies reviewed previously concur, showing lower death rates and a lower incidence of heart disease in more active men and women. Figure 1.1 shows a

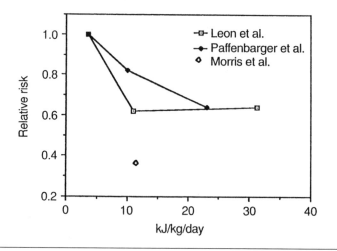

Figure 1.1   Relative risk of coronary heart disease mortality in men by energy expenditure expressed in kilojoules per kilogram of body weight per day. Data from three papers: Leon, Connett, Jacobs, & Rauramaa, 1987 (p. 2388); Paffenbarger, Hyde, Wing, & Hsieh, 1986a (p. 605); Morris, Everitt, Pollard, Chave, & Semmence, 1980 (p. 1207).

summary of some of the results on coronary heart disease death in men. Substantially lower death rates are seen in more active men. The three prospective studies reported in Figure 1.1 (Leon et al., 1987; Morris et al., 1980; Paffenbarger et al., 1986a) are characterized by careful assessment of exercise habits, with validated questionnaires, excellent surveillance systems, nearly complete follow-up, and control for possible confounding variables. Two of the studies report similar results for all-cause mortality (not shown), thereby avoiding the problem of determining the cause of death from death certificates. All the studies reinforce the inference that regular exercise protects against early mortality.

Physical Fitness

We (Blair et al., 1989) found that death rates from cardiovascular disease, as with all-cause mortality, were lower in fit men and women than in the unfit (see Figure 1.2). The greatest difference in death rates was seen between the low- and moderate-fitness categories for both sexes, but there was a further reduction between the moderate- and high-fitness categories. The death rate

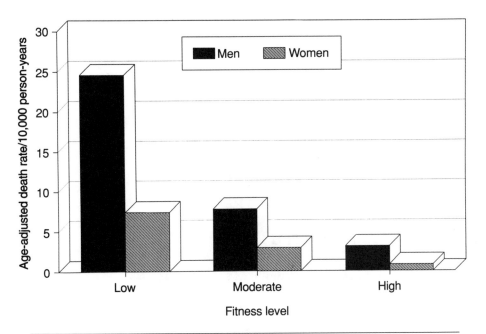

Figure 1.2   Age-adjusted cardiovascular disease death rates per 10,000 person-years for men and women by low, moderate, and high levels of physical fitness, Aerobics Center Longitudinal Study. Data from Blair, Kohl, Paffenbarger, Clark, Cooper, & Gibbons, 1989 (p. 2398).

for the highly fit men was about half that of the moderately fit, but the rate for the low-fitness group was more than 3 times that of moderately fit men. In women the death rate for the moderately fit was 3.6 times that of the highly fit, and the low-fitness group had a death rate 2.5 times higher than that of the moderately fit.

Recent data from the Lipid Research Clinics Prevalence Survey show a strong relationship between fitness and cardiovascular disease and coronary heart disease mortality. Ekelund et al. (1988) followed 3,106 healthy white men aged 30 to 69 years at baseline for an average of 8.5 years. Physical fitness was measured at baseline by a submaximal treadmill test. During follow-up 45 deaths were attributed to cardiovascular disease. Death rates for coronary heart disease and cardiovascular disease are shown by physical-fitness quartiles in Figure 1.3. The RR of death for men in the least-fit quartile, compared with that of the most-fit quartile, was high: RR of 6.5 for coronary heart disease and RR of 8.5 for cardiovascular disease. There was a striking dose-response gradient across fitness categories.

Low physical fitness is associated with increased risk of coronary heart disease and cardiovascular disease. The reported RR ratios are considerably higher (in the range of 6.5-8.0) than those from physical-activity studies (approximately 2.0). As we have stated, the relatively crude methods available to assess habitual physical activity may underestimate the true risk, whereas the more objective measurement of fitness yields a more accurate estimate of risk. Clearly, the relationship between fitness and coronary heart disease mortality supports the hypothesis of a causal relationship between regular exercise and longevity.

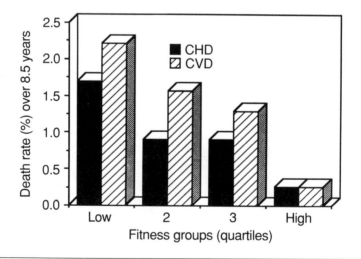

Figure 1.3 Coronary heart disease and cardiovascular disease death rates by fitness quartiles (estimated by heart rate at stage 2 of a modified Bruce submaximal exercise test) for men in the Lipid Research Clinics Prevalence Survey (*N* = 3,106). From data presented by Ekelund, Haskell, Johnson, Whaley, Criqui, & Sheps, 1988 (p. 1379).

Stroke

Although its mortality rates are well below those for heart disease and cancer, cerebrovascular disease is the third leading disease-related cause of death in the United States in both men and women (see Table 1.1). Stroke (both fatal and nonfatal) is the common endpoint for cerebrovascular disease, and it will be our focus here. Unfortunately, few studies have examined stroke in relation to physical activity.

In the generally sedentary Framingham population an inverse relationship was found between reported physical activity and the incidence of stroke in men (Kannel & Sorlie, 1979). When results were adjusted for age, however, the RR values did not achieve significance. Relative-risk values for low physical activity and cerebral stroke did reach statistical significance in the Finnish study cited (Salonen et al., 1982). In the third panel of Table 1.3, age-adjusted RR values show that low work-related physical activity was associated with increased risk of stroke in both men and women, after controlling for age, serum cholesterol, diastolic blood pressure, height, weight, and smoking.

In the Harvard Alumni Study the incidence of stroke was inversely related to the physical-activity index (Paffenbarger, Hyde, Wing, & Steinmetz, 1984). Based on 10,000 man-years of observation, the stroke rate for subjects expending less than 500 kcal · week^{-1} was 6.5; for those expending 500 to 1,999 kcal · week^{-1} it was 5.2; and for those expending more than 2,000 kcal · week^{-1} it was 2.4.

There is limited evidence that cerebral atherosclerosis, as manifested by stroke, is reduced in more active men and women. Hypertension is highly related to the development of cardiovascular diseases, including cerebrovascular disease and stroke. In fact, stroke is a common endpoint for hypertension. In the Framingham Study men with hypertension (> 160/95 mmHG) were about four times more likely to suffer a stroke than those who were normotensive (Kannel et al., 1984). In the Nurses' Health Study the RR for stroke in women with hypertension was 4.2 (Fiebach et al., 1989). The elevated risk of stroke in these women occurred at all levels of relative weight. The investigators concluded that hypertension was an independent risk factor for stroke in middle-aged women.

Studies on hypertension and activity or fitness were reviewed in a previous section. In summary, we believe that these data indirectly support the hypothesis that regular physical activity and higher levels of physical fitness reduce the risk of developing hypertension and may also reduce mortality from stroke.

Diabetes

Helmrich, Ragland, Leung, and Paffenbarger (1991) report that the incidence of non-insulin-dependent diabetes mellitus (NIDDM) is inversely related to leisure-time physical activity in 5,990 male University of Pennsylvania alumni who were followed for 14 years. The categories of lowest and highest energy expenditure studied were fewer than 500 kcal · week^{-1} and more than 3,500 kcal · week^{-1}, and the age-adjusted risk of developing NIDDM decreased 6% for each 500-kcal increase in weekly energy expenditure. Adjustment for obesity, hypertension, and parental history did not weaken the relationship. Those subjects at risk because of obesity, history of hypertension, or parental history of diabetes received the greatest apparent protection from high levels of physical activity.

Physically active women also have reduced risk of NIDDM. Manson et al. (1991) followed 87,253 women from the Nurses' Health Study cohort for 8 years and found that the age-adjusted risk for NIDDM among those who exercised vigorously at least weekly was only 67% (84% after adjustment for BMI) of the risk for sedentary women. Frequency of activity had no effect on RR, and multivariate adjustment for age, BMI, and family history did not change the beneficial effect of activity.

Cancer

Cancer is the second leading cause of death in both genders and in all age groups in the United States and the primary cause of death among women aged 35 to 54. In 1985 cancer accounted for approximately 22% of American deaths. It has recently been suggested that high levels of physical activity may offer protection from certain forms of cancer. Kohl, LaPorte, and Blair (1988) provide a recent review of the epidemiological evidence for such an association. Therefore, we will only briefly review that evidence here and will discuss some more recent contributions.

Occupational Activity

Four recent studies demonstrate a significantly reduced risk of colon cancer in people with physically active occupations (Garabrant, Peters, Mack, & Bernstein, 1984; Gerhardsson, Norell, Kiviranta, Pederson, & Ahlbom, 1986; Vena, Graham, Zielezny, Brasure, & Swanson, 1987; Vena et al., 1985). The studies varied in design, target population, statistical control, method of classifying job-related activity, time reference (follow-up period and exposure to occupational activity level), and types of cancer studied. Significant associations were not found for physical activity and rectal cancer (Garabrant et al., 1984; Gerhardsson et al., 1986; Vena et al., 1987; Vena et al., 1985) or for prostate cancer (Vena et al., 1987). The only study to include women (Vena et al., 1987) reported a significantly reduced risk of mortality from colon cancer and breast cancer in women in the highest occupational physical-activity category.

We must consider several problems before drawing a conclusion from the given evidence. One is the matter of self-selection. Another problem is that some studies did not control for smoking, which is more prevalent in blue-collar workers, who presumably have more physically active jobs than white-collar workers. Although smoking has not been associated with colon cancer per se, the lack of statistical control for smoking may have resulted in an underestimation of the true relationship between occupational physical activity and protection from colon cancer. In addition, smoking is associated with breast cancer in women and therefore should be controlled by statistical methods in the calculation of RR.

Leisure-Time Physical Activity

Paffenbarger, Hyde, and Wing (1987) report on 56,683 male alumni from the University of Pennsylvania and Harvard College who were classified as having played sports less than 5 hr a week or more than 5 hr a week while in college. The more active former students were less likely to develop rectal cancer (RR = 0.46) and more likely to develop prostate cancer (RR = 1.66). No association was found for other forms of cancer, including lung, colorectal, and colon cancer. In a second analysis the physical-activity index in kcal · week^{-1} (the same index used in the Harvard Alumni Study on coronary heart disease reported by Paffenbarger et al. [1986a]), was used to assign the post-college physical-activity levels of 16,936 male Harvard alumni to three categories (<500 kcal · week^{-1}, 500-1,999 kcal · week^{-1}, >2,000 kcal · week^{-1}). The men were followed for 12 to 16 years, during which 32% of all deaths were attributed to cancer. Results were adjusted for age, smoking behavior, and BMI, offering control of possible confounding variables. Adjusted RR for the least-active group was 1.47 for all cancers, relative to the most-active group. Results on activity and site-specific cancer were inconclusive in these analyses, but more recent data from extended follow-up are now available. Lee, Paffenbarger, and Hsieh (1991) report that highly active alumni (>2,500 kcal · week^{-1}) have approximately half the risk of developing colon cancer of their inactive counterparts. In a second paper Lee, Paffenbarger, and Hsieh (1992) show that alumni who expended 4,000 kcal · week^{-1} or more had a reduced risk of prostate cancer, but the authors find no dose-response gradient of risk across activity levels.

Frisch et al. studied the prevalence of cancers of the breast and reproductive system (1985) and non-reproductive-system cancers (Frisch, Wyshak, Albright, Albright, & Schiff, 1989) in female former college athletes and nonathletes. They obtained a history of athleticism and cancer development in 5,398 living alumnae (2,622 former college athletes and 2,776 nonathletes) aged 21 to 80 years. Relative risks were calculated for lifetime occurrence of reproductive-system cancers (ovary, uterus, cervix, vagina) and breast cancer and adjusted for the confounding effects of age, number of pregnancies, family history of cancer, age at menarche, smoking, use of oral contraceptives, and estrogen therapy at menopause. Adjusted RR (nonathletes/athletes) was 2.53 for reproductive-system cancers and 1.86 for breast cancer. The former athletes had a notably lower rate of breast cancer during the perimenopausal years. Current exercise habits were reported by 74% of the former athletes, compared with 57% of the nonathletes—evidence that many of the former athletes had maintained physically active lifestyles.

The former athletes also had a significantly lower rate of non-reproductive-system cancers (digestive system, thyroid, bladder, lung, lymphoma, leukemia, myeloma, and Hodgkin's disease) (Frisch et al., 1989). Age-adjusted RR (nonathletes/athletes) was 3.34 for these cancers. There was no significant difference between the two groups in the prevalence of skin cancer. Because these were prevalence studies in living subjects, women who had already died of cancer or other causes were not included; therefore, a selection bias may have been present. The investigators argue that the prevalence rates for both reproductive and breast cancers in nonathletes were in accord with national data, indicating there were no selection or reporting biases.

Total Physical Activity

Two recent studies merit mention. Slattery, Schumacher, Smith, West, and Abd-Elghany (1988) used a population-based case-control design to assess the effects of diet and leisure and occupational physical activity on the development of colon cancer in Utah residents. Physical activity was expressed in calories per week, and dietary data were obtained from a quantitative food-frequency questionnaire. Cases were identified through the Utah Cancer Registry and control led through a random-digit-dialing telephone sampling procedure. Multiple regression analysis controlled for age, BMI, fiber intake, and calories. The odds ratios (high quartile/low quartile) for physical activity and colon cancer were 0.70 for men and 0.48 for women. Vigorous activity appeared to have a greater protective effect. These results were not due to the confounding influences of dietary fat, protein, or total calories. The investigators concluded that high levels of physical activity reduce the risk associated with high levels of dietary intake, especially dietary fat.

The second study of total physical activity and cancer was completed by Albanes, Blair, and Taylor (1989) from data obtained by the first National Health and Nutrition Examination Survey. The cohort was first examined in 1971 through 1975, and participants were followed for cancer incidence by re-interviews in 1982 through 1984. The study sample included 5,138 men and 7,407 women aged 25 to 74 years. Inactive people had an increased risk of cancer compared with very active people (for men RR = 1.8, for women RR = 1.3). Adjustment for potential confounders did not change these findings. Men who were inactive on the job had an increased risk of lung cancer (2.0) when compared with occupationally active men. There were also suggestive but not statistically significant trends for increased rates of colorectal and prostate cancer in inactive men. Postmenopausal women who were inactive at work were somewhat more likely to develop breast cancer than active women, but the trend was opposite for premenopausal women. Inactive women were much more likely than active women to develop cervical cancer (RR = 5.2). Recreational activity (much exercise, moderate exercise, and little or no exercise) generally had a weaker relationship with cancer than did occupational activity. Men reporting little or no exercise, however, had an increased risk of prostate cancer (RR = 1.8). These results, though somewhat mixed, suggest that inactive people are more likely to develop cancer.

Physical Fitness

Blair et al. (1989) reported a pattern for reduced cancer mortality that resembled the reductions in cardiovascular disease and all-cause mortality discussed earlier. The low-fit men's risk was 4.3 times that of the highly fit and 2.8 times that of the moderately fit. Low-fit women had 16.3 times greater cancer mortality than the most fit and 1.7 times the risk of the moderately fit.

Markedly different mechanisms may influence the initiation of site-specific cancers, so it is not logical to look for a single underlying mechanism or protective factor. Several possibly protective effects have been suggested to explain the apparent inverse association between a physically active lifestyle and incidence of cancer (Calabrese, 1990; Kohl et al., 1988). For example, exercise is known to stimulate peristalsis, reducing the transit time of organic waste through the large intestine, which may provide some protection against colon cancer. Another hypothesis is that physically active people may eat differently than inactive people or that other protective habits may be associated with an active lifestyle. Some cancers (particularly those of women's reproductive organs) are known to be hormonally sensitive, and exercise may alter the hormonal milieu, although it is not clear how this occurs, the extent to which it is an acute or chronic effect, or how it could affect the initiation of cancer. Many highly active women have lower endogenous levels of estrogen (Wells, 1991), and this might protect against cancers of the reproductive organs. Still another hypothesis is that physical activity may alter the risk of cancer indirectly by affecting adiposity (for more detailed explanations of the last two hypotheses, see Frisch et al., 1985).

Whatever the mechanisms, we believe the evidence gives at least modest support for the hypothesis that regular exercise provides protection against the development of some cancers, particularly colon cancer in men and women and breast cancer in women.

Obesity

Considerable differences of opinion exist about the definition and clinical significance of obesity (Ernsberger & Haskew, 1987; National Center for Health Statistics, 1987; National Institutes of Health, 1985). Nevertheless, the report of the NIH Consensus Conference on the Health Implications of Obesity shows that in the majority opinion, obesity is a disease and is related to increased risk of morbidity and mortality from most of the chronic diseases addressed in this chapter.

It is unclear whether excess body weight or body fat per se causes the problem (Van Itallie, 1985), and no agreement exists on the point at which excess weight or fat becomes a health problem. Most studies of the relationship between obesity and health have used BMI as the measure of obesity. This may be a valid assessment of obesity and is related to health risk, but it is a poor predictor of body composition. Using BMI as an indicator of obesity in the Nurses' Health Study, Manson et al. (1990) found that being even mildly to moderately overweight increases the risk of coronary heart disease in middle-aged women.

Food intake, physical activity, basal metabolism, and adaptive thermogenesis were examined in a recent review by Shah and Jeffery (1991). They conclude that food intake is poorly related to obesity, suggesting that physical activity (the most variable component in energy balance) usually has an inverse association with body weight and fatness. However, the interrelationships between physical activity and obesity are complex. Although it is widely believed that inactivity plays a major causal role in the development of adiposity, low physical activity may also be a consequence of obesity.

Another recent review (Poehlman, Melby, & Goran, 1991) examined the effect of physical activity on energy expenditure. Metabolism not only undergoes as much as a 20-fold elevation during exercise (for short duration in fit individuals) but has also been reported to remain elevated after exercise. This elevation may last less than 10 min following exercise for 30 min at 37% of maximal aerobic power to as much as 24 hr after 65 to 90 min of exercise at 70% of maximal aerobic power. These bouts of activity accounted for an extra 9 kcal and greater than 130 kcal expended, respectively, during the recovery periods. The authors concluded that activity prescribed for the general public is likely to lead to 9 to 130 kcal in excess postexercise energy expenditure for each exercise session. Some people also respond to training with an increased resting metabolic rate and postprandial thermogenesis. Considerable individual variability exists, however, and the response may be a function of genetic factors, body composition, or state of training.

The ACSM (1991) recommends that exercise for fat loss be of an intensity, duration, and frequency sufficient to require 1,000 to 2,000 kcal $\cdot$ week^{-1}, with the assumption that fat loss occurs in proportion to increased energy expenditure. In an uncontrolled but interesting study of the efficacy of daily walking, stationary cycling, and swimming (Gwinup, 1987), little change in weight was observed until activity duration approached 30 min per session. Commonly tolerated intensities of effort may require durations of 30 min or more on a nearly daily basis to provide significant energy expenditure.

Of course, a subject's ability to endure lower-intensity activity longer means a greater energy expenditure. This seems to be confirmed by the 1,366 female and 1,257 male participants in the Canadian Fitness Survey (Tremblay et al., 1990), in whom decreased skinfold measurements and waist-to-hip ratios were associated with regular activity. The limitations of their method, however, make judgment of causality impossible, and two experimental investigations have shown intensity to have no effect on fat loss when total energy expenditure is unchanged (Ballor, McCarthy, & Wilterdink, 1990; Gaesser & Rich, 1984). Both research groups trained subjects three times per week, comparing intensities of

45% and 85% of maximal aerobic power endured for 50 and 25 min, respectively, and found no differences in body-fat changes. Gaesser and Rich studied 16 nonobese men who trained for 18 weeks, whereas Ballor and colleagues examined the combined effects of 8 weeks of exercise and a 1,200 kcal daily diet on 27 obese women.

Osteoporosis

Although osteoporosis has not been suggested as a direct cause of premature death, it has been implicated in hip and other fractures, which are often followed by hospitalization and death. Snow-Harter and Marcus (1991) suggest that the age-related decrease in bone mineral content and architectural integrity may be more a function of inactivity than of aging. Bone loss parallels losses in physical fitness, and some components of fitness have been found to predict bone mineral density better than does age.

These reviewers cite evidence that gradual stress-related bone damage stimulates a remodeling process that increases bone mass and that the magnitude of load is more important than the number of repetitions. They report the results of many studies showing an increase in or a retarded loss of bone mineral density in response to varied physical activity. The adaptation to activity seems to depend upon the initial state of the bone and the load imposed upon it. In accordance with Wolff's law, when greater than normal stress is habitually imposed, bone mass will increase and stabilize.

In apparent contradiction to the activity-induced improvement in bone mineral, Snow-Harter and Marcus also cite studies showing bone loss in response to severe endurance training in both males and females. This has been reported more frequently in females and has been inconsistently associated with low body weight or fat, irregular menstrual status or sex-hormone levels, and low caloric or red-meat intake.

In light of the evidence we have examined, it seems clear that regular, appropriate physical activity may reasonably be expected to reduce the incidence of several chronic diseases, thereby reducing overall mortality rate and increasing longevity. The dose-response relationship has become clearer over the past 3 decades. Although complete understanding will require further investigation, and differences by disease and gender exist, it appears that the risk of coronary heart disease, stroke, non-insulin-dependent diabetes mellitus, reproductive and colon cancers, obesity, and osteoporosis declines with increased physical activity.

The mechanisms whereby regular exercise exerts its healthful effects may be direct or indirect. The evidence is particularly strong in supporting a hypothesis of exercise's protective effect against athlerosclerosis. This effect is evident even after extensive multivariate modeling and adjustment for a variety of factors (such as age, diet, economic status, smoking, and other clinical risk factors). The results also hold in analyses stratified by early and late follow-up, which lessens the chance that the relationship between physical activity and mortality was due to pre-existing subclinical disease that may have reduced the activity level of those so afflicted.

Much of the activity-related reduction of risk for chronic disease seems primarily related to the average weekly energy expenditure and relatively independent of intensity and duration. The energy expenditure required to improve health probably depends upon the health risk to be reduced and present status for that factor. We believe that there is probably no minimum threshold of energy expenditure necessary to improve health, that any increase in energy expenditure is likely to improve some aspect of health, and that the magnitude of increased energy expenditure affects both the rate and degree of improvement. Risk of osteoporosis appears more related to mechanical loading than to energy expenditure per se, but reasonable risk reduction for other chronic diseases can probably be obtained by most individuals with as little as 30 min of daily walking or its equivalent in other activities.

The lowest relative risks are generally associated with the highest levels of activity; however, the reduction in risk does not appear to be linear. It is unclear whether a minimum threshold of activity must be passed in order to produce a response, but several studies indicate that most of the risk reduction occurs in response to relatively low doses of activity. In other words, the health benefits of changing one's activity from doing nothing to doing something often exceed those gained by increasing from moderate to high levels of activity. Extraordinary amounts of exercise or physical fitness are not required for subjects to gain considerable benefit. For millions of individuals, getting out of the least active and least fit groups is a worthwhile goal. The extremely sedentary and unfit may make up nearly 30% of the North American population. Such high-risk individuals number as many as 50 million adult U.S. residents. This high prevalence, in light of the strength of the physical activity–mortality relationship, constitutes a major public-health problem. Clinicians should accept the challenge of identifying and vigorously intervening with patients at high risk of premature mortality because of sedentary habits. Even if we are wrong and exercise does not increase longevity, those who undertake an active lifestyle gain important benefits. As they become more physically fit, they will have more vigor to carry out their routine activities, be less susceptible to chronic fatigue, have more energy for participating in a broad spectrum of life's activities, and gain an enhanced feeling of well-being. We believe it is the obligation of health professionals to vigorously promote regular exercise as a means of improving health and function and preventing premature mortality.

References

Albanes, D., Blair, A., & Taylor, P.R. (1989). Physical activity and risk of cancer in the NHANES I population. *American Journal of Public Health*, **79**, 744-750.

American College of Sports Medicine. (1975). *Guidelines for graded exercise testing and exercise prescription*. Philadelphia: Lea & Febiger.

American College of Sports Medicine. (1991). *Guidelines for testing and prescription* (4th ed.). Philadelphia: Lea & Febiger.

Ballor, D.L., McCarthy, J.P., & Wilterdink, E.J. (1990). Exercise intensity does not affect the composition of diet- and exercise-induced body mass loss. *American Journal of Clinical Nutrition*, **51**, 142-146.

Blair, S.N., Goodyear, N.N., Gibbons, L.W., & Cooper, K.H. (1984). Physical fitness and incidence of hypertension in healthy normotensive men and women. *Journal of the American Medical Association*, **252**, 487-490.

Blair, S.N., Kohl, H.W., Barlow, C.E., & Gibbons, L.W. (1991). Physical fitness and all-cause mortality in hypertensive men. *Annals of Medicine*, **23**, 307-312.

Blair, S.N., Kohl, H.W., Paffenbarger, R.S., Jr., Clark, D.G., Cooper, K.H., & Gibbons, L.W. (1989). Physical fitness and all-cause mortality: A prospective study of healthy men and women. *Journal of the American Medical Association*, **262**, 2395-2401.

Bouchard, C., Lesage, R., Lortie, G., Simoneau, J.A., Hamel, P., & Boulay, M.R. (1986). Aerobic performance in brothers, dizygotic and monozygotic twins. *Medicine and Science in Sports and Exercise*, **18**, 639-646.

Calabrese, L.H. (1990). Exercise, immunity, cancer, and infection. In C. Bouchard, R.J. Shephard, T. Stephens, J.R. Sutton, & B.D. McPherson (Eds.), *Exercise, fitness, and health: A consensus of current knowledge* (pp. 567-579). Champaign, IL: Human Kinetics.

Cauley, J.A., LaPorte, R.E., Sandler, R.B., Orchard, T.J., Slemenda, C.W., & Petrini, A.M. (1986). The relationship of physical activity to high density lipoprotein cholesterol in postmenopausal women. *Journal of Chronic Diseases*, **39**, 687-697.

Cooper, K.H. (1968). *Aerobics*. New York: Bantam.

Duncan, J.J., Gordon, N.F., & Scott, C.B. (1991). Walking for fitness—walking for health: How much is enough for sedentary women? *Journal of the American Medical Association*, **266**, 3295-3299.

Ekelund, L.G., Haskell, W.L., Johnson, J.L., Whaley, F.S., Criqui, M.H., & Sheps, D.S. (1988). Physical fitness as a predictor of cardiovascular mortality in asymptomatic North American men: The Lipid Research Clinics Mortality Follow-Up Study. *New England Journal of Medicine*, **319**, 1379-1384.

Ernsberger, P., & Haskew, P. (1987). Health implications of obesity: An alternative view. *Journal of Obesity and Weight Regulation*, **6**, 58-137.

Fiebach, N.H., Hebert, P.R., Stampfer, M.J., Colditz, G.A., Willett, W.C., & Rosner, B. (1989). A prospective study of high blood pressure and cardiovascular disease in women. *American Journal of Epidemiology*, **130**, 646-654.

Frisch, R.E., Wyshak, G., Albright, N.L., Albright, T.E., & Schiff, I. (1989). Lower prevalence of non-reproductive system cancers among female former college athletes. *Medicine and Science in Sports and Exercise*, **21**, 250-253.

Frisch, R.E., Wyshak, G., Albright, N.L., Albright, T.E., Schiff, I., & Jones, K.P. (1985). Lower prevalence of breast cancer and cancers of the reproductive system among former college athletes compared to nonathletes. *British Journal of Cancer*, **52**, 885-891.

Gaesser, G.A., & Rich, R.G. (1984). Effects of high- and low-intensity exercise training on aerobic capacity and blood lipids. *Medicine and Science in Sports and Exercise*, **16**, 269-274.

Garabrant, D.H., Peters, J.M., Mack, T.M., & Bernstein, L. (1984). Job activity and colon cancer risk. *American Journal of Epidemiology*, **119**, 1005-1014.

Gerhardsson, M., Norell, S.E., Kiviranta, H., Pederson, N.L., & Ahlbom, A. (1986). Sedentary jobs and colon cancer. *American Journal of Epidemiology*, **123**, 775-780.

Gwinup, G. (1987). Weight loss without dietary restriction: Efficacy of different forms of aerobic exercise. *American Journal of Sports Medicine*, **15**, 275-279.

Helmrich, S.P., Ragland, D.E., Leung, R.W., & Paffenbarger, R.S., Jr. (1991). Physical activity and reduced occurrence of non-insulin-dependent diabetes mellitus. *New England Journal of Medicine*, **325**, 147-152.

Kannel, W.B., Doyle, J.T., Ostfeld, A.M., Jenkins, C.D., Kuller, L., & Podell, R.N. (1984). Optimal resources for primary prevention of atherosclerotic diseases. *Circulation*, **70**, 157A-205A.

Kannel, W.B., & Sorlie, P. (1979). Some health benefits of physical activity. *Archives of Internal Medicine*, **139**, 857-861.

Karvonen, M., Kentala, K., & Mustala, O. (1957). The effects of training heart rate: A longitudinal study. *Annals of Medicinae Experimentalis et Biologiae Fenniae*, **35**, 307-315.

Kohl, H.W., LaPorte, R.E., & Blair, S.N. (1988). Physical activity and cancer: An epidemiological perspective. *Sports Medicine*, **6**, 222-237.

Lee, I-M., Paffenbarger, R.S., Jr., & Hsieh, C-C. (1991). Physical activity and risk of developing colorectal cancer among college alumni. *Journal of the National Cancer Institute*, **83**, 1324-1329.

Lee, I-M., Paffenbarger, R.S., Jr., & Hsieh, C-C. (1992). Physical activity and risk of prostatic cancer among college alumni. *American Journal of Epidemiology*, **135**, 169-179.

Leon, A.S., Connett, J., Jacobs, D.R., Jr., & Rauramaa, R. (1987). Leisure-time physical activity levels and risk of coronary heart disease and death: The Multiple Risk Factor Intervention Trial. *Journal of the American Medical Association*, **258**, 2388-2395.

Manson, J.E., Colditz, G.A., Stampfer, M.J., Willett, W.C., Rosner, B., & Monson, R.R. (1990). A prospective study of obesity and risk of coronary heart disease in women. *New England Journal of Medicine*, **322**, 882-889.

Manson, J.E., Rimm, E.B., Stampfer, M.J., Colditz, G.A., Willett, W.C., & Krolewski, A.S. (1991). Physical activity and incidence of non-insulin-dependent diabetes mellitus in women. *Lancet*, **338**, 774-778.

Marti, B., Tuomilehto, J., Salonen, J.T., Puska, P., & Nissinen, A. (1987). Relationship between leisure-time physical activity and risk factors for coronary heart disease in middle-aged Finnish women. *Acta Medica Scandinavica*, **222**, 223-230.

Morris, J.N., Clayton, D.G., Everitt, M.G., Semmence, A.M., & Burgess, E.H. (1990). Exercise in leisure time: Coronary attack and death rates. *British Heart Journal*, **63**, 325-334.

Morris, J.N., Everitt, M.G., Pollard, R., Chave, S.P.W., & Semmence, A.M. (1980). Vigorous exercise in leisure-time: Protection against coronary heart disease. *Lancet*, **2**, 1207-1210.

Morris, J.N., Heady, J.A., Raffle, P.A.B., Roberts, C.G., & Parks, J.W. (1953). Coronary heart disease and physical activity of work. *Lancet*, **ii**, 1053-1057, 1111-1120.

National Center for Health Statistics. (1987). *Anthropometric reference data and prevalence of overweight, United States, 1976-80. Vital and health statistics* (Series 11, No. 238; DHHS Publication No. PHS 87-1688). Washington, DC: U.S. Government Printing Office.

National Institutes of Health. (1985). Health implications of obesity: National Institutes of Health Consensus Development Conference statement. *Annals of Internal Medicine*, **103**, 1073-1077.

Paffenbarger, R.S., Jr., Hyde, R.T., & Wing, A.L. (1987). Physical activity and incidence of cancer in diverse populations: A preliminary report. *American Journal of Clinical Nutrition*, **45**, 312-317.

Paffenbarger, R.S., Jr., Hyde, R.T., Wing, A.L., & Hseih, C.C. (1986a). Physical activity, all-cause mortality, and longevity of college alumni. *New England Journal of Medicine*, **314**, 605-613.

Paffenbarger, R.S., Jr., Hyde, R.T., Wing, A.L., & Hsieh, C.-C. (1986b). Physical activity and longevity of college alumni [Letter to the editor]. *New England Journal of Medicine*, **315**, 400-401.

Paffenbarger, R.S., Jr., Hyde, R.T., Wing, A.L., & Steinmetz, C.H. (1984). A natural history of athleticism and cardiovascular health. *Journal of the American Medical Association*, **252**, 491-495.

Poehlman, E.T., Melby, C.L., & Goran, M.I. (1991). The impact of exercise and diet restriction on daily energy expenditure. *Sports Medicine*, **11**, 78-101.

Powell, K.E., Thompson, P.D., Caspersen, C.J., & Kendrick, J.S. (1987). Physical activity and the incidence of coronary heart disease. *Annual Review of Public Health*, **8**, 253-287.

Salonen, J.T., Puska, P., & Tuomilehto, J. (1982). Physical activity and risk of myocardial infarction, cerebral stroke and death: A longitudinal study in Eastern Finland. *American Journal of Epidemiology*, **115**, 526-537.

Seals, D.R., Hagberg, J.M., Hurley, B.F., Ehsani, A.A., & Holloszy, J.O. (1984). Effects of endurance training on glucose tolerance and plasma lipid levels in older men and women. *Journal of the American Medical Association*, **252**, 645-649.

Shah, M., & Jeffery, R.W. (1991). Is obesity due to overeating and inactivity, or to a defective metabolic rate? A review. *Annals of Behavioral Medicine*, **13**(2), 73-81.

Slattery, M.L., Schumacher, M.C., Smith, K.R., West, D.W., & Abd-Elghany, N. (1988). Physical activity, diet, and risk of colon cancer in Utah. *American Journal of Epidemiology*, **128**, 989-999.

Snow-Harter, C., & Marcus, R. (1991). Exercise, bone mineral density, and osteoporosis. In J.O. Holloszy (Ed.), *Exercise and sport sciences reviews* (Vol. 19) (pp. 351-388). Baltimore: Williams & Wilkins.

Tremblay, A., Despres, J-P., Leblanc, C., Craig, C.L., Ferris, B., & Stephens, T. (1990). Effect of intensity of physical activity on body fatness and fat distribution. *American Journal of Clinical Nutrition*, **51**, 153-157.

Van Itallie, T.B. (1985). Health implications of overweight and obesity in the United States. *Annals of Internal Medicine*, **103**, 983-988.

Vena, J.E., Graham, S., Zielezny, M., Brasure, J., & Swanson, M.K. (1987). Occupational exercise and risk of cancer. *American Journal of Clinical Nutrition*, **45**, 318-327.

Vena, J.E., Graham, S., Zielezny, M., Swanson, M.K., Barnes, R.E., & Nolan, J. (1985). Lifetime occupational exercise and colon cancer. *American Journal of Epidemiology*, **122**, 357-365.

Verbrugge, L.M., & Wingard, D.L. (1987). Sex differentials in health and mortality. *Women and Health*, **12**, 103-145.

Wells, C.L. (1991). *Women, sport, and performance: A physiological perspective* (2nd ed.). Champaign, IL: Human Kinetics.

Wenger, N.K. (1985). Coronary disease in women. *Annual Review of Medicine*, **36**, 285-294.

Whitehurst, M., & Menendez, E. (1991). Endurance training in older women. *Physician and Sportsmedicine*, **19**(6), 95-103.

CHAPTER 2

Exercise and Mental Health in Clinical and Free-Living Populations

Egil W. Martinsen
Thomas Stephens

This chapter examines several major questions concerning the relationship between exercise and mental health:

- Does evidence exist for a causal association?
- What, if any, are the principal mental-health effects?
- Does the association apply regardless of age, sex, and health status?
- What key dimensions of exercise (e.g., type, intensity, frequency) are associated with psychological benefits?

We start with the assumption that there is indeed an association between exercise and mental health, and evidence for this is reviewed in this chapter. The real issue is whether there is sufficient evidence to claim that exercise alleviates mental illness or promotes good mental health. If it does, this strengthens the argument for exercise adherence at the individual and population levels.

This chapter examines these issues from clinical and population perspectives. Clinical studies investigate interventions with patients in health-care settings, whereas population studies typically describe relatively healthy individuals who are not exposed to interventions. The distinction is important because recent reviews have concluded that the mental-health benefits of exercise are largely limited to more distressed individuals (Brown, 1990; Harris, Caspersen, De-Friese, & Estes, 1989; Sime, 1990), although this benefit may stem from the fact that patients are usually subjected to more deliberate exercise interventions than free-living subjects. This gives particular importance to the small number of controlled trials on normal subjects in nonclinical settings.

An overview of the evidence for mental-health benefits of exercise follows a brief discussion of methods and definitions; the chapter concludes with a discussion of the implications for therapy, health promotion, and future research. Each of these topics is treated from both clinical and population perspectives.

Methodological Considerations in Clinical Studies

A series of instruments has been developed to assess the various aspects of mental disorders, symptoms, cognitions, behavior, and level of function, and these instruments are widely used in clinical studies. Most patients seek therapy to get help from distressing symptoms, and most scales and inventories are developed to assess their symptom level. In most clinical studies, standardized scales, in which the psychometric properties have been shown to be satisfactory, are used.

Exercise

According to the American College of Sports Medicine (1980), physical exercise may be divided into three main categories: aerobic capacity and endurance; muscular strength and endurance; and flexibility, coordination, and relaxation. Most intervention studies have been performed with aerobic exercise, and in a few studies aerobic exercise has been compared with other forms.

Sample Representativeness

Modern criteria-based diagnostic systems in psychiatry have greatly increased diagnostic reliability, thus increasing the probability that independent researchers will agree in the classification of a given patient. The Research Diagnostic Criteria, or RDC (Spitzer, Endicott, & Robins, 1978), and the Diagnostic and Statistical Manual of Mental Disorders, or DSM-III (American Psychiatric Association, 1980), are commonly used. The use of such diagnostic systems makes it easier for researchers to compare results across studies.

In some rating scales, such as the Beck Depression Inventory, or BDI (Beck, Ward, Mendelson, Mock, & Erbaugh, 1961), normal ranges for the item scores are given. These instruments may be used to identify cases or patients in population studies. In some exercise-intervention studies, the score on such scales is the sole means of classification, and no formal diagnoses are made. This is not satisfactory because it makes comparing results across studies difficult.

The effects of exercise may vary between the sexes, between old and young people, and among the social classes. In order for researchers to make general conclusions, information about these factors should be reported in clinical studies.

Design

Nonexperimental studies are useful in the early phases of research in a new field. Exploratory studies without control groups are cheap and easy to perform and are useful for generating hypotheses. If no measurable effects are found in an exploratory study, there is little merit in performing controlled studies on the same topic. If positive effects are found, however, these must be verified in controlled and preferably randomized studies with adequate sample size.

Methodological Considerations in Population Studies

The dimensions of mental health typically examined in population studies are affective states and mood, including anxiety, depression, stress reactivity, and general well-being. Because such studies deal by definition with normal populations, the manifestations of mental distress are generally mild. Standardized scales such as the CES-D depression scale (Radloff & Locke, 1986) and the State-Trait Anxiety Inventory are sometimes used, but this is by no means the norm. New or nonstandardized scales are still common, even in studies that are otherwise well designed (e.g., Camacho, Roberts, Lazarus, Kaplan, & Cohen, 1991), whereas secondary analysis of survey data is often hampered by an absence of good outcome measures (e.g., Stephens, 1988).

Standardized or not, interviews and pencil-and-paper tests are the usual techniques for assessing mental health in population surveys. Most of the large population studies that have provided evidence on the association of exercise and mental health have been general-health surveys that examined a range of health practices and dimensions of health status. Thus, detail on mental health (and exercise) has been limited.

Exercise

The form of physical activity most often studied in population research is voluntary leisure-time exercise; studies of occupational physical activity are relatively rare. Interviews or self-administered questionnaires are generally used to assess exercise. These are the most feasible means for population studies, but their validity and reliability are often untested (Caspersen, 1989). Population studies typically measure only energy expenditure; distinctions between aerobic, strengthening, and flexibility exercise are seldom obtained. The cost of large-scale population studies usually dictates that they be multi-purpose, and sometimes the detail collected on exercise is extremely sparse, consisting at minimum of three ordered levels of exercise (e.g., Farmer et al., 1988). Even such simple measures of the independent variable can be useful, however, as they have been in studies of the effect of exercise on coronary heart disease (Powell, Thompson, Caspersen, & Kendrick, 1987).

Sample Representativeness

The strength of population studies is the representative nature of their samples, although they are not by nature representative. Some useful studies of free-living individuals, notably the population-based experiments of Steptoe and colleagues (Moses, Steptoe, Mathews, & Edwards, 1989; Steptoe, Edwards, Moses, & Mathews, 1989) are based on samples as small as 34. At the other extreme are large-scale surveys whose purpose was an assessment of population health status. When they cover mental health and exercise habits on a national level, as has been done in some surveys in the United States and Canada, the samples number in the thousands and can adequately represent entire noninstitutionalized populations (Stephens, 1988).

Correlation Versus Causation

Cross-sectional population studies can provide evidence only of correlations between exercise and mental health. Although they offer good evidence of such correlations (Ross & Hayes, 1988; Stephens, 1988), such studies leave open the questions of whether exercise improves mental health, whether only people in good mental health engage in physical activity, or whether some third factor, such as higher social status, is connected to both exercise and mental health.

Longitudinal population studies help resolve this chicken-and-egg question and establish the correct time sequence by measuring exercise at Time 1 and mental health at Time 2. Although the evidence from such studies can never be as unequivocal as that from random intervention studies, such population data provide important information about the generality of effects seen in special groups such as patients and older adults. Three important longitudinal studies have been reported since the most recent reviews of this literature, and all support the conclusions for mental health benefits inferred from research in clinical settings. A later section reviews this evidence.

Evidence for an Association in Clinical Studies

Depression

Two quasi-experimental and eight experimental exercise-intervention studies in clinically depressed patients have been published. Sime (1987) used a multiple-baseline single-case design in a study of 15 subjects with no formal diagnosis but with a moderately elevated score on the BDI. Depression scores did not significantly change during a screening phase and a 2-week pre-exercise period but dropped significantly during the 10-week exercise period. Doyne, Chambless, and Beutler (1983) used the same design in a study of four women with RDC major depressive disorder. A significant reduction in depression scores was obtained during the 6-week exercise period, and this reduction was significantly larger than what occurred in the pre-exercise screening phase.

The first experimental study was performed by Greist, Klein, Eischens, Gurman, and Morgan (1979). Running was compared with two forms of individual psychotherapy in the treatment of 28 patients with RDC minor depression. No significant differences were found in treatment outcome for those with the various conditions after 12 weeks; significant reductions in depression scores were obtained in all groups.

Rueter, Mutrie, and Harris (1982) studied 18 subjects with elevated scores on the BDI. These subjects were randomly assigned to counseling alone or supervised running in addition to counseling. Reductions in BDI scores were significantly larger in the combined running and counseling group than in the counseling-alone group.

Klein et al. (1985) studied 74 patients with RDC major or minor depression. Patients were randomly assigned to running, meditation-relaxation, or group psychotherapy. After 12 weeks significant reductions in depression scores were obtained in each treatment group, but there were no significant differences among the groups. Follow-up results indicated better outcomes for the exercise and meditation groups.

McCann and Holmes (1984) randomly assigned 41 women with elevated BDI scores to aerobic exercise, relaxation training, or a waiting-list control group. After 10 weeks significant reductions in depression scores occurred in each treatment group, but the reduction in the aerobic-exercise group was significantly larger than that in the two other groups.

Freemont and Craighead (1987) studied 49 people with elevated BDI scores who were randomly assigned to cognitive therapy, aerobic exercise, or a combination of the two. After 10 weeks significant reductions in depression scores were obtained in each treatment group, but no significant differences were seen among the groups.

Martinsen, Medhus, and Sandvik (1985) randomly assigned 49 hospitalized patients of both sexes with DSM-III major depression to aerobic training or a control group. Training patients exercised aerobically for 1 hr three times a week for 6 to 9 weeks, whereas those in the control group attended occupational therapy. Patients in both groups received individual psychotherapy and milieu therapy as well. The increase in physical work capacity (PWC) and the reduction in depression scores (BDI) were significantly larger in the training group, indicating that aerobic exercise and improved fitness were associated with an antidepressive effect in these patients.

Doyne et al. (1987) compared aerobic exercise (running) with nonaerobic exercise (weight training) in the treatment of outpatients with RDC minor or major depression. This random study showed that in both exercise groups the reductions in depression scores were larger than those in a waiting-list control group. The differences between the two forms of exercise were minimal and not statistically significant.

Sexton, Mære, and Dahl (1989) compared running and walking in a randomized trial comprising 25 hospitalized patients with DSM-III depression diagnoses. In both groups there were significant reductions in symptom scores, but the differences between groups were small and not statistically significant.

Martinsen, Hoffart, and Solberg (1989b) studied 99 inpatients of both sexes (mean age 41) with DSM-III-R major depression, dysthymic disorder, or depressive disorder not otherwise specified. They were randomly assigned to aerobic exercise (jogging or brisk walking) or nonaerobic exercise (training of muscular strength, relaxation, and flexibility) for 1 hr three times a week for 8 weeks. Patients in the aerobic group achieved a significant increase in PWC, whereas those in the nonaerobic group were unchanged on this variable. Both groups achieved significant reductions in depression scores, but the differences between the groups were small and not statistically significant.

Prevention

Only two studies have examined whether exercise can prevent the occurrence of depression in vulnerable individuals and prevent relapse in those who have recovered from a depressive episode. Gøtestam and Stiles (1990) studied Norwegian soldiers exposed to a stressful real-life situation. They found that soldiers actively engaged in sports were significantly less depressed 12 weeks after exposure to the stress, compared with the sedentary ones. Martinsen, Sandvik, and Kolbjørnsrud (1989) found that previous adult experience with exercise and sports predicted a smaller chance of relapse in patients treated in hospital, and ongoing exercise at follow-up was also associated with lower depression scores.

Exercise and Medication

Two studies have addressed whether exercise may potentiate the effects of antidepressant medication and vice versa. In the first study Martinsen (1987) found that exercise and medication had no better effect than exercise alone. In the second study a nonsignificant trend was found, indicating a better result for the combination of exercise and medication compared with the result for exercise alone (Martinsen et al., 1989b). No study has yet compared exercise and medication.

Anxiety

Few studies have addressed the value of physical exercise in the treatment of patients with anxiety disorders. Orwin (1974) used physical exercise in the treatment of phobias by asking patients to run to near-exhaustion before exposure to the anxiety-provoking stimulus. The idea was that the autonomic excitation caused by the exercise would inhibit the situational anxiety. By this method he reported success in the treatment of 8 patients with agoraphobia and 1 patient with a simple phobia. In a later study Muller and Armstrong (1975) reported that the same method was successful in the treatment of 1 patient with elevator phobia. Johnsgård (1989) reported several clinical examples in which exercise was successfully used to treat patients with phobias as well as panic disorder.

Martinsen et al. (1989) followed patients with anxiety disorders through an 8-week inpatient treatment program whose main ingredient was daily sessions of aerobic exercise. During the patients' hospital stay, mean anxiety scores in all diagnostic subgroups were significantly reduced. At 1-year follow-up, patients with panic disorder with agoraphobia (23 subjects) had lost their gains, whereas those with generalized anxiety disorder (6 subjects) and agoraphobia without panic disorder (2 subjects) remained well. Patients with social phobia (5 subjects) were almost unchanged at discharge and at follow-up.

In a controlled experiment Martinsen, Hoffart, and Solberg (1989a) studied 79 inpatients with DSM-III-R anxiety disorders. These subjects were randomly assigned to aerobic exercise (jogging or brisk walking) or nonaerobic exercise (training of muscular strength, relaxation, and flexibility) for 1 hr three times a week for 8 weeks. Patients in the aerobic group achieved a significant increase in aerobic fitness, whereas those in the nonaerobic group were unchanged in aerobic fitness. Patients in both groups achieved significant reductions in anxiety scores. The differences between the groups were small and not statistically significant.

In a randomized trial of 21 hospitalized patients with DSM-III anxiety disorders, Sexton et al. (1989) found similar reductions in anxiety symptoms following walking and jogging.

Somatoform Disorders

Exercise intervention may have beneficial effects in conversion disorder (Delargy, Peatfield, & Burt, 1986) and somatoform pain disorder (Martinsen et al., 1989), but it does not seem to influence the course of hypochondriasis and somatization disorder (Martinsen et al., 1989). Exercise intervention in body dysmorphic disorder has not been studied.

Substance Abuse and Dependence

Exercise is commonly included in comprehensive treatment programs of substance abuse and dependence. A few studies indicate that exercise intervention may be useful in treating patients for alcohol abuse and dependence (Martinsen et al., 1989; Taylor, Sallis, & Needle, 1985), but no controlled studies exist.

Psychotic Disorders

Chamove (1988) studied the short-term effect of exercise intervention in 40 long-term schizophrenic patients from two Scottish psychiatric hospitals. Exercise was introduced at irregular intervals, and patients and nurses made daily ratings of symptoms and behavior. Nurses were not aware whether patients had exercised. Both patients and nurses rated patients as improved on the days patients had exercised. They showed fewer psychotic features and movement disorders; were less irritable, depressed, retarded, and tense; and showed more social interest and competence. The less disturbed patients made the greatest improvements.

Eating Disorders

Vigorous exercise to prevent weight gain is included as a diagnostic criterion in DSM-III-R bulimia nervosa, and it is often seen in anorexia nervosa as well. Such patients often exercise alone, intensively, and for long periods, causing a high caloric expenditure. The motivation for exercise seems to be twofold: Exercise prevents weight increase and reduces inner tension, giving a feeling of well-being. During treatment this vigorous exercise must often be stopped or reduced, at least for a period.

Moderate exercise might seem useful for patients with anorexia and bulimia. Many of these patients are depressed, and exercise might help alleviate their depression. For the moment, however, empirical evidence supporting this hypothesis is lacking.

Another important point is that vigorous exercise and competitive sports may induce eating disorders in vulnerable individuals. This phenomenon is most often seen in weight-dependent sports such as wrestling, aesthetic sports such as gymnastics, and endurance sports such as long-distance running and cross-country skiing.

Evidence for an Association in Population Studies

Several major population surveys in the United States and Canada have measured exercise and various dimensions of mental health. Although only one, the Canada Fitness Survey Follow-Up (Stephens & Craig, 1989), was designed to examine the health effects of exercise, all provide some evidence regarding the association and its generality.

Cross-Sectional Evidence

Stephens (1988) carried out an extensive secondary analysis of four national surveys and concluded that level of leisure physical activity is positively associated with general well-being and mood and negatively associated with depression and anxiety. These relationships were found in all four surveys, which covered two national populations over 10 years, used four techniques to measure exercise, and employed six scales of various dimensions of mental health. The analyses were controlled for social status (education level) and physical health so that the positive relationship between exercise and mental health could not be dismissed as the result of associations with these confounding variables. The relationship was demonstrated for both sexes and younger and older adults but was particularly strong for women and people age 40 or older. Because these data were cross-sectional, however, it was not possible to conclude whether exercise preceded good mental health. For this purpose, three longitudinal studies that address this point are particularly valuable.

Longitudinal Evidence

The first evidence comes from the U.S. National Health and Nutrition Examination Survey Epidemiologic Follow-Up Study. Farmer and co-workers (1988) measured depression at Time 2 (1982-1984) with the CES-D scale and concluded that physical inactivity at Time 1 (1971-1975) may be a risk factor for depressive symptoms. White women who were not depressed at Time 1 were twice as likely to be depressed at Time 2 if sedentary than women who reported much or moderate physical activity. White men who were depressed and sedentary at baseline were 12 times as likely to be depressed at follow-up as initially depressed men who were physically active. Although promising, this study suffered from a crude classification of physical activity—a simple self-rating that might have been affected by the respondent's mood. Moreover, no association between exercise and mental health was found in men who were not depressed at the start of the study.

The second major longitudinal population study is from Alameda County, California (Camacho et al., 1991). A custom-designed scale with acceptable reliability was used to assess depression, and a physical-activity index was constructed, based on reported frequency of five recreational activities. Both men and women who were inactive at baseline were found to have a significantly higher risk for later depression than those who were active at Time 1. This relationship diminished somewhat but did not disappear when the results were adjusted for physical health, social status, social supports, and life events. Interestingly, after the data were adjusted for these important covariates, there was no difference between the mental-health benefits experienced by those at moderate and high levels of activity. This fact suggests a possible threshold at the level of moderate exercise. Unfortunately, the construction of the physical-activity index makes it impossible to equate this threshold to an exercise dose defined by frequency, intensity, and duration of exercise or kilocalories expended.

The most recent large-scale longitudinal study to examine exercise and mental health is the 1988 follow-up to the 1981 Canada Fitness Survey (Stephens &

Craig, 1989). This study's dependent measures were the CES-D depression scale and Bradburn's Affect Balance Scale. The latter was also used in the baseline study and was thus available for adjusting Time 1 scores. The Bradburn scale consists of subscales that reflect positive and negative mood (Bradburn, 1969), thus providing a conceptualization of mental health as something more than the absence of mental illness.

Two independent variables have been used in analysis of this study to date:

1. Total kilocalorie expenditure at Time 1 (1981), based on detailed reports of type, frequency, and duration of leisure physical activity over the previous 12 months
2. 1981 through 1988 changes in total energy expenditure

Analyses of variance with data from approximately 2,500 people aged 25 and over at follow-up were carried out, with controls for several potential confounders of the exercise–mental health relationship, namely, age, sex, social status (education), baseline physical health, and baseline psychological status. A significant relationship in the expected direction between exercise at Time 1 and mental health at Time 2 was found in five of eight comparisons. Future analyses will examine the contribution of exercise frequency, duration, and type.

Type of exercise is of particular interest because it not only provides information about intensity and thus aerobic requirements but also may reveal something about the psychological characteristics of the activity. Cross-sectional analyses comparing leisure activities with household chores requiring the same energy expenditure reveal that the former are much more likely than the latter to be associated with positive mental health (Stephens, 1988). This suggests, not surprisingly, that the mechanism underlying mental-health benefits is not strictly physiological.

Experimental Evidence

Although the three studies just reviewed provide the only longitudinal population data that bear on the association of exercise and mental health, another promising line of research deserves mention, as it bridges the gap between clinical and population research. A British team of researchers (Moses et al., 1989) conducted controlled trials with healthy sedentary adult volunteers from the community. Subjects were assigned to exercise programs or placebo conditions for 10 weeks, and pre- and post-training measures of anxiety, depression, and coping ability were taken. Subjects in the moderate-exercise condition experienced psychological benefits in such areas as anxiety/tension, confusion, and coping, while there were no such benefits for subjects in the two control conditions or in the high-exercise group. In a smaller study using community volunteers who were initially anxious, Steptoe et al. (1989) found evidence of benefits similar to those found in the study by Moses et al.

These results are consistent with those of Goldwater and Collis (1985), who found modest reductions in anxiety and improvements in psychological well-being in healthy students randomly assigned to a cardiovascular conditioning program, compared with those in a nonaerobic exercise program. Hughes, Casal, and Leon (1985) found no benefits in anger, tension, mood, depression, and other states, however, when testing a small sample with a crossover design, nor were improvements in depression observed in two recent controlled trials of exercise (King, Taylor, Haskell, & DeBusk, 1989; Lennox, Bedell, & Stone, 1990).

Conclusions

Exercise intervention in clinical psychiatric populations is a young and relatively undeveloped field of research. Few studies have been published, and of those, a minority reach a satisfactory level of scientific rigor. The best studies have addressed a subgroup of depressive disorders—unipolar depression without psychotic or melancholic features. Although these studies also vary in sample size and methodological strength, their results point in the same direction. Aerobic exercise is more effective than no treatment and not significantly different in effectiveness from other forms of treatment, including psychotherapy.

The studies' samples vary greatly, including outpatients and inpatients, males and females, and people from age 17 to 60. Studies have been performed in the United States and in Norway. The same trend is seen in all studies, indicating that the antidepressant effect associated with exercise is a general one.

No good studies have addressed the value of exercise intervention in psychotic depression or melancholia or in the prevention of bipolar disorders. Clinical experience, however, indicates that exercise has limited value in these disorders. In such cases exercise may be a supplement to traditional treatment.

The results of uncontrolled studies on panic disorder and agoraphobia are conflicting. There may be a positive effect on generalized anxiety disorder and on simple phobia. Exercise intervention in post-traumatic stress disorder has not been studied. No controlled exercise-intervention study with patients with anxiety disorders has been performed, so our knowledge is limited.

The evidence is also weak for any effect of exercise on the other psychiatric disorders. Exploratory studies suggest that exercise intervention might be useful in conversion and somatoform pain disorders, cases of alcohol abuse and dependence, and chronic schizophrenia. None of these disorders, however, have been studied with controlled experiments. We have interesting hypotheses and promising clinical experience but little empirical evidence.

Similar effects are obtained with aerobic and other forms of exercise. Increases in aerobic fitness do not seem necessary, as patients without physiological gains have psychological effects similar to those of subjects who have improved their fitness. This has been shown in four methodologically sound, controlled studies of patients with anxiety and depressive disorders, and we consider it a relatively strong and consistent finding.

Exercise is associated with reduced depression scores in sedentary individuals. During vigorous exercise in athletes, however, one might observe a phenomenon called staleness, which is caused by overtraining (Morgan, Costill, Flynn, Raglin, & O'Connor, 1988). Staleness is similar to depression and in our opinion may be looked upon as a form of exercise-induced depression. This teaches us that the dose of exercise is important: Too much or too little may cause harm.

Good population studies of the mental-health benefits of exercise are still rare and recent. Only three longitudinal population studies of note have been conducted, but they are consistent in identifying at follow-up various psychological benefits associated with exercise at baseline. These studies clearly indicate that such benefits are independent of age, sex, social status, physical health, and initial psychological health. The issue of self-selection into the exercise group remains a problem for these studies, however, and this places particular importance on the randomized exercise trials of healthy, normal subjects. Unfortunately, this line of research is still too new for definitive conclusions, and as yet it has provided only limited support for the hypothesis that exercise is of long-term benefit to the mental health of well individuals. Moreover, the key dimensions of exercise that are related to mental-health benefits remain unclear because gains are associated with both aerobic and nonaerobic exercise.

Hypotheses About Mechanisms.   Physiological, biochemical, and psychological mechanisms have been suggested to explain the psychological effects of exercise. Although several hypotheses have been put forward, little empirical evidence supports them. The mechanisms mediating the psychological effects are still unknown.

Vigorous exercise is accompanied by a transient increase in body temperature. Morgan (1984) has proposed this as a possible mechanism mediating the psychological effects of exercise, calling it the pyrogen hypothesis. During endurance exercise, the circulating beta-endorphin concentrations increase (Carr et al., 1981). An increase in concentrations of monoamines in the brain has also been postulated to accompany exercise (Ransford, 1982). The psychological hypotheses commonly mention such factors as mastery (White, 1959), self-efficacy (Bandura, 1977), and distraction (Bahrke & Morgan, 1978).

Implications and Issues for Psychiatric Treatment

The beneficial psychological effects of exercise are best documented for those with nonbipolar, nonpsychotic depressive disorders. For such patient groups, exercise may be considered a supplement or alternative to traditional treatment. For the effects of exercise among patients in other diagnostic categories, the scientific evidence is much weaker. There are indications that a therapeutic effect may be achieved in some anxiety disorders, conversion and somatoform pain disorder, schizophrenia, and alcohol abuse and dependence, but the empirical evidence is weak. In the treatment of these disorders exercise may be considered a potentially useful approach.

The need for treatment in psychiatry can never be fully met by health professionals. There is, therefore, a great need for simple strategies, which individuals may adopt themselves or with a little help from instructors, to help patients cope more effectively with their mental problems. Exercise is one such strategy for some patient groups.

Most exercise-intervention studies have used aerobic exercise, but similar psychological effects may be achieved with other forms of exercise as well. This fact has important implications for training. For people to make psychological gains, the important thing seems to be participation in exercise, not the acquisition of a fitness effect. Individuals may choose activities that suit them and need not focus on the aerobic element of training.

Implications and Issues for Health Promotion and Future Research

The scientific evidence does not suggest that widespread and substantial mental-health benefits will accrue from promoting exercise among the general population. It is apparent, however, that exercise has benefits for depressed, anxious, and stressed individuals and may have some protective effect for those disposed to psychological distress. Because a good deal of transient distress exists in the population and increasing numbers of mentally ill individuals in North America are in community rather than institutional settings, a case may be made for exercise promotion as the best means of reaching needy individuals who are not in therapy. In short, the promotion of exercise may well be sound public policy, as long as expectations of the extent and depth of psychological benefits are not exaggerated.

This conclusion is strengthened by the fact that

- moderate exercise has never been shown to cause psychological harm, and
- moderate to vigorous exercise results in considerable physical health benefits (Bouchard, Shephard, Stephens, Sutton, & McPherson, 1989).

This conclusion is consistent with the position taken recently in a report for the U.S. Preventive Services Task Force (Harris et al., 1990)—that evidence for the effectiveness of routine exercise interventions in clinical practice is weak, but interventions may nevertheless be encouraged on other grounds.

Clinical Populations

The number of studies on clinical populations is still limited, and there is a great need for well-designed research. Controlled studies have examined only depression. Exploratory studies, indicating potential therapeutic effects for other diagnostic groups, should be followed by new studies with larger samples and with experimental designs, if possible, including random assignment of subjects.

A few studies have compared the effectiveness of exercise to that of psychotherapy and counseling in the treatment of depression, finding them about equal. This opens interesting possibilities and should spur new, well-designed studies. In cases of depression, medication is considered the standard treatment. No study has yet compared exercise and medication in the treatment of depression. More studies are also needed to test the preliminary findings that exercise may prevent relapse in successfully treated patients and prevent depression in vulnerable individuals.

In exercise-intervention studies the type of exercise should be carefully described, as well as the frequency, duration, and intensity of each session and the duration of the whole program. If possible, measurements of fitness should also be included, so that researchers may assess whether the intervention has induced the expected physiological effect. The identification of effective elements within an exercise program is another topic of interest. An increase in fitness does not seem essential for psychological effects. Other potentially important factors may be the patients' subjective experience of altered fitness rather than objectively measured fitness. Changes in self-concept or body image and experiences of mastery and group cohesiveness are other alternatives.

The mechanisms mediating the beneficial effects of exercise on mental status are unknown, although various hypotheses have been forwarded for this complicated but important area of research. In the field of psychiatry, the status of exercise intervention is low. In our opinion this is partly due to the fact that the intervention is so simple. Most therapists spend years learning a therapeutic technique. Some feel provoked when someone tells them that the same results may be achieved with exercise. If researchers were able to identify the mechanisms by which the psychological effects of exercise are mediated, the prestige of exercise treatment, as well as practitioners' interest in it, would increase.

Population Studies

It is apparent that more work is needed for researchers to progress beyond reliance on cross-sectional data. Longitudinal studies are costly in many respects, and when they involve large populations, they are unlikely to focus on exercise or mental health. Thus, it becomes important to have valid, reliable, inexpensive, and brief measures of exercise that can be incorporated into epidemiological studies on other topics. Further developmental work on such measures remains a priority, although there has been definite improvement in the past 10 years (Stephens & Caspersen, 1994). Another priority is research into the importance of the various dimensions of exercise—type, intensity, frequency, duration, and so forth. Without such specification, we may never be able to understand conflicting research results or to establish an exercise prescription.

Population research has focused on milder versions of the same psychological outcomes as have studies in clinical settings. The study of other important potential outcomes of an active lifestyle, such as quality of life of older adults, is held back by an absence of suitable measures (Stewart & King, 1991). Measuring this and other positive outcomes is particularly important in population studies because, in contrast to clinical studies, most members of the population will exhibit little or no mood disturbance, thus limiting the apparent potential of exercise to improve their condition.

References

American College of Sports Medicine. (1980). *Guidelines for graded exercise testing and exercise prescription* (2nd ed.). Philadelphia: Lea & Febiger.

American Psychiatric Association. (1980). *Diagnostic and statistical manual of mental disorders* (3rd ed.). Washington, DC: American Psychiatric Association.

Bahrke, M.S., & Morgan, W.P. (1978). Anxiety reduction following exercise and meditation. *Cognitive Therapy and Research*, **2**, 323-333.

Bandura, A. (1977). Self-efficacy: Toward a unifying theory of behavioral change. *Psychological Reviews*, **84**, 191-215.

Beck, A.T., Ward, C.H., Mendelson, M., Mock, J., & Erbaugh, H. (1961). An inventory for measuring depression. *Archives of General Psychiatry*, **4**, 561-571.

Bouchard, C., Shephard, R.J., Stephens, T., Sutton, J.R., & McPherson, B.D. (Eds.) (1990). *Exercise, fitness, and health: A consensus of current knowledge*. Champaign, IL: Human Kinetics.

Bradburn, N.M. (1969). *The structure of psychological well-being*. Chicago: Aldine.

Brown, D.R. (1990). Exercise, fitness, and mental health. In C. Bouchard, R.J. Shephard, T. Stephens, J.R. Sutton, & B.D. McPherson (Eds.), *Exercise, fitness, and health: A consensus of current knowledge* (pp. 607-626). Champaign, IL: Human Kinetics.

Camacho, T.C., Roberts, R.E., Lazarus, N.B., Kaplan, G.A., & Cohen, R.D. (1991). Physical activity and depression: Evidence from the Alameda County Study. *American Journal of Epidemiology*, **134**, 220-231.

Carr, D.B., Bullen, B.A., Skrinar, G.S., Arnold, M.A., Rosenblatt, M., Beitens, I.Z., Martin, J.B., & McArthur, J.W. (1981). Physical conditioning facilitates the exercise-induced secretion of beta-endorphin and beta-lipoprotein in women. *New England Journal of Medicine*, **305**, 560-563.

Caspersen, C.J. (1989). Physical activity epidemiology: Concepts, methods, and applications to exercise science. *Exercise and Sports Sciences Reviews*, **17**, 423-473.

Chamove, A. (1988, October). Exercise effects in psychiatric populations: A review. In *Proceedings of the Sport, Health, Psychology and Exercise Symposium*. Buckinghamshire, England.

Delargy, M.A., Peatfield, R.C., & Burt, A.A. (1986). Successful rehabilitation in conversion paralysis. *British Medical Journal*, **292**, 1730-1731.

Doyne, E.J., Chambless, D.L., & Beutler, L.E. (1983). Aerobic exercise as a treatment for depression in women. *Behavior Therapy*, **14**, 434-440.

Doyne, E.J., Ossip-Klein, D.J., Bowman, E.D., Osborn, K.M., McDougall-Wilson, I.B., & Neimeyer, R.A. (1987). Running versus weight-lifting in the treatment of depression. *Journal of Consulting and Clinical Psychology*, **55**, 748-754.

Farmer, M.E., Locker, B.Z., Moscicki, E.K., Dannenberg, A.L., Larson, D.B., & Radloff, L.S. (1988). Physical activity and depressive symptoms: The NHANESI Epidemiologic Follow-Up Study. *American Journal of Epidemiology*, **128**, 1340-1351.

Freemont, J., & Craighead, L.W. (1987). Aerobic exercise and cognitive therapy in the treatment of dysphoric moods. *Cognitive Therapy and Research*, **2**, 241-251.

Goldwater, B.C., & Collins, M.L. (1985). Psychological effects of cardiovascular conditioning: A controlled experiment. *Psychomatic Medicine*, **47**, 174-181.

Gøtestam, K.G., & Stiles, T.C. (1990). *Physical exercise and cognitive vulnerability: A longitudinal study*. Paper presented at the annual meeting of the Association for the Advancement of Behavior Therapy, San Francisco.

Greist, J.H., Klein, M.H., Eischens, R.R., Gurman, A.S., & Morgan, W.P. (1979). Running as treatment for depression. *Comprehensive Psychiatry*, **20**, 41-54.

Harris, S.S., Caspersen, C.J., DeFriese, G.H., & Estes, H., Jr. (1989). Physical activity counseling for healthy adults as a primary preventive intervention in the clinical setting. *Journal of the American Medical Association*, **261**, 3590-3598.

Hughes, J.R., Casal, D.C., & Leon, A.S. (1985). Psychological effects of exercise: A randomized cross-over trial. *Journal of Psychosomatic Research*, **30**, 355-360.

Johnsgård, K.W. (1989). *The exercise prescription for depression and anxiety*. New York: Plenum Press.

King, A.C., Taylor, C.B., Haskell, W.L., & DeBusk, R.F. (1989). Influence of regular aerobic exercise on psychological health: A randomized, controlled trial of healthy middle-aged adults. *Health Psychology*, **8**, 305-324.

Klein, M.H., Greist, J.H., Gurman, A.S., Neimeyer, R.A., Lesser, D.P., Bushnell, N.J., & Smith, R.E. (1985). A comparative outcome study of group psychotherapy versus exercise treatments for depression. *International Journal of Mental Health*, **13**, 148-177.

Lennox, S.S., Bedell, J.R., & Stone, A.A. (1990). The effect of exercise on normal mood. *Journal of Psychosomatic Research*, **34**, 629-636.

Martinsen, E.W. (1987). The role of aerobic exercise in the treatment of depression. *Stress Medicine*, **3**, 93-100.

Martinsen, E.W., Hoffart, A., & Solberg, Ø. (1989a). Aerobic and nonaerobic forms of exercise in the treatment of anxiety disorders. *Stress Medicine*, **5**, 115-120.

Martinsen, E.W., Hoffart, A., & Solberg, Ø. (1989b). Comparing aerobic and nonaerobic forms of exercise in the treatment of clinical depression: A randomized trial. *Comprehensive Psychiatry*, **30**, 324-331.

Martinsen, E.W., Medhus, A., & Sandvik, L. (1985). Effects of aerobic exercise on depression: A controlled study. *British Medical Journal*, **291**, 109.

Martinsen, E.W., Sandvik, L., Kolbjørnsrud, O.B. (1989). Aerobic exercise in the treatment of nonpsychotic mental disorders. An exploratory study. *Nordic Journal of Psychiatry*, **43**, 521-529.

McCann, I.L., & Holmes, D.S. (1984). Influence of aerobic exercise on depression. *Journal of Personality and Social Psychology*, **46**, 1142-1147.

Morgan, W.P. (1984). Physical activity and mental health. In H.M. Eckhert & H.J. Montoye (Eds.), *Exercise and health* (pp. 132-145). Champaign, IL: Human Kinetics.

Morgan, W.P., Costill, D.L., Flynn, M.G., Raglin, J.S., & O'Connor, P.J. (1988). Mood disturbance following increased training in swimmers. *Medicine and Science in Sports and Exercise*, **20**, 408-414.

Moses, J., Steptoe, A., Mathews, A., & Edwards, S. (1989). The effects of exercise training on mental well-being in the normal population: A controlled trial. *Journal of Psychosomatic Research*, **33**, 47-61.

Muller, B., & Armstrong, H.E. (1975). A further note on the "running treatment" for anxiety. *Psychotherapy Theory, Research and Practice*, **12**, 385-387.

Orwin, A. (1974). Treatment of situational phobia—a case for running. *British Journal of Psychiatry*, **123**, 95-98.

Powell, K.E., Thompson, P.D., Caspersen, C.J., & Kendrick, J.S. (1987). Physical activity and the incidence of coronary heart disease. In L. Breslow, J.E. Fielding, & L.B. Lave (Eds.), *Annual review of public health*, **8**. Palo Alto, CA: Annual Reviews.

Radloff, L.S., & Locke, B.Z. (1986). The community mental health assessment survey and the CES-D scale. In M.M. Weisman, J.K. Myers, & C.E. Ross (Eds.), *Community surveys of psychiatric disorders*. New Brunswick, NJ: Rutgers University Press.

Ransford, C.P. (1982). A role for amines in the antidepressant effect of exercise. *Medicine and Science in Sports and Exercise*, **14**, 1-10.

Ross, C.E., & Hayes, D. (1988). Exercise and psychologic well-being in the community. *American Journal of Epidemiology*, **127**, 762-771.

Rueter, M., Mutrie, N., & Harris, D. (1982). *Running as an adjunct to counseling in the treatment of depression*. Unpublished manuscript, Pennsylvania State University, University Park.

Sexton, H., Mære, Å., & Dahl, N.H. (1989). Exercise intensity and reduction in neurotic symptoms. *Acta Psychiatrica Scandinavica*, **80**, 231-235.

Sime, W.E. (1987). Exercise in the treatment and prevention of depression. In W.P. Morgan & S.E. Goldston (Eds.), *Exercise and mental health*. Washington, DC: Hemisphere.

Sime, W.E. (1990). Discussion: Exercise, fitness, and mental health. In C. Bouchard, R.J. Shephard, T. Stephens, J.R. Sutton, & B.D. McPherson (Eds.),

Exercise, fitness, and health: A consensus of current knowledge (pp. 627-633). Champaign, IL: Human Kinetics.

Spitzer, R.L., Endicott, J., & Robins, E. (1978). Research diagnostic criteria: Rationale and reliability. *Archives of General Psychiatry*, **35**, 773-782.

Stephens, T. (1988). Physical activity and mental health in the United States and Canada: Evidence from four population surveys. *Preventive Medicine*, **17**, 35-47.

Stephens, T., & Caspersen, C.J. (1994). The demography of physical activity. In C. Bouchard, R.J. Shephard, & T. Stephens (Eds.), *Physical activity, fitness, and health: International proceedings and consensus statement* (pp. 204-213). Champaign, IL: Human Kinetics.

Stephens, T., & Craig, C.L. (1989). *The well-being of Canadians: Highlights of the 1988 Campbell's Survey*. Ottawa, ON: Canadian Fitness and Lifestyle Research Institute.

Steptoe, A., Edwards, S., Moses, J., & Mathews, A. (1989). The effects of exercise training on mood and perceived coping ability in anxious adults from the general population. *Journal of Psychosomatic Research*, **33**, 537-547.

Stewart, A.L., & King, A.C. (1991). Evaluating the efficacy of physical activity for influencing quality-of-life outcomes in older adults. *Annals of Behavioral Medicine*, **13**, 108-116.

Taylor, C.B., Sallis, J.F., & Needle, R. (1985). The relation of physical activity and exercise to mental health. *Public Health Reports*, **100**, 105-109.

White, R.W. (1959). Motivation reconsidered: The concept of competence. *Psychological Reviews*, **66**, 297-333.

CHAPTER *3*

International Physical Activity Patterns: A Methodological Perspective

Carl J. Caspersen
Robert K. Merritt
Thomas Stephens

Physical activity has a significant effect on public health because of its influence on many chronic diseases and conditions (Harris, Caspersen, DeFriese, & Estes, 1989). International consensus exists regarding the importance of physical activity for preventing and controlling coronary heart disease (CHD) (Bijnen, Mosterd, & Caspersen, 1994) and many other chronic physical and emotional conditions (Bouchard, Shephard, & Stephens, 1994). Therefore, assessing and understanding physical activity levels within populations has become a critical public-health function internationally.

In this chapter we describe international physical activity patterns and trends, presenting an overview of physical-activity surveillance, primarily from the physical activity epidemiologist's perspective. We also focus on important methodological issues to help readers interpret relevant population-based physical activity data. We restrict this chapter to a review of four countries that have undertaken physical activity surveillance over the past decade using a generally consistent methodology. We make comparisons between countries mainly to point out methodological issues. We also compare similarities in activity trends between countries, especially for certain demographic groups. Finally, we outline a number of important uses for and desirable features of physical activity surveillance systems.

Surveillance as Part of Physical Activity Epidemiology

Only recently has physical activity epidemiology been defined as a scientific subspecialty, with physical activity surveillance serving as a significant part of that subspecialty (Caspersen, 1989). The Centers for Disease Control and Prevention (CDC) has created the following definition of surveillance, extending a prior definition by Langmuir (1963):

> Epidemiologic surveillance is the ongoing systematic collection, analysis, and interpretation of health data essential to the planning, implementation, and evaluation of public health practice, closely integrated with the timely dissemination of these data to those who need to know. The final link in the surveillance chain is the application of these data to prevention and control. A surveillance system includes a functional capacity for data collection, analysis, and dissemination linked to public health programs. (Thacker & Berkelman, 1988, p. 164)

Clearly, surveillance systems must be ongoing and specifically linked to public-health activities to qualify as public-health surveillance (Thacker & Berkelman, 1988). In this chapter we consider two repeated surveys as constituting surveillance, although the two Canadian surveys we report would not qualify together as an example of a surveillance system or public-health surveillance.

Historically, surveillance has arisen from the need to prevent and control communicable diseases (Langmuir, 1963). As part of physical activity epidemiology, surveillance can be extended to monitor the prevalence and incidence of chronic diseases, conditions, or health events; the prevalence of physical activity patterns; and even the prevalence of behavioral determinants of physical activity.

Physical activity epidemiologists may wish to monitor the incidence and distribution of selected chronic diseases and conditions (e.g., CHD, obesity, injuries) according to selected demographic and geographic variables. A balanced view of the impact of physical activity would include the monitoring of untoward events or consequences.

Primarily, however, physical activity epidemiologists conduct surveillance of physical activity patterns. Such monitoring may include examining patterns of total amounts or specific types of physical activity. With such data, epidemiologists can estimate levels of undesirable or desirable amounts of physical activity thought to be linked to health outcomes. Detailed reports also may include prevalence estimates for different sociodemographic subgroups within the population. With extended surveillance, epidemiologists can assess behavior changes for the total population and for demographic groups.

Finally, surveillance can be extended to monitor the determinants of physical activity (e.g., community facilities, activity participation with friends or relatives, stages of behavior change). These types of data can be compared with data from physical activity patterns as part of the same or another surveillance system. Such data may be used to develop promotional efforts and guide the allocation of limited resources and as part of policymaking.

Ideally, surveillance data should be used to guide the development of public-health promotions, evaluate the outcomes of public-health interventions to promote physical activity, and determine whether programs have helped people in need or those who are the most difficult to reach.

International Trends in Physical Activity

Evidence from various sources published before the mid-1980s strongly suggests that North America had experienced an "exercise boom" (Stephens, 1987). Since the mid-1980s few countries have conducted surveillance to monitor national patterns of physical activity in representative population surveys. Such data do not exist in developing countries, and they are limited to a single point in time in other countries, such as England (Activity and Health Research, 1992).

This review considers Australia, Canada, Finland, and the United States because they have used large, generally representative samples, as well as consistent modes of survey administration, sampling frames, and physical activity surveys. Moreover, they have generally presented their data using the same scoring procedures for the period under observation. Because these four countries differ vastly, we can make few meaningful comparisons regarding the prevalence of physical activity. Nonetheless, we can describe the basic nature of changes between countries by assuming that each is, for the most part, internally consistent. An in-depth report about other national survey data from these and other countries—focusing not on trends but on recent survey results—provides additional details (Stephens & Caspersen, 1994).

The characteristics of each country's data system differ somewhat (see Table 3.1). The calendar years covered by these systems span from 1981 for Canada to 1991 for Finland, with periods covered ranging from 2.5 years for Australia to 9 years for Finland. Australia has recently conducted an extensive survey for the city of Adelaide, using activity questions similar to those used for all of Australia (Department of Arts, Sport, the Environment, Tourism and Territories, 1992). We did not include the estimates because they do not represent the entire country. The U.S. data are limited to 26 states with trend data, but estimates are not thought to vary substantially from estimates from all 50 states (Caspersen & Merritt, 1994).

Collection periods range from monthly for the ongoing U.S. surveys to yearly (essentially in one season) for the Finnish and Canadian surveys (see Table 3.1). The data from Australia excluded July 1985 (Bauman, Owen, & Rushworth, 1990). The survey samples were smallest for Finland and largest for the 1981 Canadian and U.S. surveys. Each country has surveyed males and females ranging from age 7 in Canada to 65 and over in Canada and the United States. All countries except Canada contacted new, independent samples after the initial

Table 3.1 Characteristics of Data Systems for Leisure-Time Physical Activity Surveillance Used in Selected Countries

Country and survey name	Survey year	Months[a] of surveying JFMAMJJASOND	Study sample characteristics[b] number/sex/age	Survey method[c]	Recall period	Total survey items	Method of activity probing	Nature[d] and detail of survey data	Activity summary score
Australia									
Department of Arts, Sport, Environment, Tourism and Territories	1984	- - - - - J - - - - -	3,502/M+F/14-50+	PI	2 weeks	5	open-ended	F/I/T/D	kcal
	1985	J - - - - - - - - - -	3,483/M+F/14-50+						
	1986	J - - - - - - - - - -	3,359/M+F/14-50+						
	1986	- - - - - J - - - - -	3,699/M+F/14-50+						
	1987	J - - - - - - - - - -	3,594/M+F/14-50+						
Canada									
Canada Fitness Survey	1981	- F M A M J J - - - -	9,006/M -/7-65+	SAQ/PI	past year	20	list-specific	F/I/T/D	kcal
	1981	- F M A M J J - - - -	11,174/- F/7-65+						
	1988	- - M A M - - - - - -	1,977/M -/10-65+	SAQ/PI	past year	19	list-specific	F/I/T/D	kcal
	1988	- - M A M - - - - - -	2,192/- F/10-65+						
Finland									
National Public Health Institute	1982	- - - A M J - - - - -	2,068/M -/15-64	Mail	usual week	1	generic	combination of F/I/T/D	3 groups
	1982	- - - A M J - - - - -	1,869/- F/15-64						
	1985	- - - A M J - - - - -	1,617/M -/15-64						
	1985	- - - A M J - - - - -	1,755/- F/15-64						
	1988	- - - A M J - - - - -	1,857/M -/15-64						
	1988	- - - A M J - - - - -	1,969/- F/15-64						
	1991	- - - A M J - - - - -	1,765/M -/15-64						
	1991	- - - A M J - - - - -	2,001/- F/15-64						

United States

Behavioral Risk Factor Surveillance System (26 states)

			TI	past month	10	open-ended	F/I/T/D	4 groups
1986	JFMAMJJASOND	14,318/M - -/18-65+						
1986	JFMAMJJASOND	20,482/- - F/18-65+						
1987	JFMAMJJASOND	17,633/M - -/18-65+						
1987	JFMAMJJASOND	24,513/- - F/18-65+						
1988	JFMAMJJASOND	18,408/M - -/18-65+						
1988	JFMAMJJASOND	25,477/- - F/18-65+						
1989	JFMAMJJASOND	18,932/M - -/18-65+						
1989	JFMAMJJASOND	26,570/- - F/18-65+						
1990	JFMAMJJASOND	20,746/M - -/18-65+						
1990	JFMAMJJASOND	28,000/- - F/18-65+						

[a]JFMAMJJASOND = January, February, March, April, May, June, July, August, September, October, November, December.

[b]M = males; F = females.

[c]PI = personal interview.

SAQ = self-administered questionnaire.

Mail = mail survey.

TI = telephone interview.

[d]F = frequency; I = intensity; T = type; D = duration.

Data from Bauman et al. (1990), Berg et al. (1992), Stephens and Craig (1990), Caspersen and Merritt (1994) and Stephens et al. (1986).

survey (the first wave). In Canada the 1988 survey was a longitudinal follow-up to the 1981 baseline survey.

The methods of survey included personal interviews in Australia, mail questionnaires in Finland, telephone interviews in the United States, and a combination of self-administered questionnaires and personal interviews in Canada (see Table 3.1). Canada assessed household and work activity, and Finland queried people about their transportation-related activities to and from work (Berg, Peltoniemi, & Puska, 1992; Stephens & Craig, 1989). We restrict this review to leisure-time physical activity.

The period for physical activity recall ranged from the past 2 weeks for Australia to the past year for Canada, to a usual week in the past year for Finland. The number of physical activity questions ranged from 1 for Finland to 20 for Canada, and the type of elicitation ranged from open-ended queries for Australia and the United States to list-specific probing for Canada.

The Finnish question asked the frequency of any and all activities performed for at least 30 minutes that resulted in at least light sweating. The other three countries probed for the frequency and duration of individual activity participation. Australia ascertained the intensity of physical activity on a 4-point scale (i.e., not at all vigorous, not very vigorous, fairly vigorous, and very vigorous). Canada and the United States used published estimates for the intensity of each individual activity; however, the United States used a velocity-correction procedure to create intensity codes for walking, jogging, and swimming (Caspersen & Merritt, unpublished data, 1994).

The physical activity summary score varied from a kilocalorie score for Australia and Canada to a three-group categorization (estimated by the authors) for the Finnish survey and a four-group categorization for the United States (see Table 3.1). The Australian and Canadian scores were published in three categories.

Table 3.2 presents the definitions for three levels of the summary scores used for each of the four countries. We present each definition in a standardized manner rather than list the exact words used in each paper (see Table 3.2). This should enable readers to make comparisons among the activity definitions. No review can fully capture the complexity of each data system. Hence, we strongly encourage readers to carefully review the primary sources to more fully appreciate the details of the activity definitions, survey methods, and sampling frames.

Australia presented data for only the lowest and highest activity levels by creating cutoff points for kcal $\cdot$ week^{-1} for activities thought to be at least moderately aerobic (see Table 3.2, footnote a) and that had a self-reported intensity level of fairly vigorous or very vigorous (Bauman et al., 1990). We subtracted to estimate the moderate activity value. This energy expenditure score was different from Canada's score, which was based on all activities regardless of intensity (Stephens & Craig, 1990).

In our review of the data from Finland, we classified all participants performing activities that resulted in at least light sweating as being at the highest level (two or more times per week), the moderate level (between one time per week and two to three times per month), or the lowest level (a few times per year or less, including

Table 3.2 Definitions, Recent Prevalence Estimates, and Temporal Changes of Physical Activity Levels Used in Selected Countries

	Physical activity level								
	Lowest			Moderate			Highest		
		Prevalence (%)			Prevalence (%)			Prevalence (%)	
Country, survey name, and years of surveillance	Description of activity definition	Most recent	Total change	Description of activity definition	Most recent	Total change	Description of activity definition	Most recent	Total change
Australia									
Department of Arts, Sport, Environment, Tourism and Territories (1984-87)	No aerobic physical activity reported over 2 weeks[a]	26.5	–5	> 0 to < 1,600 kcal/week over 2 weeks of aerobic activities	56	+1.5	> 1,600 kcal/week over 2 weeks of aerobic activity	17.5	+3.5
Canada									
Canada Fitness Survey (1981-1988)	0-1.4 kcal/kg/day (<600 kcal/week)	43	–15	1.5-2.9 kcal/kg/day of any intensity activity (>~600 to <~1,250 kcal/week)	24	+7	3+ kcal/kg/day of any intensity activity (>~1,250 kcal/week)	33	+8
Finland									
National Public Health Institute (1982-1991)	A few times a year or less of physical activity to produce light sweating or cannot exercise	16.1	–6.6	1 time/week or 2-3 times/month of physical activity to produce light sweating	33.3	–0.7	2+ times/week and 30+ min/occasion of physical activity to produce light sweating	51.3	+7.3

(continued)

Table 3.2 (*continued*)

Country, survey name, and years of surveillance	Lowest			Moderate			Highest		
	Description of activity definition	Prevalence (%) Most recent	Total change	Description of activity definition	Prevalence (%) Most recent	Total change	Description of activity definition	Prevalence (%) Most recent	Total change
United States									
Behavioral Risk Factor Surveillance System (26 states) (1986-1990)	No physical activity reported during the past month	30.5	-2.3	3+ times/week and 20+ min/occasion of physical activity either not reaching 60% of age- and sex-specific maximum cardiorespiratory capacity or not involving rhythmic contractions of large muscle groups[b]	31.9	+0.5	3+ times/week and 20+ min/occasion of physical activity at 60%+ of age- and sex-specific maximum cardiorespiratory capacity involving rhythmic contractions of large muscle groups	9.1	+2.1

[a]The Australian survey estimated an energy expenditure score as derived from "aerobic" activities such as cricket/football, jogging/running, calisthenics, aerobics, swimming or bicycling for exercise, netball/basketball, squash, etc.

[b]The BRFSS has another category between the lowest and moderate activity levels, which had a 1990 prevalence of 28.5%, reflecting a decrease of 0.3% over the 5-year period.

Data from Bauman et al. (1990), Berg et al. (1992), Stephens and Craig (1990), Caspersen and Merritt (1994), and Stephens et al. (1986).

those who reported they cannot exercise). In an earlier review we excluded people who were unable to exercise (Stephens & Caspersen, 1994). In this review we departed from the earlier convention because anyone performing an activity two or more times per week at an intensity greater than that resulting in light sweating would be at the highest activity level. (This departure from the earlier convention points to the limitation of using a single question for surveillance purposes.) We also made this change in order to completely classify all segments of the Finnish sample.

Some readers might argue that people who are unable to exercise cannot be fairly assessed. We included them in the lowest category because it most likely reflected their level of activity. Furthermore, to separate such people as a distinct group is less a matter of describing population-based activity levels and more one of ascribing the determinants of existing activity levels. A similar convention was adopted recently for elderly Dutch men (Caspersen, Bloemberg, Saris, Merritt, & Kromhout, 1991). Addressing the issue of determinants is beyond the scope of this review.

The U.S. survey uses four activity categories as a summary score (see Table 3.1). We did not assign one of these categories to the three activity levels (see Table 3.2). The unassigned category would fit between the lowest and moderate activity levels. We did so because we wanted to adhere to the convention of keeping the inactive at the lowest level (Caspersen, Christenson, & Pollard, 1986). One might include this category with the moderate activity level in order to group the entire sample into three levels, but we could not justify doing so. We used the three activity levels for didactic purposes. Forcing the unassigned U.S. category into the lowest or moderate level, however, would have defeated the purpose of the scoring procedure (Caspersen et al., 1986). Conversely, we were unable to assign data from Canada and Finland to four physical activity levels.

Recent prevalence estimates for the three activity levels reveal considerable diversity between countries, with values ranging from 16.1% to 43% for the lowest level, from 24% to 56% for the moderate level, and from 9.1% to 51.3% for the highest level (see Table 3.2). In 1990 the missing category for the United States had a prevalence of 28.5% and a decrease of 0.3% during the 5-year period (Caspersen & Merritt, 1994).

The broad range of estimates between countries stems from the differing survey and sample methodologies and is not attributable solely or even mainly to cultural or geographic differences. The only reasonable way to interpret international trend data is to evaluate activity trends within each country, using consistent survey and sample methods.

One way to compare trends between countries is to look at the total change in prevalence within an activity level for the period of monitoring. The total change in prevalence ranged from a 0.5% increase for the moderate activity level in the United States to a 15% decrease for the lowest activity level in Canada (see Table 3.2). Because the total change in activity prevalence is influenced by the number of years monitored for each country, a better way to compare trends between countries is to calculate average yearly changes by dividing the total change in prevalence by the total years of monitoring (Figure 3.1). We calculated that Australia and Canada had the greatest yearly changes for lowest and highest activity levels.

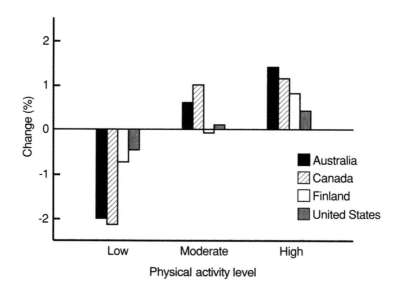

Figure 3.1   Average yearly change in physical activity levels in selected countries. Data from Bauman et al. (1990), Berg et al. (1992), Caspersen and Merritt (1994), Stephens and Craig (1990), and Stephens et al. (1986).

The declines in lowest activity levels were compensated for by changes in the other activity levels within each country. Australia and Canada showed gains in both the moderate and highest levels, whereas Finland and the United States showed their greatest gains in the highest activity level. We had difficulty fully interpreting the Canadian trend data because the months of surveying changed from 1981 and 1988 (see Table 3.1); the 1988 survey included a higher net number of activity-specific probes than the 1981 survey; and the published population prevalence included people aged 20 years and over in 1981 but included those aged 10 years and over in 1988 (Stephens & Craig, 1990; Stephens, Craig, & Ferris, 1986). Cohort analyses, however, suggest increases for the highest activity levels for both males and females—increases lower than the cross-sectional increases for males (see Figure 3.2).

In most countries the number of sedentary people has declined during the past decade. It is not clear, however, whether all countries made a transition to both more intensive and less intensive activities. Transitions from one level of activity to another are complex (Prochaska & Marcus, chapter 6, this volume) and beyond the scope of this review.

Patterns of Physical Activity Trends by Demographic Characteristics

We compared the prevalence and trends for the lowest and highest physical-activity levels according to sex, age, and educational level (see Tables 3.3, 3.4, &

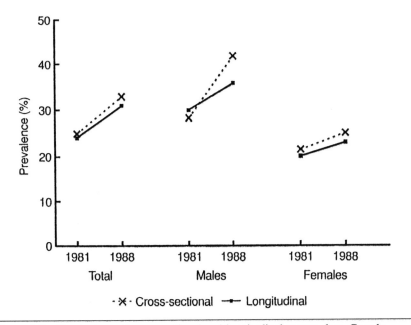

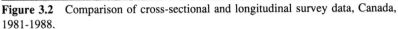

Figure 3.2   Comparison of cross-sectional and longitudinal survey data, Canada, 1981-1988.
Data from Stephens and Craig (1990) and Stephens, Craig, and Ferris (1986).

3.5). We used prevalence differences for each group to emphasize the direction and size of demographic disparities. We excluded Australian data because the authors did not report national trends for demographic groups (Bauman et al., 1990).

Over the past decade declines in the lowest activity levels have varied by sex. In Canada women had smaller decreases than men, in Finland women had greater decreases than men, and in the United States women and men had very similar decreases. Changes by sex in the highest activity levels have also varied. In Canada women had smaller increases than men, and in Finland and the United States women had somewhat greater increases than men.

The prevalence differences over time suggest that sex disparities vary by country (see Table 3.3). We observed an apparent widening sex disparity for Canada but relative stability for the United States. For Canada the widening disparity in the lowest activity levels was paralleled by a widening disparity for the highest activity levels. Furthermore, Canadian males had increasingly more favorable activity profiles than females did. American males originally had greater values for highest activity levels than females; this difference diminished and was virtually eradicated by the end of the monitoring period. The near equivalence for the sexes in the United States might be explained by the age- and sex-specific scoring of activities to identify the highest activity levels (Caspersen & Merritt, 1994). Finnish sex differences were much greater than those for the two other

Table 3.3 Differences in Prevalence Estimates for Two Physical Activity Levels Over Time According to Sex Groups

Country and survey name	Survey year	Physical activity level							
		Lowest				Highest			
		Prevalence (%)				Prevalence (%)			
			Sex				Sex		
		Total	Male	Female	Difference	Total	Male	Female	Difference
Canada									
Canada Fitness Survey	1981	57.8	53.9	61.6	−7.7	24.9	28.3	21.4	+6.9
	1988	43.0	36.0	49.0	−13.0	33.0	42.0	25.0	+17.0
Finland									
National Public Health	1982	22.7	23.2	22.2	+1.0	44.0	43.9	44.0	+0.1
Institute	1985	20.1	20.2	19.9	+0.3	46.3	38.1	44.4	+3.7
	1988	17.0	20.4	13.7	+6.7	49.3	47.2	51.4	−4.2
	1991	16.1	19.0	13.4	+5.6	51.3	50.0	52.5	−2.5
United States									
Behavioral Risk Factor	1986	32.8	31.2	34.3	−3.1	7.0	8.2	5.9	+2.3
Surveillance System	1987	31.8	29.6	33.9	−4.3	7.3	7.9	6.8	+1.1
(26 states)	1988	29.6	27.5	31.5	−4.0	8.8	9.2	8.5	+0.7
	1989	31.3	28.8	33.6	−4.8	8.8	9.0	8.7	+0.3
	1990	30.5	28.6	32.3	−3.7	9.1	9.0	9.2	−0.2

Data from Berg et al. (1992), Stephens and Craig (1990), Caspersen and Merritt (1994), and Stephens et al. (1986).

Table 3.4 Differences in Prevalence Estimates for Two Physical Activity Levels Over Time According to Age Groups

Country and survey name	Survey year	Physical activity level							
		Lowest				Highest			
		Total	Prevalence (%) Age group[a]		Difference	Total	Prevalence (%) Age group		Difference
			Young	Old			Young	Old	
Canada									
Canada Fitness Survey	1981	57.8	55.8	63.9	-8.1	24.9	26.5	19.6	+6.9
	1988	43.0	39.5	47.0	-7.5	33.0	36.5	32.5	+4.0
Finland									
National Public Health	1982	22.7	13.8	32.8	-19.0	44.0	52.9	47.5	+5.4
Institute	1985	20.1	10.9	24.9	-14.0	46.3	55.8	50.6	+5.2
	1988	17.0	11.6	17.9	-6.3	49.3	58.0	60.0	-2.0
	1991	16.1	9.2	19.7	-10.5	51.3	60.0	55.5	+4.5
United States									
Behavioral Risk Factor	1986	32.8	24.3	39.2	-14.9	7.0	5.1	9.2	-4.1
Surveillance System	1987	31.8	22.6	39.1	-16.5	7.3	5.2	9.2	-4.0
(26 states)	1988	29.6	21.4	35.1	-13.7	8.8	5.6	11.9	-6.3
	1989	31.3	23.1	36.6	-13.5	8.8	4.4	11.8	-4.4
	1990	30.5	22.5	34.5	-12.0	9.1	6.0	13.3	-7.3

[a]For Canada in 1981, young = 20-29 years, and old = 65+ years; in 1988, young = 24-29 years, and old = 65+ years. For Finland, young = 15-24 years, and old = 55-64 years. For the United States, young = 18-29 years, and old = 65+ years.
Data from Berg et al. (1992), Stephens and Craig (1990), Caspersen and Merritt (1994), and Stephens et al. (1986).

Table 3.5 Differences in Prevalence Estimates for Two Physical Activity Levels Over Time According to Educational Groups

Country and survey name	Survey year	Physical activity level							
		Lowest				Highest			
		Total	Prevalence (%) Education[a]		Difference	Total	Prevalence (%) Education		Difference
			Low	High			Low	High	
Canada									
Canada Fitness Survey	1981	57.8	—	—	—	24.9	—	—	—
	1988	43.0	52.0	33.0	+19.0	33.0	27.0	41.0	−14.0
Finland									
National Public Health	1982	22.7	—	—	—	44.0	—	—	—
Institute	1985	20.1	—	—	—	46.3	—	—	—
	1988	17.0	—	—	—	49.3	—	—	—
	1991	16.1	—	—	—	51.3	53.0	51.0	+2.0
United States									
Behavioral Risk Factor	1986	32.8	50.6	21.4	+29.2	7.0	4.2	11.9	−7.7
Surveillance System	1987	31.8	50.4	18.8	+31.6	7.3	3.9	12.5	−8.6
(26 states)	1988	29.6	48.6	19.5	+29.1	8.8	4.8	13.9	−9.1
	1989	31.3	51.6	19.4	+32.2	8.8	4.9	14.7	−9.8
	1990	30.5	51.5	17.9	+33.6	9.1	4.6	14.3	−9.7

[a]For Canada, low = < high school, and high = university degree or higher. For Finland, low = < 8 years, and high = 12 years or higher. For the United States, low = < high school, and high = college degree or higher.

Data from Berg et al. (1992), Stephens and Craig (1990), Caspersen and Merritt (1994), and Stephens et al. (1986).

countries. For example, when compared with females, Finnish males were more sedentary and less likely to be at the highest activity levels, especially during the later years of the survey.

When we assessed differences between young and old demographic groups, we found that each year the prevalence of lowest activity levels was highest among older segments of the population (see Table 3.4). The opposite was true for the highest activity level, with the exception of the United States (this too was likely a result of the age- and sex- scoring procedure).

The direction and magnitude of the prevalence differences between young and old groups varied by country. In Canada the age disparity for the lowest activity level was fairly stable in contrast to a somewhat decreasing age disparity for the highest activity level. The age comparison for Canada was not fully consistent over time, however, because the young group was defined in 1981 as people aged 20 to 29 years and in 1988 as people aged 24 to 29 years (Stephens & Craig, 1990; Stephens et al., 1986). In Finland and the United States the values and prevalence differences decreased over time for the lowest activity level. In Finland this was countered by generally increasing values but stable prevalence differences for younger and older people at the highest activity level. The Finnish data suggest a compensatory widening age disparity for people at the moderate activity level. For U.S. adults the age disparity for people at the lowest activity level decreased, and the age disparity for those at the highest activity level widened. However, the age disparity generally favored older adults over time.

Canadian data reveal that only females under age 20 did not increase in the highest levels of physical activity over time (Stephens & Craig, 1990). In Finland males under age 55 and females under age 44 had smaller decreases in the lowest activity level than did older people. In the United States males and females younger than age 45 had smaller or no declines in the lowest activity level, relative to older adults (who often had substantial gains in the highest activity level) (Caspersen & Merritt, 1992; Merritt & Caspersen, 1992). Although this pattern in young people is disturbing, the trend among older people of the three industrialized countries is encouraging.

Only the United States supplied information about educational differences for each year of monitoring (see Table 3.5). Canada and Finland reported educational data for the final year. The Canadian and United States data clearly show that the educational gap is quite pronounced for both activity extremes. Moreover, U.S. data suggest the gap is expanding but favoring the more highly educated. In Canada surveys in 1985 and 1990 indicate a modest narrowing of the education disparity for the most active group (Stephens, 1993). Data from these two countries support the results of earlier reviews of national physical-activity data (Stephens, 1987; Stephens & Caspersen, 1994; Stephens, Jacobs, & White, 1985). The Finnish data are unique because they indicate that people with lower levels of education were slightly more likely to be at the highest activity levels. This difference remains unexplained but probably arises from younger persons having lower educational levels and higher activity levels.

Most educational data (and most data in general) are not age-standardized (Stephens & Caspersen, 1994). Hence, with older and less active adults, who as a cohort traditionally have lower educational levels, we might find a spurious association between education levels and physical inactivity. Age-stratification by younger- and older-adult status, however, suggests that the educational disparity for physical inactivity is not age-dependent (see Figure 3.3) (Caspersen & Merritt, 1992; Merritt & Caspersen, 1992).

Some countries have provided physical activity trend data in a fairly consistent fashion for the past decade. Although Australia and Canada used an energy-expenditure score, their distributions across the three activity levels varied considerably. Almost 6 in 10 Australians were at the moderate activity level, and 3 in 10 were at the lowest activity level. Almost 1 in 4 Canadians were at the moderate activity level, and 4 in 10 were at the lowest activity level. In contrast, Finland used a single activity question to assess the frequency of sustained moderately intensive activity, and roughly half of its population was classified as having the highest activity level. In the United States only about 1 in 10 adults regularly engaged in intensive activities for at least 20 min per occasion, and about 3 in 10 Americans were categorized into 1 of 3 levels of activity (less intensive, less frequent or of shorter duration, or completely inactive). Similar results have been obtained by countries that have more recently adopted such conventions of measuring regular and intensive activity (Activity and Health Research, 1992; Bauman et al., 1990; Department of Arts, Sport, the Environment, Tourism and Territories, 1992; Stephens & Craig, 1990; Stephens et al., 1986).

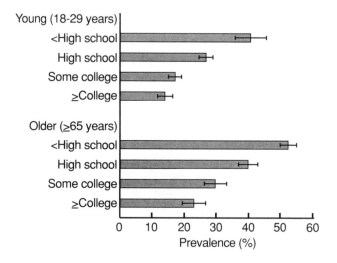

Figure 3.3   Estimated prevalence and 95% confidence intervals of physical inactivity among adults, compared by educational level, in 26 states participating in the 1990 Behavioral Risk Factor Survey.
Data from Merritt and Caspersen (1992) and Caspersen and Merritt (1992).

Although we had limited information on which to base international comparisons, we were able to compare activity trends between countries. Trend data for these four countries suggest a decrease in the lowest levels and an increase in highest levels over the past decade, with Australia having the most pronounced and most favorable changes. Patterns of exercise levels pertaining to sex and age are more similar than different between the countries. One exception for sex differences was apparent (i.e., the United States) when we used summary scores to adjust for individual cardiorespiratory capacity. Also, Finland had different patterns of activity for educational levels than the other countries. For most countries women, older adults, and people with higher levels of education have tended to gain the most favorable activity profiles.

Factors Influencing the Interpretation of Physical Activity Surveillance Data

Many factors can influence the interpretation of physical activity surveillance data. We consider defining physical activity as it relates to health: setting cutoff points for intensity, time, and number of activities as part of physical activity ascertainment; estimating the survey error variances; using single-item physical activity surveys; dealing with the effect of seasonality; scoring physical activity data to make survey data more comparable; and taking steps to ensure the reliability and validity of the data. A more thorough understanding of these factors will aid readers in using or collecting surveillance data.

Definitions of Health-Related Dimensions of Physical Activity

The physical activity epidemiologist must define and measure health-related aspects of physical activity when conducting surveillance for public health purposes. Five health-related dimensions of physical activity—ranging from caloric expenditure to muscular strength—have been defined (Caspersen, 1989) (see Table 3.6). Other dimensions will evolve as scientific research identifies more health-related effects of increased physical activity.

Surveillance of a given health-related dimension may require a distinctly different operational definition for measures used in physical activity surveillance (see Table 3.6) because each dimension may involve a different mechanism to influence diseases or conditions (Caspersen, 1989). The mechanisms range from physiological, as with energy utilization, to physical, as with the force generated by skeletal muscles to produce strength. Hence, the diseases affected may vary from chronic diseases and conditions such as CHD and diabetes mellitus to obesity and physical disability.

The surveillance definitions chosen to reflect those dimensions include kilocalorie scores, total time scores, estimated patterns of regular and sustained

Table 3.6   Dimensions of Physical Activity With Proposed Mechanism of Effect, Diseases or Conditions Affected, and Potential Surveillance Definitions

Physical activity dimension	Possible mechanisms	Diseases or conditions affected[a]	Potential operational definitions for surveillance purposes
Caloric expenditure	Energy use	CHD, NIDDM, obesity, cancer	Kilocalorie score; total time spent in or pattern of regular, sustained activities
Aerobic intensity	Enhanced cardiac function	CHD, NIDDM, cancer	Kilocalorie score; total time spent in or pattern of intensive activities
Weight-bearing	Gravitational force	Osteoporosis	Total time spent in or pattern of weight-bearing activities
Flexibility	Range of motion	Disability	Total time spent in or pattern of activities that promote or require flexibility
Muscular strength	Muscle force generation	Disability	Total time spent in or pattern of activities that promote or require muscular strength

[a]CHD = coronary heart disease; NIDDM = non-insulin-dependent diabetes mellitus.
Data from Caspersen (1989).

physical activity participation, and energy expenditure assessments. In addition, estimates of time spent performing specific activities requiring or promoting muscular strength and assessments of activity patterns may serve as surveillance definitions.

Note that in physical activity surveillance, few health-related dimensions are unique to a single type of activity (Caspersen, 1989). This fact must be taken into account because when physical activities such as running and lap swimming are used as an index of aerobic intensity, that index may also be highly correlated (albeit incompletely) with energy expenditure.

As noted, estimates of physical activity levels vary greatly between countries, especially estimates for the highest levels (see Table 3.2, Figure 3.4). One cause of this difference is selection of the health-related dimension of physical activity for monitoring. Australia and Canada used energy expenditure scores, although Australia examined only activities that were at least moderately aerobic. The

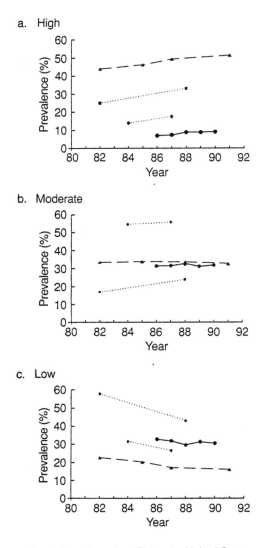

Figure 3.4   Prevalence of highest, moderate, and lowest physical activity levels in selected countries by year.
Data from Bauman et al. (1990), Berg et al. (1992), Caspersen and Merritt (1994), and Stephens and Craig (1990).

United States used a score for regular intensive activity and thus measured aerobic intensity. Both the U.S. score for the moderate activity level and the Finnish query of the frequency of at least mildly demanding activity focused on modest amounts of energy expenditure. Hence, the dimensions of physical activity, as well as the cutoff points for frequency, duration, and intensity, varied by country.

Energy expenditure estimates, even when restricted to vigorous activity, result in greater prevalence estimates than do estimated patterns of regular and intensive physical activity participation. This overestimation occurs when activities occur for long durations but at irregular or suboptimal frequencies (e.g., a 2-hr bicycle ride or 4 hr of yard work on a weekend day).

Until now no country had conducted surveillance of the other health-related dimensions of physical activity. The year 2000 objectives for the United States, however, call for surveillance of physical activity linked to muscular strength and flexibility (U.S. Department of Health and Human Services, Public Health Service, 1991).

The Effect of Intensity Ascertainment on Physical Activity Estimates

Epidemiologists have at least two ways to set an individual intensity level beyond which improvement or maintenance of cardiorespiratory fitness is assured (Caspersen et al., 1986). Each method influences prevalence estimates. The first method is to set an intensity level of 60% of maximal cardiorespiratory capacity at 6 METs or an individually estimated criterion level (see Figure 3.5). Six METs is equivalent to 6 times resting metabolism and has been correctly proposed by investigators studying men aged 35 to 57 years (Taylor, Jacobs, Schucker, Leon, & DeBacker, 1978). The second method is to use sex-specific regression equations

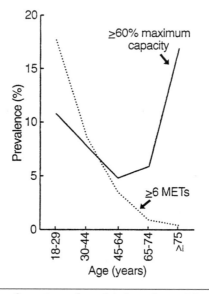

Figure 3.5   Prevalence of a pattern of regular, intensive activity among U.S. men, compared by intensity definition, from the 1985 National Health Interview Survey. Data from Caspersen et al. (1988).

with age as a predictor variable because 6 METs is too low for younger adults and too high for older adults (Caspersen, Pollard, & Pratt, 1988).

Prevalence estimates for the proportion of adults performing physical activity are more equitably derived when a 60% criterion level is based on individually estimated maximal cardiorespiratory capacity than on the 6-METs level (see Figure 3.5). This point is especially important in studies of older people, who tend to have reduced functional capacity associated with advancing age (Caspersen, Pollard, & Pratt, 1988).

The process of estimating the prevalence of regular and vigorous physical activity is analogous to the process of how exercise has traditionally been prescribed (King, chapter 7, this volume). That is, each process makes use of the fact that an individual's age and sex will influence their maximal cardiorespiratory capacity, which, in turn, influences the amount of physical activity that can be performed.

The Effect of Time Parameters on Physical Activity Estimates

Time parameters for a physical activity summary score should correspond with the health-related dimensions of physical activity. Ideally, such cutoff points should reflect the dose-response relationship of that dimension with health outcomes; unfortunately, this relationship is not always clear (Blair, Wells, Weathers, & Paffenbarger, chapter 1, this volume).

The selection of cutoff points for frequency and duration will affect prevalence estimates for physical activity levels. Activity prevalence estimates will decrease from 67% to 32% as the criterion for participation increases from 5 to 20 times per month and from 63% to 24% as it increases from 5 to 20 hr per month (Goodman, Baker, Powell, & Sayre, 1988).

The Effect of Total Activity Ascertainment on Physical Activity Estimates

Goodman and colleagues (1988) have shown that increasing the number of physical activities one must perform as a qualifying criterion also influences physical activity prevalence. The authors found that 23% of people performed no physical activity, 77% performed one activity, and 50% performed at least two activities. Furthermore, the prevalence of being termed sedentary or inactive may be as low as 5% when recreational activities are ascertained in older adults who have a considerable amount of leisure time (Caspersen et al. 1991).

Estimates of Survey Error Variance

Survey data always include errors in prevalence estimates, and such errors are primarily affected by survey sample size and sampling frame characteristics. In general, the larger the sample, the smaller the error variance. Estimating the error variance for prevalence estimates is critical if meaningful comparisons are to be made between demographic groups as part of cross-sectional data or if the significance of changes in activity levels as part of trend analyses is to be established. Australian total population estimates had 95% confidence intervals for error variances ranging between 2.4% and 3.2% (Bauman et al., 1990). The U.S. total population estimates had 95% confidence intervals for error variances ranging from 0.4% to 0.8% but as high as 3.7% for smaller demographic subgroups (Caspersen & Merritt, 1994). Moreover, estimates of physical inactivity for younger or older adults having some college education did not differ significantly from estimates for those possessing a college degree or higher education (Figure 3.3) (Caspersen & Merritt, 1992; Merritt & Caspersen, 1992).

Single-Item Physical Activity Surveys

The ideal situation for epidemiologic research is to use a single question or a limited battery of questions to ascertain levels of physical activity (Caspersen, 1989). Several single-question surveys exist (Washburn, Adams, & Haile, 1987; Washburn, Goldfield, Smith, & McKinley, 1990; Weiss et al., 1990). A limited battery of two questions has been used to create three categories of participation in strenuous work or leisure activity (Haskell, Taylor, Wood, Schrott, & Heiss, 1980).

Although using a single question has some validity, it also has several inherent limitations. For example, the global self-report (e.g., self-assessed rating of general activity level compared with that of others of the same age) has commonly been used in the National Health Interview Survey (National Center for Health Statistics, 1982). This measure is easy to use and has some validity (Caspersen & Pollard, 1988; Weiss et al., 1990). Very different physical activity profiles are obscured, however, when people of different ages and sexes report the same rating (Caspersen & Pollard, 1988). Physical activity is a complex behavior with many dimensions differentially associated with various disease and health effects (Caspersen, 1989). Hence, a single question might not be useful in assessing specific dimensions of health-related activity, aside from aerobic intensity, which can be assessed in that manner with some validity (Washburn et al., 1987, 1990).

As noted, the Finnish survey used a single question to assess physical activity (Berg et al., 1992). Some unexpected results on educational levels were found (Table 3.5). A greater richness of data would have been helpful in disentangling that perplexing finding. This example highlights the desirability of detail on specific activities when describing population-based levels of physical activity and related trends.

Future research must establish the reliability and validity of such simple single questions as they relate to the varied health-related dimensions of physical activity (LaPorte, Montoye, & Caspersen, 1985). Some progress has been made in establishing a simple battery of questions for use in older adult populations (DiPietro,

Caspersen, Ostfeld, & Nadel, 1993). Until better evidence of validity is provided, use of the single question should be limited to epidemiological studies that simply adjust (albeit incompletely) for the confounding influence of physical activity when exploring associations of greater interest (Caspersen, 1989).

Seasonality

Monthly participation in selected activities in Canada (Stephens & Craig, 1989) and the percentage of Scottish people who are physically active (Uitenbroek & McQueen, 1992) reveal wide seasonal variations (see Figure 3.6). Although Canadian estimates of activity did not include winter sports (e.g., skating, alpine and cross-country skiing), the similarity between the two sets of data is remarkable. Although activity prevalence in Australia did not differ significantly between winter and summer, the data suggested some seasonal variation (Bauman et al., 1990).

Seasonal variation has required survey measures to appropriately classify activity levels for populations. Australians measured activity in January and July (see Table 3.1). Canadians used a 12-month time frame for activity recall. Finns asked about the usual amount of activity participation, perhaps neutralizing the effect of seasonality. Finally, Americans asked about physical-activity participation in the past month, which resulted in individual misclassification for other seasons of the year. To overcome the seasonal effect, population estimates are weighted by month of survey administration.

The Canadian and Finnish surveys may be suitable for classifying individuals as part of epidemiological research. Such classification, however, is not critical

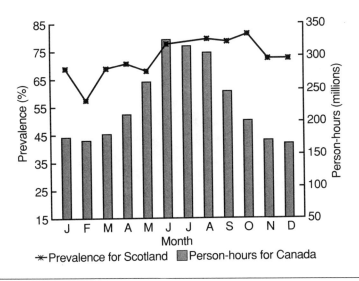

Figure 3.6   Seasonal variation in physical activity in Canada and Scotland.
Data from Stephens and Craig (1989) and Uitenbroek and McQueen (1992).

for a surveillance system that must estimate population levels of physical activity. For example, individuals have difficulty recalling details over a 12-month period (Stephens & Craig, 1989). Also, the Canadian 12-month recall data may have been influenced by seasons because people may have averaged their activity frequency and duration differently when surveyed in the more active spring and summer months than in the fall and winter months. To overcome that problem, one would have to conduct the survey 12 months of the year.

Scoring Physical Activity Data to Make Survey Data More Comparable

Comparing estimates from different surveys is difficult (Stephens et al., 1985), even when the same survey method is used (Caspersen, 1989; Caspersen et al., 1988). Factors such as survey and sampling methodologies may account for most of the differences between countries. Even with nearly identical styles of data collection, however, summary scores may differ even though they are formulated similarly. Such is the case with energy expenditure estimates, which derive from the summation of frequency, duration, and intensity parameters for individual activities (Taylor et al., 1978). Surveys that ask about more activities will generate greater energy expenditure scores than those that probe for fewer activities. Hence, the Australian and Canadian energy expenditure scores differ, in part, because of the differences in the number of survey items, which render the scores incomparable.

One advantage of using a scoring system that identifies patterns of physical activity is that estimates from different surveys using this system are comparable (see Figure 3.7). When 1985 National Health Interview Survey (NHIS) data and 1986 Behavioral Risk Factor Surveillance System (BRFSS) data are scored similarly, the resulting activity estimates are nearly identical across surveys for people classified as physically inactive; irregularly active; regularly active, not intensive; and regularly active, intensive (Caspersen et al., 1986; Caspersen & Merritt, 1994). This is remarkable because the two data systems have dissimilar survey items, methods of probing, and modes of survey administration. We are unaware of any other scoring technique that has achieved this level of comparability. It may be possible to compare surveys that are even more disparate and achieve fairly uniform results.

Reliability and Validity

Many methods are used to assess physical activity (Caspersen, 1989; LaPorte et al., 1985). Surveys are the most suitable for epidemiological research and the method of choice for surveillance. At minimum, each survey should have established acceptable repeatability to assure that people's self-reports will be consistent. Validity is the extent to which the survey instrument measures what it intends to measure. To ensure high validity, a survey should individually validate each health-related dimension of

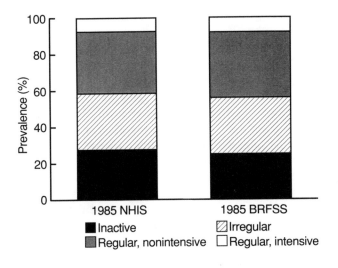

Figure 3.7   Comparison of results from the 1985 National Health Interview Survey (NHIS) and the 1986 Behavioral Risk Factor Surveillance System (BRFSS) to assess four physical activity patterns in the United States.
Data from Caspersen et al. (1986) and Caspersen and Merritt (1994).

physical activity that it intends to measure, using a different criterion for each (Caspersen, 1989). For example, estimates of maximal oxygen consumption may be used to assess aerobic intensity (Washburn et al., 1990), whereas the doubly labeled water technique has been used to assess caloric expenditure (Westerterp, Saris, Bloemberg, Kempen, Caspersen, and Kromhout, 1992).

All of the countries considered in this review except Finland have provided some insight into the reliability and validity of their surveys (Department of Arts, Sport, the Environment, Tourism and Territories, 1992; Shea, Stein, Lantigua, & Basch, 1991; Stephens & Craig, 1989). Additional evidence is needed, however.

Survey data are limited by their reliance on self-reported behavior, respondent cooperation, and memory. Furthermore, physical activity survey procedures are rarely examined for demographic subgroups, either cross-culturally, by age, or by sex (LaPorte et al., 1985). Hence, culturally sensitive physical activity probing might be necessary to assure accurate assessment within selected subgroups (Haskell et al., 1992). In addition, a fruitful area of research would be the examination of how cognitive factors such as encoding, storage, and retrieval of memory influence responses and the quality of data in physical activity surveys (Baranowski, 1988).

Issues in Using Physical Activity Surveillance Data

Researchers must consider a number of factors before using physical activity surveillance data: making comparisons across age groups, understanding and plotting geographic variation in activity patterns, caveats in data analyses, and using surveillance data for physical activity policy development.

Comparisons Across Age Groups

An analysis of the three activity levels by age group in the final year of monitoring in Canada, Finland, and the United States reveals that with increases in cross-sectional age, the prevalence of lowest activity levels increases; the prevalence of moderate activity levels generally decreases; and the prevalence of highest activity levels shows a U-shaped pattern in Finland and Canada and a slight increase in the United States (see Figure 3.8). Finnish and Canadian data, reflecting energy expenditure summary scores, support the contention of earlier reviews that physical activity declines and sedentariness increases with cross-sectional age (Stephens, 1987; Stephens et al., 1985). U.S. data differ from Finnish and Canadian data, however, because the latter two countries' definitions of activity reflect regular conditioning-related behavior (i.e., activities that are intensive for the individual) that seems to increase with age.

In assessing age-related differences in the two summary scores, we observed distinct differences between both types of definitions for high levels of physical activity (see Figure 3.9) (Caspersen et al., 1988). Specifically, we observed a generally increasing prevalence in people manifesting a regularly active, intensive pattern. It may seem paradoxical that an index of physical activity might increase with age. The explanation is as follows: The amount of time and energy devoted to physical activity declines with age (Caspersen et al., 1988; Schoenborn, 1986). Time spent in activities considered light to moderate for young adults increases for older adults at retirement age and declines continuously with further increases in age (Caspersen & Merritt, 1994; Caspersen et al., 1988; Folsom et al., 1985). Also, with increasing age virtually any activity is harder to perform (Caspersen et al., 1988). Hence, activities such as brisk walking may produce a conditioning stimulus for older adults but not for younger adults, thereby creating a need to adjust for age-related declines in capacity when estimating regular and intensive activity participation (Caspersen et al., 1988). Thus with increasing age older adults expend less time and energy participating in physical activities than younger adults, yet even small amounts of regular and intensive activities can be seen as high levels of physical activity, thus increasing older adults' prevalence in this category (Caspersen & Merritt, 1994).

Few surveillance systems use the same survey for persons under age 18 and for older adults. This practice may stem from the need to use different modes of survey administration and sampling frames in assessing different age groups. It may also arise from the need for context-specific questions to aid memory recall, which varies for youths, adults, and older adults (Baranowski, 1988).

Two of the countries included adolescent populations that might be compared with older segments of the population. Although the Finnish question was asked of adolescents as young as age 15 (Berg et al., 1992), the data presented do not

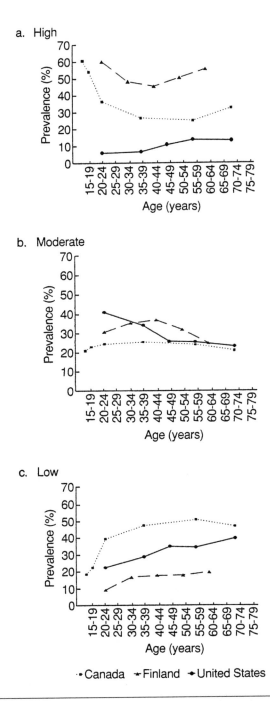

a. High

b. Moderate

c. Low

•·Canada ▲Finland •United States

Figure 3.8 Prevalence of highest, moderate, and lowest physical-activity levels in selected countries, by age group.
Data from Berg et al. (1992), Stephens and Craig (1990), and Caspersen and Merritt (1994).

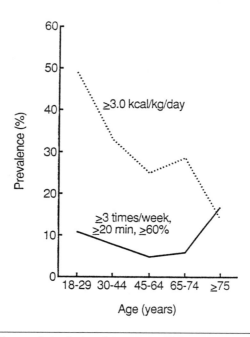

Figure 3.9   Prevalence of physical activity among U.S. men according to two definitions, from the 1985 National Health Interview Survey.
Data from Caspersen et al. (1988).

differentiate between people under and over age 18. On the other hand, the Canadian survey found little difference between males aged 7 to 14 years and 15 to 19 years for the highest activity level (each at around 70%), but it showed a pronounced decrease—to 47%—for males aged 20 to 24 years. Females decreased their activity level from 49% for those aged 7 to 14 years and 39% for those aged 15 to 19 years to 26% for those aged 20 to 24 years. Hence, Canadian data suggest that the pattern of decreasing activity for females begins in adolescence and continues after high school age, whereas males show a dramatic decline only after reaching college age (Stephens & Craig, 1990). Recent data offer a view of the change from more active to less active states as cross-sectional age increases (Caspersen et al., 1991). Among people beyond retirement age, older Dutch men showed the greatest decline in sports and active hobbies, with surprisingly strong preservation of gardening and walking behaviors. We would like to see future surveys carefully examine the entire age–developmental spectrum and the pattern of activity decline.

Geographic Variation

Canadian data from 1981 showed a general increase in energy expenditure for males and females from east to west after adjustments for the effects of age and education (Stephens et al., 1986). Similarly, data for 22 states participating in the 1985 BRFSS showed a decrease in sedentary lifestyle from the southwestern and mountain states to the southeastern states (Centers for Disease Control, 1987). We do not fully understand this observation, although the Canadian data suggest it cannot be attributed to age and sex differences or to climate (Stephens et al., 1986).

Geographic variations in physical activity may be presented in a variety of ways. The simplest, most intuitive, and most visually appealing way is to present geographically diverse physical activity prevalence rates directly on a map, making use of county, state, region, or province boundaries (see Figure 3.10). This may be done by using different colors, shades, or patterns. The 1990 BRFSS data for physical inactivity (Caspersen & Merritt, 1993) are presented, with darker patterns and shades for higher levels of physical inactivity (see Figure 3.10a). A disadvantage to this approach is that it does not indicate prevalence values for each state, making interstate comparisons difficult. This might be overcome by plotting the values within the boundaries of each state. For small states, however, this may compete with the visual effect. Another approach is to plot the values for each state, from low to high (see Figure 3.10b). The advantage is that the viewer can get a sense of the lowest and highest values, allowing better comparisons of state values. The disadvantage is that in noting regional differences, one loses the visual impact of the geographic map. A third approach is to use the box plot for presenting prevalence values for each region (see Figure 3.10c). This approach gives the reader an immediate sense of the range of values for each region, the measure of central tendency, and the statistical significance of regional differences (in this case, they were not statistically significant). Each approach has its pros and cons, and the data can also be presented in numerous other ways (e.g., bar charts). By trying these approaches, readers may be able to better interpret others' results or select the best approach for presenting their own data.

Caveats in Analyses of Data

The physical activity epidemiologist must often conduct secondary analyses of surveillance data. Such analyses are important if researchers are to make full use of existing data in order to gain new insights or generate new hypotheses. Problems arise when researchers do not completely understand the nuances of the data. For example, Jacobs and coworkers described leisure-time physical activity for parts of the upper Midwest from 1980 to 1987, using a "rigorous surveillance methodology held scrupulously constant over time" (Jacobs, Folsom, et al., 1991, p. 316; Jacobs, Hahn, et al., 1991). The authors concluded that physical activity increased during that period (see Figure 3.11). Using BRFSS data for 1984 to 1988 for Minnesota, Yeager and coworkers challenged the study, suggesting that a large increase in sedentary behavior had instead occurred (Yeager, Macera, Eaker, & Merritt, 1991). Unfortunately, the BRFSS survey changed slightly between 1984 and 1985 and

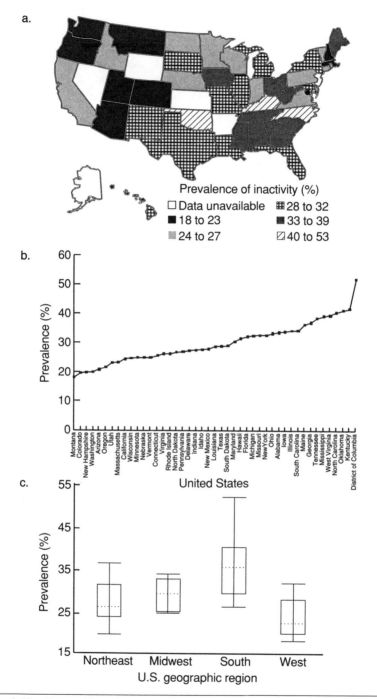

Figure 3.10 Geographic variation in prevalence of physical inactivity in 45 states participating in the 1990 Behavioral Risk Factor Survey, presented in a map, a graph, and a box plot.

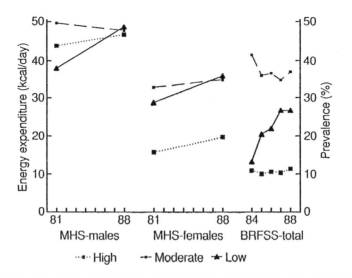

Figure 3.11 Comparison of the prevalence of highest, moderate, and lowest physical activity levels from the Minnesota Heart Surveys (MHS), 1980-1982 and 1985-1987, and the Minnesota Behavioral Risk Factor Surveillance System (BRFSS), 1984-1988 (Jacobs, Hahn et al., 1991; Yeager et al., 1991).

again between 1986 and 1987, and these changes were the most likely cause of the discrepant results (Jacobs, Folsom, et al., 1991). Yeager et al. (1991) might have avoided making the erroneous assertion by becoming familiar with the objectives for the development of the BRFSS physical activity survey and scoring procedures and becoming aware of the subtle changes that occurred in the surveillance system over time. Awareness of such factors is critical for any physical activity epidemiologist conducting analyses of surveillance data.

Using Surveillance Data for Physical Activity Policy Development

In 1990 the United States released *Healthy People 2000*, which proposes 300 measurable objectives within 22 priority areas to improve Americans' length and quality of life (U.S. Department of Health and Human Services, Public Health Service, 1991). One priority area—physical activity and fitness—relies on or calls for surveillance of two health status objectives, five risk reduction or behavioral objectives, and five services and protection objectives. The health status objectives pertain to the monitoring of CHD and reducing obesity. The risk reduction objectives are linked to the health status objectives and represent behavioral patterns of physical activity (light to moderate physical activity; vigorous activity; inactivity; activities pertaining to muscular strength, endurance, and flexibility; and combined activity and dietary behaviors for the purpose of reducing overweight). Finally, the services and protection objectives pertain to overarching determinants of physical activity (the amount and the quality of physical education within schools, worksite physical activity promotion, physician-based activity assessment and counseling, and community facilities). The use of surveillance with respect to the year 2000 objectives helps to quantify progress made toward each objective (U.S. Department of Health and Human Services, Public Health Service, 1991).

The United States developed a four-category scoring procedure primarily to estimate the nation's progress in meeting the 1990 Objectives for Physical Fitness and Exercise (Caspersen et al., 1986; Public Health Service, 1981). Those objectives called for the promotion of "appropriate physical activity," defined as "exercise which involves large muscle groups in dynamic movement for periods of 20 minutes or longer, 3 or more days per week, and which is performed at an intensity of 60% or greater of an individual's cardiorespiratory capacity" (Public Health Service, 1981, p. 79). When these objectives were developed more than a decade ago, this behavioral focus was considered useful because such exercise would lead to improvements in cardiorespiratory fitness that could be "cardioprotective" (Caspersen et al., 1986, p. 588). The highest activity level (see Table 3.2) was developed to assess "appropriate physical activity." The other three categories were developed because it seemed necessary to recognize other levels of physical activity participation, some of which could lead to disease prevention and improved health. Moreover, the four categories reflected stages of behavior that could lead to improvements in or maintenance of cardiorespiratory fitness. In essence, these categories reflected the behaviors of four types of people, who required different media messages regarding physical activity.

The lowest physical activity level has served as the basis of comparison for a year 2000 objective of reducing the prevalence of leisure-time physical inactivity. This objective's emphasis shifts from physical fitness and exercise to the promotion of physical activity and, thereafter, fitness. This focus is more realistic, given the sedentary nature of Americans. To our knowledge, the scoring procedure for the United States is the only one that not only had the purpose of monitoring progress on an old set but also had the capacity to model a new set of national policy objectives for physical activity. The NHIS (Caspersen et al., 1986) and the BRFSS (Caspersen & Merritt, 1994) data systems have distinguished themselves as public health surveillance systems relative to physical activity epidemiology.

Desirable Features of Physical Activity Surveillance Systems

An effective physical activity surveillance system must use a number of questions related to each health-related dimension it seeks to measure. Although single-question physical activity surveys are appealing, their validity appears to be elusive for all but the aerobic-intensity dimension. Furthermore, survey items should include estimates of specific forms of physical activity, if only as a means of establishing internal consistency. Survey questions should allow for the influence of seasonality by extending the time frame of recall across seasons or by adjusting monthly or seasonal estimates to overcome seasonal effects in creating population estimates. Ideally, surveyors should test and establish reasonable estimates of reliability and validity. Each data system should employ a quality control method that includes procedures for training interviewers and for ensuring realistic estimates of time and intensity parameters. This will ensure the cleanest possible data.

Surveillance summary scores should reflect the health-related dimension of interest as closely as possible and should be used for public health purposes. In the case of assessing aerobic intensity, age- and sex-specific adjustments of individual capacity should be made. Summary scores should reflect distinct patterns of physical activity (e.g., as used by the United States) because such patterns help identify groups of individuals in need of physical activity promotion. Moreover, scores reflecting distinct patterns better lend themselves to the development and tracking of policy objectives for physical activity promotion. Lowest activity levels should pertain to those who report no leisure-time physical activity—a straightforward and almost uncontestable definition of inactivity.

Sampling procedures should ensure that the sample represents the intended population as well as possible, and efforts should be made to ensure adequate survey response rates. When systematic departures from the population exist, they should be described and reported. Some statistical procedure should calculate error variances in prevalence estimates to ensure meaningful comparisons for cross-sectional or trend data.

Trend analyses of data from different systems have been conducted (Brooks, 1988), but we advise against such analyses unless comparability of summary scores can be ensured. For trend analyses, the sampling frame, the survey instrument, the mode of administration, and quality control, data editing, and scoring procedures must be consistent. Hence, unless researchers have compelling reasons to make alterations, surveys and surveillance systems should remain immutable if their goal is to present physical activity trends.

This last point is critical. One of the most vexing and confounding problems in interpreting surveillance data is the result of changes in activity surveys over time. For example, alterations in the BRFSS survey designs from 1984 to 1985 and from 1986 to 1987 created the appearance of major activity changes, when the actual changes were minor or nonexistent (see Figure 3.11). Even when analyses clarify what might have transpired had the survey remained unchanged, such changes may be made at the expense of precise prevalence estimates. For example, Uitenbroek and McQueen (1992) used a logistic regression procedure to re-estimate the prevalence of sedentary status to overcome a wording change in their questionnaire (see Figure 3.12). Although the researchers artfully re-estimated the prevalence, they stipulated that "caution should be observed in attaching too much value to any precise estimate of the decrease [in sedentary prevalence] as it is dependent on the regression procedure utilized and may be influenced by chance fluctuation and seasonal effects" (Uitenbroek & McQueen,

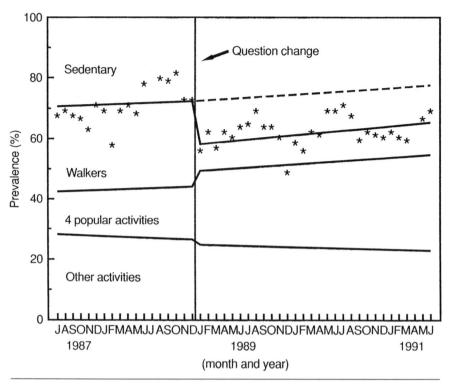

Figure 3.12 Seasonal variation in physical activity and the effect of a change in questionnaire's wording (the dashed line shows the prevalence of sedentary behavior that might have occurred without the change, the asterisks show the actual monthly prevalence). Scotland, 1987-1991.
Adapted from Uitenbroek and McQueen (1992).

1992, p. 117). Furthermore, they would have considerable difficulty explaining the results of such a procedure to health professionals or policymakers who must use the data.

Summary

We have described physical activity patterns and trends for four countries that have used fairly consistent methodology over time. We have specifically examined selected demographic data to better understand population-based physical activity levels for the people of each country.

We have also presented several methodological issues associated with physical activity surveillance, primarily from the perspective of the physical activity epidemiologist. Moreover, we have described a number of desirable features for physical activity surveillance systems. This discussion should help readers in the interpretation, use, and collection of physical activity surveillance data.

Finally, we have presented a specific example of the use of physical activity surveillance data as part of policy development that can help promote physical activity among populations.

References

Activity and Health Research. (1992). *Allied Dunbar National Fitness Survey: Main findings*. London: The Sports Council and the Health Education Authority.

Baranowski, T. (1988). Validity and reliability of self-report measures of physical activity: An information processing perspective. *Research Quarterly for Exercise and Sport, 59*, 314-327.

Bauman, A., Owen, N., & Rushworth, R.L. (1990). Recent trends and socio-demographic determinants of exercise participation in Australia. *Community Health Studies, 14*, 19-26.

Berg, M.A., Peltoniemi, J., & Puska, P. (1992). *Health behaviour among Finnish adult population, spring, 1991*. National Public Health Institute. Helsinki: Government Printing Center, Kampin Office.

Bijnen, F.C.H., Mosterd, W., & Caspersen, C.J. (1994). Physical inactivity: A risk factor for coronary heart disease. *Bulletin of the World Health Organization, 74*, 1-4.

Bouchard, C., Shephard, R.J., & Stephens, T. (Eds.) (1994). *Physical activity, fitness, and health: International proceedings and consensus statement*. Champaign, IL: Human Kinetics.

Brooks, C. (1988). Adult physical activity behavior: A trend analysis. *Journal of Clinical Epidemiology, 41*, 385-392.

Caspersen, C.J. (1989). Physical activity epidemiology: Concepts, methods, and applications to exercise science. *Exercise and Sport Sciences Reviews, 17*, 423-473.

Caspersen, C.J., Bloemberg, B.P.M., Saris, W.H.M., Merritt, R.K., & Kromhout, D. (1991). The prevalence of selected physical activities and their relation with coronary heart disease risk factors in elderly men: The Zutphen Study, 1985. *American Journal of Epidemiology, 133*, 1079-1092.

Caspersen, C.J., Christenson, G.M., & Pollard, R.A. (1986). Status of the 1990 Physical Fitness and Exercise Objectives—Evidence from the NHIS 1985. *Public Health Reports, 101*, 587-592.

Caspersen, C.J., & Merritt, R.K. (1992). Trends in physical activity patterns among older adults: The Behavioral Risk Factor Surveillance System, 1986-1990. *Medicine and Science in Sports and Exercise, 24*, S26.

Caspersen, C.J., & Merritt, R.K. (1994). [Trends in physical activity participation: Evidence from the Behavioral Risk Factor Surveillance System, 1986-1990.] Unpublished data.

Caspersen, C.J., & Pollard, R.A. (1988). Validity of global self-reports of physical activity in epidemiology. *CVD Epidemiology Newsletter, 43*, 15.

Caspersen, C.J., Pollard, R.A., & Pratt, S.O. (1988). Scoring physical activity data with special consideration for elderly populations. *Proceedings of the 21st National Meeting of the Public Health Conference on Records and Statistics: Data for an Aging Population* (pp. 30-34). (DHHS Publication No. PHS 88-1214). Washington, DC: U.S. Government Printing Office.

Centers for Disease Control. (1987). Sex-, age-, and region-specific prevalence of sedentary lifestyle in selected states in 1985: The Behavioral Risk Factor Surveillance System. *Morbidity and Mortality Weekly Report*, **36**, 195-204.

Department of Arts, Sport, the Environment, Tourism and Territories (1992). *Pilot survey of the fitness of Australians.* Canberra, Australia: Government Publishing Service.

DiPietro, L., Caspersen, C., Ostfeld, A., & Nadel, E. (1993). A survey for assessing physical activity among older adults. *Medicine and Science in Sports and Exercise*, **25**, 628-642.

Folsom, A.R., Caspersen, C.J., Taylor, H.L., Jacobs, D.R., Jr., Luepker, R.V., Gomez-Marin, O., Gillum, R.F., & Blackburn, H. (1985). Leisure-time physical activity and its relationship to coronary risk factors in a population-based sample. The Minnesota Heart Survey. *American Journal of Epidemiology*, **121**, 570-579.

Goodman, R.A., Baker, D.B., Powell, K.E., & Sayre, J.W. (1988). Estimating the prevalence of leisure-time physical activity. *Journal of Sports Medicine and Physical Fitness*, **28**, 360-366.

Harris, S.S., Caspersen, C.J., DeFriese, G.H., & Estes, E.H. (1989). Physical activity counseling for healthy adults as a primary preventive intervention in the clinical setting. *Journal of the American Medical Association*, **261**, 3588-3598.

Haskell, W.L., Leon, A.S., Caspersen, C.J., Froelicher, V.F., Hagberg, J.M., Harlan, W., Holloszy, J.O., Regensteiner, J.G., Thompson, P.D., Washburn, R.A., & Wilson, P.W.F. (1992). Cardiovascular benefits and assessment of physical activity and fitness in adults. *Medicine and Science in Sports and Exercise*, **24** (Suppl.), S201-S220.

Haskell, W.L., Taylor, H.L., Wood, P.D., Schrott, H., & Heiss, G. (1980). Strenuous physical activity, treadmill exercise test performance and plasma high-density lipoprotein cholesterol: The Lipid Research Clinics Program Prevalence Study. *Circulation*, **62**(Suppl. 4), 53-61.

Jacobs, D.R., Jr., Folsom, A.R., Hannan, P.J., Sprafka, J.M., McGovern, P.G., & Salem, N. (1991). Time trends in leisure-time physical activity: Another perspective [Author's reply]. *Epidemiology*, **4**, 315-316.

Jacobs, D.R., Jr., Hahn, L.P., Folsom, A.R., Hannan, P.J., Sprafka, J.M., & Burke, G.L. (1991). Time trends in leisure-time physical activity in the upper Midwest, 1957-1987: University of Minnesota Studies. *Epidemiology*, **2**, 8-15.

Langmuir, A.D. (1963). The surveillance of communicable diseases of national importance. *New England Journal of Medicine*, **268**, 182-192.

LaPorte, R.E., Montoye, H.J., & Caspersen, C.J. (1985). Assessment of physical activity in epidemiologic research: Problems and prospects. *Public Health Reports*, **100**, 131-146.

Merritt, R.K., & Caspersen, C.J. (1992). Trends in physical activity patterns among young adults: The Behavioral Risk Factor Surveillance System, 1986-1990. *Medicine and Science in Sports and Exercise*, **24**, S26.

National Center for Health Statistics. (1988). Health promotion and disease prevention, United States, 1985. *Vital and Health Statistics, Series 10* (No. 163), pp. 37 and 86, (DHHS Publication No. PHS 88-1591). Washington, DC: U.S. Government Printing Office.

Public Health Service. (1981). *Promoting health/preventing disease: Objectives for the nation*. Washington, DC: U.S. Government Printing Office.

Schoenborn, C.A. (1986). Health habits of U.S. adults, 1985: The "Alameda 7" revisited. *Public Health Reports*, **101**, 571-580.

Shea, S., Stein, A.D., Lantigua, R., & Basch, C.E. (1991). Reliability of the Behavioral Risk Factor Survey in a triethnic population. *American Journal of Epidemiology*, **133**, 489-500.

Stephens, T. (1987). Secular trends in adult physical activity: Exercise boom or bust? *Research Quarterly for Exercise and Sport*, **58**, 94-105.

Stephens, T. (1993). Leisure-time physical activity. In T. Stephens & D. Fowler-Graham (Eds.), *Canada's Health Promotion Survey, 1990: Technical report* (pp. 139-150), (Catalogue No. H39-263/2-1990). Ottawa, ON: Minister of Supply and Services.

Stephens, T., & Caspersen, C.J. (1994). The demography of physical activity. In C. Bouchard, R.J. Shephard, & T. Stephens (Eds.), *Physical activity, fitness, and health: International proceedings and consensus statement* (pp. 204-213). Champaign, IL: Human Kinetics.

Stephens, T., & Craig, C.L. (1989). Fitness and activity measurement in the 1981 Canada Fitness Survey. In T. Drury (Ed.), *Assessing physical fitness and physical activity in population-based surveys* (pp. 401-432), (DHHS Publication No. PHS 89-1253). Hyattsville, MD: Public Health Service.

Stephens, T., & Craig, C.L. (1990). *The well-being of Canadians: Highlights of the 1988 Campbell's Survey*. Ottawa, ON: Canadian Fitness and Lifestyle Research Institute.

Stephens, T., Craig, C.L., & Ferris, B.F. (1986). Adult physical activity in Canada: Findings from the Canada Fitness Survey I. *Canadian Journal of Public Health*, **77**, 285-290.

Stephens, T., Jacobs, D.R., & White, C.C. (1985). A descriptive epidemiology of leisure-time physical activity. *Public Health Reports*, **100**, 147-158.

Taylor, H.L., Jacobs, D.R., Schucker, B., Leon, A.S., & DeBacker, G. (1978). A questionnaire for the assessment of leisure time physical activities. *Journal of Chronic Diseases*, **31**, 741-755.

Thacker, S.B., & Berkelman, R.L. (1988). Public health surveillance in the United States. *Epidemiologic Reviews*, **10**, 164-190.

Uitenbroek, D.G., & McQueen, D.V. (1992). Leisure-time physical activity in Scotland: Trends 1987-1991 and the effect of question wording. *Sozial und Praventivmedizin*, **37**, 113-117.

U.S. Department of Health and Human Services, Public Health Service. (1991). *Healthy people 2000: National health promotion and disease prevention objectives* (DHHS Publication No. [PHS] 91-50212). Washington, DC: U.S. Government Printing Office.

Washburn, R.A., Adams, L., & Haile, G. (1987). Physical activity assessment for epidemiologic research: The utility of two simplified approaches. *Preventive Medicine*, **16**, 636-646.

Washburn, R.A., Goldfield, S.R.W., Smith, K.W., & McKinley, J.B. (1990). The validity of self-reported exercise-induced sweating as a measure of physical activity. *American Journal of Epidemiology*, **132**, 107-113.

Weiss, T.W., Slater, C.H., Green, L.W., Kennedy, V.C., Albright, D.L., & Wun, C.C. (1990). The validity of single-item, self-assessment questions as measures of adult physical activity. *Journal of Clinical Epidemiology*, **43**, 1123-1129.

Westerterp, K.R., Saris, W.H.M., Bloemberg, B.P.M., Kempen, K., Caspersen, C.J., & Kromhout, D. (1992). Validation of the Zutphen Physical Activity Questionnaire for the elderly with doubly labeled water. *Medicine and Science in Sports and Exercise*, **23**, S68.

Yeager, K.K., Macera, C.A., Eaker, E., & Merritt, R.K. (1991). Time trends in leisure-time physical activity: Another perspective. *Epidemiology*, **4**, 313-315.

The authors would like to gratefully acknowledge Ms. Jane Grimsley for her help in the preparation of this manuscript and Dr. Rick Hull for his editorial suggestions and written contributions. Their invaluable assistance has helped to greatly improve the quality of this chapter.

PART II

Theory and Determinants of Physical Activity

CHAPTER *4*

Social-Cognitive Models

Gaston Godin

At the beginning of the 1980s few authors had noted that most studies of adherence to physical activity were atheoretical, the information obtained concerning the motives for exercising being generally descriptive and guided by researcher bias. Dishman (1982) in particular was critical of the atheoretical nature of research into compliance. Sonstroem (1982) also suggested that the understanding of exercise behavior was limited by the theoretical framework adopted, but more often by the absence of one, and that researchers would benefit from reference to attitudinal theories such as the theory of reasoned action developed by Fishbein and Ajzen (1975). Similarly, Godin and Shephard (1983) have shown that assessing the effectiveness of physical-fitness-promotion programs in modifying exercise behavior was extremely difficult because most programs implemented during the 1970s were developed without reference to theoretical models of human behavior. In summary, for all of the authors named, the absence of a theoretical approach to the study of exercise behavior was seen as a possible explanation for the poor understanding of exercise adherence at that time and, consequently, for the low level of adherence to regular physical activity among North Americans.

The first authors to study exercise behavior in reference to a theoretical approach were Heinzelmann and Bagley (1970), who used some of the health-belief model variables to study exercise adherence in a group of individuals at risk of coronary heart disease; Wankel and Beatty (1975), who applied one of the earlier versions of Fishbein's model to the study of attendance in an organized exercise program; and Riddle (1980), who used Fishbein and Ajzen's theoretical framework to predict jogging in an adult population. Since then, however, a number of authors have applied different theoretical frameworks to the study of exercise behavior among different segments of the population.

I examine here the main social-cognitive models, and more specifically the attitude-behavior models, that have been used to analyze exercise behavior to date. I explain and define the most popular theoretical frameworks used by researchers in the field of exercise adherence, summarize available findings, and consider their implications for future research on exercise adherence and the development of new exercise-promotion programs. My review concerns all studies that provided information concerning one or more of the variables included in a theoretical social-cognitive model. Given this book's focus on exercise promotion and health, however, I excluded studies conducted on sport and competition.

Health-Belief Model

The health-belief model (HBM; Becker & Maiman, 1975) postulates that the likelihood of adopting a behavior appropriate to the prevention or control of some disease depends on the individual's perception of a threat to personal health and a conviction that the recommended action will reduce this threat (see Figure 4.1). The perception of a health threat is determined by the strength of two underlying beliefs: personal susceptibility to a given disease and the potential severity of its impact on the individual's life. Such perceptions can be awakened or strengthened by such occurrences as the death of a close friend. The perceived efficacy of the recommended preventive action depends on

- a personal assessment of the perceived benefits of the proposed behavior (in reducing the susceptibility to or the severity of the condition) and
- real or perceived barriers to initiation or continuation of the suggested behavior.

According to the HBM, an individual should decide to exercise regularly if a sedentary lifestyle is perceived as a threat to some aspect of health and if regular physical activity is seen as decreasing that risk. For example, in the context of ischemic heart disease, the perception of a significant threat is influenced by

- a belief in personal vulnerability to coronary heart disease,
- a belief that the consequences of a coronary episode will be severe, or
- the occurrence of an unanticipated event, such as a myocardial infarction, in a close friend who has also been sedentary.

The HBM has to date found relatively little application in attempts to augment physical activity among sedentary individuals. Heinzelmann and Bagley (1970) noted that the exercise participation of middle-aged men prone to coronary heart disease was related to their perception that exercise involvement would reduce their risk of heart disease. Men who had been exercising for some time perceived that they had become less susceptible to heart disease than they had been before joining the program. Mirotznik, Speedling, Stein, and Bronz (1985) compared recruits in a cardiovascular-fitness program with individuals who had chosen not

| Individual perceptions | Modifying factors | Likelihood of action |

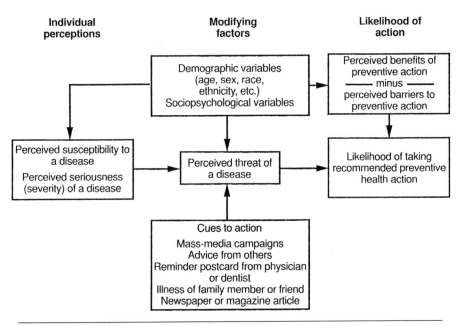

Figure 4.1   Elements of the health-belief model.
Reprinted from Becker and Maiman (1975).

to join the program. Those recruited were more concerned about their health and more likely to see an improvement in health as benefitting other areas of their lives.

Some authors have been less supportive of the HBM as a means of explaining habitual exercise behavior. In their study of physical-activity patterns between regular joggers and sedentary individuals, Slenker, Price, Roberts, and Jurs (1984) showed that perceived susceptibility to health problems was a relatively weak factor in discriminating between the physical-activity patterns of regular joggers and of those who chose not to exercise. Joggers and sedentary individuals both tended to believe that regular jogging would decrease susceptibility to certain health problems, and both groups believed that such problems would have a major impact on their future health. A cross-sectional study of factors influencing recruitment in an employee fitness program also found that many workers had firm beliefs about heart attacks and their relationship to lack of physical activity. Such beliefs, however, were unrelated to the regular practice of exercise or to the fitness status of individuals entering the program (Shephard, P. Morgan, Finucane, & Schimmelfing, 1980). Further reports noted no significant associations between the HBM variables and exercise behavior among adults (Mullen, Hersey, & Iverson, 1987) or adolescents (O'Connell, Price, Roberts, Jurs, & McKinley, 1985). Lindsay-Reid and Osborn (1980) even reported that in a population of fire fighters the initial perception of susceptibility to ischemic heart disease and to general illnesses was negatively associated with subsequent adherence to regular exercise. Perceptions of risk of illness apparently did not motivate this population to take up physical activity. P.P. Morgan, Shephard, Finucane, Schimmelfing, and Jazmaji (1984) likewise observed that those who initially perceived themselves as healthy were more likely to maintain their regular participation in an exercise program than those who did not perceive themselves as healthy.

Since the HBM is concerned with perceptions of disease, one might postulate that it would provide a more satisfactory framework for the study of exercise behavior in a population already affected by ischemic heart disease. Unfortunately, the results are ambiguous. One of four such studies found an association between health beliefs and compliance with a fitness program (Holm, Fink, Christman, Reitz, & Ashley, 1985), a second found no significant association between the period of continued participation in a cardiac exercise program and HBM variables (Muench, 1987), a third investigation showed that those who perceived themselves as the most susceptible to a further coronary incident were the least compliant (Tirrell & Hart, 1980), and a fourth study found that perceived severity of disease distinguished compliers from dropouts of the cardiac-rehabilitation program but in a direction opposite to that hypothesized by the HBM (Oldridge & Streiner, 1990).

Hence, existing data provide no clear indication that the HBM is appropriate for the study of exercise behavior. The likely explanation lies in the diversity of motives for exercising (Dishman, Sallis, & Orenstein, 1985). For example, many people start exercising in order to lose weight, but relatively few people attempt to reduce their body mass simply for health reasons. An attempt to improve personal appearance is more commonly the main factor initiating their behavior.

Protection Motivation Theory

The protection motivation theory (PMT; Rogers, 1975) is similar to the HBM. More recently, Maddux and Rogers (1983) and Rogers (1983) incorporated components of the self-efficacy theory (Bandura, 1977) into the PMT, proposing that the intention to protect oneself depends upon four factors:

1. The perceived severity of a threatened event (e.g., a heart attack)
2. The perceived probability of the occurrence (in our example, the perceived vulnerability of the individual to a heart attack)
3. The efficacy of the recommended preventive behavior (the perceived response efficacy)
4. The perceived self-efficacy (i.e., the level of confidence in one's ability to undertake the recommended preventive behavior)

Wurtele and Maddux (1987) applied the PMT to exercise behavior. They found that perceived susceptibility to cardiovascular problems and perceived self-efficacy enhanced intentions to exercise among a group of female undergraduates. But perhaps because the subjects were young adults and the prospect of disease was correspondingly distant, the perceived severity of the disease failed to influence intentions, and intention was the only significant predictor of exercise behavior. Desharnais, Godin, and Jobin (1987) confirmed these observations in a population of adults. Regardless of perceived susceptibility, all subjects who were exposed to persuasive communication increased their intention to exercise. Subjects with a poor fitness level who had been convinced of a high rather than a low susceptibility to disease, however, proved more likely to maintain their initial intention to exercise over a 3-month period. Godin, Cox, and Shephard (1983) found that one type of persuasive communication (a physical-fitness evaluation, with subsequent exercise and health counseling) did not significantly change the intention to exercise of subjects who had elected to visit an athletic center for the purpose of fitness testing. Finally, contrary to the hypothesis of the PMT, perceived severity of and perceived vulnerability to having another myocardial infarction exerted no influence on intention to exercise among CHD individuals (Godin, Valois, Jobin, & Ross, 1991).

In general, messages conveying a persuasive threat seem effective in enhancing participants' intention to change their behaviors, but they are less effective in inducing and sustaining changes in behavior. Thus, Godin, Desharnais, Jobin, and Cook (1987) showed that subjects who had their physical fitness evaluated reported a stronger intention to exercise over the next 3 months than those who did not have a fitness appraisal. The positive behavioral effect of the fitness evaluation, however, disappeared after 3 months. Moreover, knowledge that the objectively measured fitness level differed from the individual's self-perception of fitness had no impact on a person's exercise behavior over the 3-month period (Godin & Desharnais, 1987).

The PMT thus has limited usefulness for the study of exercise behavior. The positive findings reported to date support the influence of self-efficacy variables (Bandura, 1977) rather than the variables of the PMT (Stanley & Maddux, 1986), and some authors are now integrating the self-efficacy theory into the PMT in a manner analogous to researchers' recent modifications of the HBM (Rosenstock, Strecher, & Becker, 1988).

Self-Efficacy Theory

Bandura (1977) writes that all behavioral changes are mediated by a common cognitive mechanism termed self-efficacy, namely, a belief that one can successfully perform the desired behavior. A belief in self-efficacy is learned in various ways, including personal experiences (good or bad) and the example provided by others (modeling). Perceived self-efficacy can determine

- whether an individual attempts a given task,
- the degree of persistence when the individual encounters difficulties, and
- ultimate success.

Self-efficacy theory (SET) distinguishes between expectations of self-efficacy and of outcome. The expectation of outcome is the individual's "estimate that a given behavior will lead to certain outcomes'' (Bandura, 1977, p. 193). In contrast, an expectation of self-efficacy is "the conviction that one can successfully execute the behavior required to produce the outcomes" (p. 193). Bandura (1977, 1982) indicates that an expectation of self-efficacy is a more central determinant of subsequent behavior than the expectation of outcome, but in many situations both are important.

According to SET, attempts to increase exercise behavior would be influenced by

- self-judgment of the expected benefits of regular exercise and
- perceived ability to exercise regularly.

Desharnais, Bouillon, and Godin (1986) confirmed that in the context of a formal exercise program offered to healthy young adults, an expectation of self-efficacy was a more central determinant of adherence than the expectation of outcome, although both variables were significant cognitive mediators of exercise adherence. At the outset of an 11-week program, subsequent dropouts displayed less certainty than adherents about their capacity to attend regularly and higher expectations of increased benefits (physical, social, psychological) from participation. Dzewaltowski (1989) found similar results among a group of undergraduate students enrolled in physical-education skills classes for 8 weeks. Individuals who were confident they could adhere to an exercise program, despite possible barriers, exercised more days per week; outcome expectations did not account for a significant amount of the variance in behavior. Dzewaltowski, Noble, and Shaw (1990) subsequently examined the ability of the SET to predict the physical-activity participation of undergraduates enrolled in a course on concepts of physical education. Again, perceived self-efficacy was the best variable at explaining variation in energy expenditures over a 4-week period.

McAuley and Jacobson (1991) found that self-efficacy, defined as the capability to successfully continue an exercise regimen in the face of potential barriers, was a significant predictor of exercise levels over an 8-week low-impact aerobic fitness program designed for sedentary adult females. McAuley, Wraith, and Duncan (1991) also showed that intrinsic motivation for aerobic dance was partly explained by self-efficacy. Finally, Stanley and Maddux (1986) showed that the intention to participate in an exercise program was influenced by both perceived ability to undertake the required behaviors and expected outcome of participation.

Three other community studies support the SET in the context of spontaneously adopted physical activity. Wurtele and Maddux (1987) showed that undergraduate women who had higher perceptions of their ability to adopt a personal exercise program indicated stronger intentions to do so than those with lower perceptions of this ability. Similarly, Sallis et al. (1986) found that both adoption and maintenance of vigorous activity by adults were positively influenced by an expectation of ability to undertake vigorous activity. Finally, Sallis et al. (1989) found that the strongest correlate with exercise behavior among adults was self-efficacy, expressed as confidence in one's ability to exercise in specific situations.

Therefore, the SET has been successfully applied in explaining exercise behavior. The perceived ability to participate and to exercise regularly in a structured program seems to be the variable of prime importance. As we will discuss later, few authors have reported the superiority of self-efficacy to predict exercise behavior over and above the influence of important variables included in other theoretical frameworks. Moreover, the cumulative evidence of positive associations between expectations of self-efficacy and the adoption of various health-related behaviors has persuaded promoters of the HBM and the PMT to integrate this variable into their models.

The Theory of Reasoned Action

The primary goals of the theory of reasoned action (TRA; Fishbein & Ajzen, 1975) are to understand and predict social behaviors. Predictions must be conducted in a closely defined context. The behavior must be clearly specified, volitional in type, and performed in a given situation. In addition, it is assumed that the immediate and sole determinant of the behavior in question is the intention to perform or not perform that behavior. Consequently, this theory interprets social behavior at the level of individual decision-making.

According to the TRA, the proximate determinants of the intent to adopt a given behavior are the individual's attitude about performing the behavior and the influence of social factors (such as the perceived beliefs of the spouse) upon performance of the behavior (see Figure 4.2). The basic Fishbein and Ajzen model can thus be represented symbolically as follows:

$$B \approx I = (Aact)w_1 + (SN)w_2 \qquad (1)$$

where B is the behavior, I is the behavioral intention, *Aact* is the attitude toward the behavior, *SN* is a measure of a person's perception that the majority of "significant others" think that he or she should adopt the behavior, and w_1 and w_2 are empirical weights determined by multiple regression analysis. According to the TRA, the weighting coefficients (w_1 and w_2) should show intersituational and interindividual differences. For some behaviors the attitudinal component (*Aact*) is the major determinant of intentions, whereas for other behaviors the normative component (*SN*) is dominant.

The personal attitude toward the behavior, *Aact*, is a function of beliefs concerning the perceived consequences of carrying out a specific action, *B*, and a personal evaluation of these consequences. In essence, the subject evaluates as a summed product the probability that performance of the behavior will cause each of the anticipated consequences, and a measure of these assessments is multiplied by an evaluation of the corresponding anticipated consequences.

Generally speaking, people have between 5 and 10 readily identified beliefs with respect to a given action. For example, a person may believe that regular exercise will improve physical appearance and lower the risk of sustaining a

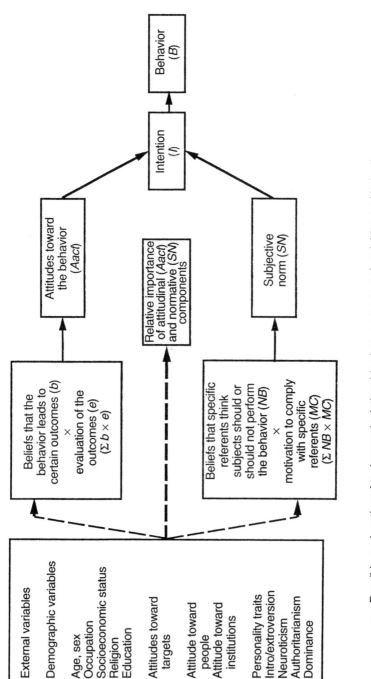

Figure 4.2 Schematic representation of Fishbein and Ajzen's model. Adapted from Ajzen and Fishbein (1980).

Behavior (B)

Intention (I)

Attitudes toward the behavior (Aact)

Subjective norm (SN)

Relative importance of attitudinal (Aact) and normative (SN) components

Beliefs that the behavior leads to certain outcomes (b) × evaluation of the outcomes (e) (Σ b × e)

Beliefs that specific referents think subjects should or should not perform the behavior (NB) × motivation to comply with specific referents (MC) (Σ NB × MC)

External variables

Demographic variables

Age, sex
Occupation
Socioeconomic status
Religion
Education

Attitudes toward targets

Attitude toward people
Attitude toward institutions

Personality traits
Intro/extroversion
Neuroticism
Authoritarianism
Dominance

- - - ▶ Possible explanations for observed relationships between external variables and behavior

——▶ Stable theoretical relationships linking beliefs to behavior

heart attack as well as take time away from the family. In the shaping of behavior each person evaluates the consequences attached to these beliefs. Thus, an individual can attribute a personal value to the improvement of physical appearance, the decreased risk of sustaining a heart attack, and time taken away from the family. The characteristic attitude of the individual is quantified as the summed product of belief times evaluation and is expressed as

$$Aact = \Sigma \, b \times e \tag{2}$$

The second component, *SN*, is determined by the perceived expectations of salient referent individuals or groups (the normative belief, NB) and by the individual's motivation to comply (MC) with the expectations of these significant others (friends, spouse, family physician, etc.). For example, the spouse may be perceived as thinking that the subject should exercise a few times a week. The subject in question may or may not be inclined to act according to such perceived beliefs, however. In the formation of *SN*, each NB is thus attenuated by a corresponding measure of MC. Thus, the summed product of normative belief times motivation to comply represents the subjective norm (*SN*) for the individual and is expressed as

$$SN = \Sigma \, NB \times MC \tag{3}$$

A further element of Fishbein and Ajzen's basic model is the supposition that external variables are related to behavior only when they affect variables specified in the model. It is assumed that most human behavior of interest to social specialists is under a degree of volitional control and hence is determined by behavioral intent. Thus, personality and other sociocultural variables influence behavior only by influencing attitudinal and normative considerations.

The basic assumptions of the TRA have been verified frequently. In an extensive review of the theories of attitude and attitude change, Cooper and Croyle (1984) concluded that Fishbein and Ajzen's theory of reasoned action has been the basis of most of the progress in the field of social psychology and that their model is now considered one of the most integrated theories of social behavior. Moreover, a recent meta-analysis (Sheppard, Hartwick, & Warshaw, 1988) of more than 87 separate studies (selected because of the quality of their operational definition of the theory) with a total sample of 11,566 subjects showed that the frequency-weighted average correlation for the prediction of behavior was .53 ($p < .01$) and .66 for the prediction of intention ($p < .001$).

A number of investigators have applied the TRA to the study of exercise behavior (see the review by Godin & Shephard, 1990). Overall, the TRA has proved very helpful in clarifying the decision-making process that underlies exercise behavior. Where such information has been provided by the investigators, approximately 30% of the variance in intention to exercise seems explained by the individual's attitudes. This observation deserves emphasis because researchers who have used less specific indicators of attitude, such as the Kenyon Attitude Inventory (Kenyon, 1968a, 1968b) and the Physical Estimation and Attraction

Scales (Sonstroem, 1974), have claimed that attitudinal scores do not predict exercise behavior (Dishman & Gettman, 1980; Dishman, Ickes, & N.P. Morgan, 1980). When attitude is measured within a proper theoretical framework, it seems an important determinant of exercise behavior (Godin & Shephard, 1986; Kendzierski & Davis Lamastro, 1988).

Subjective norm is less consistently associated with intention to exercise and does not appear to be a stable variable for the interpretation of exercise behavior. Some authors have suggested that part of the apparent ambiguity concerning the importance of SN could be attributed to the present operational definition of this construct (Miniard & Cohen, 1981). Nevertheless, even when the influence of SN has proven statistically significant, SN has always had less effect on exercise than attitude. This is perhaps to be expected; Valois, Desharnais, and Godin (1988) found that individuals believed the decision to exercise or not was their own responsibility.

A few studies have suggested that external variables can influence intentions independently of the primary TRA constructs (Bentler & Speckart, 1981; Godin et al., 1983; Godin & Shephard, 1986; Godin, Valois, Shephard, & Desharnais, 1987; Godin, Vézina, & Leclerc, 1989). Past behavior, or habit of exercising, seems particularly important. The intention to exercise is probably stronger for someone who already has the habit of exercising, and it is easier for such a person to apply the TRA variables to further encourage regular exercise. In contrast, individuals who have a habit of being sedentary find it difficult to change their habit, and the decision to begin an exercise program requires a more conscious effort of will.

Intention is an important predictor of exercise behavior. However, some external variables have a significant influence on the translation of intention into behavior. In particular, past behavior and exercise habit seem to be reliable predictors of exercise behavior (Godin, Valois, et al., 1987; Valois et al., 1988). Some social theorists also argue that real or perceived barriers have a substantial impact on the translation of intention into behavior (Ajzen, 1985; Triandis, 1977).

Fishbein and Ajzen (1975) postulated that intention was the sole predictor of behavior. Nonetheless, the basic variables in Fishbein and Ajzen's model account for only a fraction of the total variance in exercise behavior. The implication is that measurement techniques need further refinement or factors other than intention are involved. In support of the latter view, Godin, Valois, et al. (1987) reported that a measure of exercise habit significantly improved the accuracy of exercise predictions, using the TRA model. Although Fishbein and Ajzen's basic model has considerable value, the search should continue for more complete descriptors of exercise behavior.

The Theory of Interpersonal Behavior

The theory of interpersonal behavior (Triandis, 1977) specifies that the likelihood of undertaking a given behavior is a function of

- the habit of performing the behavior,
- the intention to perform the behavior, and
- the conditions facilitating or discouraging performance of the behavior (see Figure 4.3).

In contrast to a basic doctrine of Fishbein and Ajzen (1975), Triandis proposed that some behaviors were not the outcome of conscious and systematic analysis. The Triandis relationship can be expressed by the equation

$$B = (I \times F)w_{i.f} + (H \times F)w_{h.f} \tag{4}$$

where B is a given behavior, I is the individual's intention to perform or not perform the behavior, H is an evaluation of the habit or the number of times the individual has performed the behavior, F is the evaluation of conditions facilitating or discouraging performance of the behavior, and $w_{i.f}$ and $w_{h.f}$ are the corresponding regression coefficients.

Triandis writes that some behaviors become automatic and can be performed with little conscious intervention (e.g., driving a car along a familiar street or purchasing a particular brand of toothpaste). Thus, the number of times a behavior has been performed (i.e., the strength of the habit) is an important factor in predicting behavior under specific circumstances. For example, a person who has extremely sedentary living habits may fail to begin exercising despite an apparently strong intention to do so, whereas a person who has already formed the habit of exercising regularly may attend exercise sessions without any deliberate planning or obvious intention of being active. The degree of novelty of the action in question thus influences the relative importance of intention and habit to the prediction of behavior. The first experiences of a given behavior are largely under the control of intention, but with repetition the habit of undertaking the behavior progressively replaces the role of intention. Conditions that facilitate or discourage performance of a behavior are also important to its prediction, moderating the influence of both habit and intention.

Triandis (1977) indicates that intention is shaped by four elements:

1. A cognitive component
2. An affective component
3. A social component
4. A personal normative belief

The cognitive component reflects a subjective analysis of the advantages and disadvantages of adopting a behavior. As is the case with the TRA, the cognitive component is a function of perceived consequences and the value attributed to those consequences. It is estimated as the summed product benefit times the value.

The affective dimension includes the individual's emotional response to the thought of adopting a behavior and the feelings elicited by the change in behavior (pleasant or unpleasant, interesting or boring, etc.). This component is shaped by the memory of previous positive and negative experiences, with positive feelings engendering a desire to repeat the behavior.

124

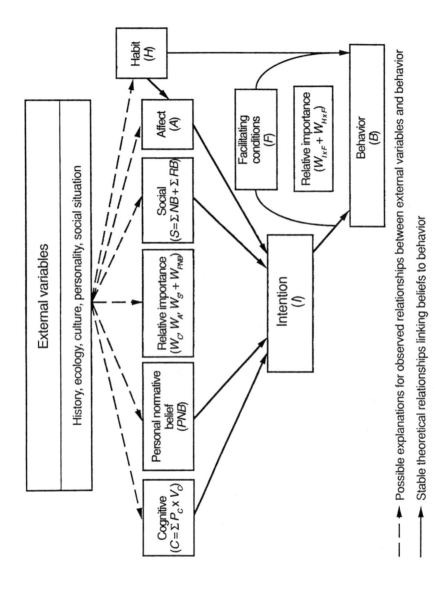

Figure 4.3 Schematic representation of the Triandis model.
Adapted from Triandis (1977) and Godin and Shephard (1990).

- - - → Possible explanations for observed relationships between external variables and behavior

——→ Stable theoretical relationships linking beliefs to behavior

The social component reflects relationships between the individual and other people. It includes both normative and role beliefs, which are formed through a subjective analysis of the attitudes of other people or groups toward performance of the given behavior. Normative beliefs consist of individual evaluations of the appropriateness of performing the behavior. Different individuals could be perceived as having differing opinions on the appropriateness of a given exercise for an individual of a given age or sex. Role beliefs represent the perceived appropriateness of the behavior for a person occupying a specific social position. For example, is it appropriate for a physical-education teacher to be sedentary or overweight? Normative and role beliefs differ among societies and situations according to the perceived consequences of violating cultural norms.

Personal normative belief is a measure of the individual's felt obligation to perform the behavior in question. This component carries a connotation of self-responsibility and a willingness to behave according to personal principles and independently of cultural norms.

The Triandis model has not been tested as extensively as that of Fishbein and Ajzen. Nonetheless, it has been applied successfully to predict exercise (Valois et al., 1988). Moreover, several studies, although not designed to test the full Triandis model, support the importance of considering certain variables incorporated into it (Godin, 1987; Godin et al., 1991; Godin, Valois, et al., 1987; Godin et al., 1989): for example, habit, the affective dimension of attitude, the conditions that facilitate or discourage exercise, and personal normative beliefs.

It is now clear that past exercise behavior is an important determinant of current exercise behavior (Godin, Valois, et al., 1987). If the established habit is being sedentary, any plan for the promotion of exercise should take this fact into consideration. Exercising is rarely a fully established habit and it is unlikely that people's exercise behavior will be regulated by habit alone. Adoption of the behavior typically requires an effort of will.

Applications of the Triandis model suggest that the affective dimension of attitude is more important than the cognitive dimension. Godin (1987) has shown that affect, that is, the perceived enjoyment related to exercise, is the main attitudinal dimension associated with intentions. Thus, it is important to ensure that exercise programs—for children or adults—offer a positive experience. Excessively rigorous programs should be avoided, and participants' enjoyment should be given high priority (Wankel, 1985).

The Triandis model adds to the basic TRA the concepts of role beliefs and personal normative beliefs. In pregnant women, role beliefs about exercise were significantly associated with the number of months that had elapsed since the onset of pregnancy (Godin et al., 1989), whereas in a group of university employees personal normative beliefs contributed to the prediction of exercise intentions (Valois et al., 1988).

Other variables that are not included in the Triandis model or the TRA appear to be associated with both intention and actual behavior. For example, perceived barriers to action influence both intention (Godin & Gionet, 1991; Godin et al., 1991; Godin et al., 1989) and behavior (Slenker et al., 1984). The theory of planned behavior (Ajzen, 1985) is among the theories that include these other variables.

The Theory of Planned Behavior

Ajzen (1985, 1988) observed that TRA (Ajzen & Fishbein, 1980) was particularly valuable when describing behaviors that were totally under volitional control. Most behaviors, however, fall somewhere along a continuum that extends from total control to complete lack of control. The individual has total control when there are no practical constraints to the adoption of a given behavior. At the opposite extreme, the individual has a complete lack of control if adoption of the behavior requires opportunities, resources, or skills that are lacking. To take account of such barriers, real or perceived, Ajzen has added a third concept of perceived behavioral control (PBC) to the original Fishbein and Ajzen model. Thus, the theory of planned behavior extends beyond the theory of reasoned action by including the concept of PBC. A simplified model, taken from Ajzen and Madden (1986) is presented in Figure 4.4.

If an individual has limited control of a behavior, the investigator should examine not only the subject's intention but also his or her perceived control over the behavior (Ajzen, 1985, 1988). PBC can influence intention (I), as can attitude ($Aact$) and subjective norm (SN). It can also predict behavior (B) directly, in concert with the potential influence of intention (I) in situations where behavior (B) is not under the total control of the individual. The following equation summarizes the theory:

$$B \sim I = (Aact)w_1 + (SN)w_2 + (PBC)w_3 \qquad (5)$$

The notion of PBC is similar to Bandura's concept of self-efficacy beliefs (Ajzen & Madden, 1986) and Triandis's concept of "facilitating conditions" (F) in his model of interpersonal behavior (Ajzen, 1985, p. 30). It reflects personal beliefs about how easy or difficult adoption of the behavior will be and how beliefs about resources and opportunities may be viewed as underlying perceived behavioral control.

The first two components of the theory (Aact and SN) are defined precisely as they were in the theory of reasoned action. The third component, PBC, was recently defined by Ajzen (1991). It is determined by the perceived presence or absence of required resources and opportunities and of anticipated obstacles; the control belief (e.g., "What is the probability it will rain this weekend?"); and by the perceived power (p) of a particular control factor to facilitate or inhibit performance of the behavior (e.g., "If it rains this weekend, what are the chances that I will participate in the planned cycling tour with my friends?"). In the formation of PBC, each control belief (c) is thus attenuated by a corresponding measure of perceived power (p). Therefore, the summed product control belief times perceived power represents the PBC for the individual and is expressed as

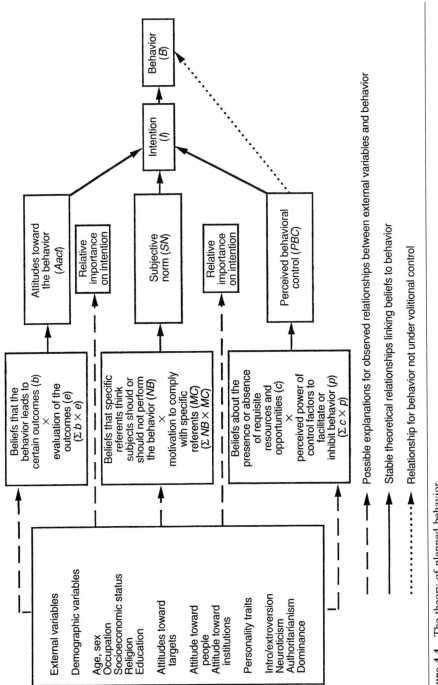

Figure 4.4 The theory of planned behavior.
Adapted from Ajzen and Madden (1986), Ajzen and Fishbein (1980) and Ajzen (1991).

127

$$PBC = \Sigma \, c \times p \qquad\qquad (6)$$

Nonetheless, in the first presentation of the theory (Ajzen, 1985, 1988; Ajzen & Madden, 1986), perceived behavioral control was not defined this way. Perceived barriers to a given behavior were first presented as a means of measuring PBC. In this regard, a few reports have suggested that perceived barriers to action influence both exercise intention and behavior. Slenker and his associates (1984) indicated that nearly 40% of the variance in exercise behavior among joggers and nonexercisers was attributable to perceived barriers to action. Godin, Colantonio, Davis, Shephard, and Simard (1986) suggested that perceived behavioral control influenced the exercise behavior of a subgroup of lower-limb disabled adults who had become disabled as a consequence of trauma. Godin and associates (1989) found that perceived barriers to exercise were a key factor in explaining differences between nulliparous and multiparous women in their intention to exercise after giving birth. Tappe, Duda, and Ehrnwald (1989) found that adolescent females and males differed in perceived barriers to exercise. Finally, Sallis et al. (1989) found that perceived barriers to exercise were significantly correlated with behavior in both younger and older subjects.

Studies examining the relevance of the theory of planned behavior to exercise adherence are beginning to emerge. Gatch and Kendzierski (1990) found that perceived behavioral control contributed to the prediction of the intention to do aerobics regularly among a group of undergraduate females; behavior was not measured. Similar results were found by Dzewaltowski and co-workers (1990) for the prediction of intention to participate in physical activity; the more positive an individual's perceived behavioral control over physical-activity participation, the stronger the intention to perform physical activity. PBC did not contribute, however, to the prediction of behavior expressed as total energy expenditure over the observed 4-week period. Godin and Gionet (1991) and Godin et al. (1991) have also observed the influence of perceived behavioral control on intention to exercise among employees of an electric power commission and individuals who suffer from coronary heart disease. Finally, in two prospective studies, Godin, Valois, and Lepage (1993) found that for adults in the general population and pregnant women, perceived behavioral control contributed to prediction of intention to exercise but not to prediction of exercising behavior.

The results in a number of studies (Dzewaltowski et al., 1990; Godin & Gionet, 1991; Godin 1991; Godin et al., 1993) reinforce the conclusion that the habit of exercising is one of the best predictors of behavior. Recently, Ajzen (1988) has suggested that the observed contribution of the habit to the prediction of behavior is the expression of one's temporal stability (consistency across time and contact). Ajzen writes:

> Most likely, temporal stability is the result of the stability in the causal antecedents of the behavior under consideration. Certain factors will have led people to perform or not to perform the behavior in the past. To the extent that these factors persist over time they will continue to exert their influence and thus produce the same behavior later on. (p. 101)

Moreover, Ajzen writes, perceived behavioral control should be an important mediator of the effect of habit upon the behavior because those individuals who have performed a behavior should have developed a feeling of control over performing it. This hypothesis formulated by Ajzen derives from an interpretation that the influence of habit on a given behavior might in many studies have masked the influence of other important variables associated with maintenance of current behavior, such as perceived behavioral control. Nonetheless, the influence of perceived behavioral control does not seem masked by habit, nor does it mediate the full influence of habit upon behavior. This finding agrees with previous observations of the effects of habit and perceived behavioral control (or facilitating conditions, in the Triandis model) in the prediction of exercise behavior among a group of 166 adults of both sexes (Valois et al., 1988). In this study, habit had a significant influence on exercise behaviors but perceived behavioral control had no influence. The identification of other important variables that could be masked by the strong influence of habit will require further investigation.

The results of these studies provide partial support for the usefulness of the theory of planned behavior in illuminating exercise behavior. In all the studies an additional portion of intention variance is explained by perceived behavioral control. This is not the case, however, for exercise behavior. One explanation for perceived behavioral control's lack of influence on exercise behavior is that exercising is a behavior under volitional control. Therefore, the theory of planned behavior will be useful in the study of exercise as it helps researchers understand the formation of intention and identify the beliefs (behavioral, normative, and control) among subgroups of the population (Ajzen, 1988) that should be targeted in interventions aimed at modifying exercise behavior.

The Social-Cognitive Models

The theories we have presented illustrate some of the ways social-cognitive scientists have sought to explain individual differences in the propensity to adopt a social behavior, such as exercising. Whereas the health-belief model and the protection motivation theory postulate that health-related behaviors can be understood in relation to their potential to protect against disease or to improve health, the other theories regard health-related behaviors as comparable to other forms of volitional behavior, analyzing them in terms of their social dimensions. According to the second category of theories, there is no essential difference in the decision-making process underlying such behaviors as attending a movie, voting for a political party, or exercising regularly.

In other words, examples can be cited in which factors other than a preoccupation with the optimization of health have a strong influence on an individual's decision to exercise. Expectations of self-efficacy, attitudes toward exercising (affect), perceived barriers, and past behavior all influence intention and thus shape behavior. Moreover, in some cases the variables explaining intention also directly influence behavior as well as indirectly influence intention.

A number of questions have emerged from the debate on the usefulness of social-cognitive theories for the understanding of exercise behavior. Is one theory better? What theoretical construct, such as attitude, perceived barriers, self-efficacy, or intention, is the best predictor of behavior? Unfortunately, there is no clear answer to such questions. Part of the ambiguity might be the result of methodological flaws in a few of the published studies. These flaws include a lack of respect for the theoretical assumptions underlying a given theory and problems in the operational definition of variables.

The study published by Mullen et al. (1987) offers an example of the first kind of methodological problem. In their study Mullen and co-workers concluded that the Fishbein and Ajzen model performed less effectively in predicting exercise behavior than the health-belief model and an ''integrative'' model that included variables in categories such as social network and demographics. Unfortunately, in this study none of the assumptions underlying the Fishbein and Ajzen theory had been respected. The operational definition of the variables, for example, intention, did not include the necessary action, context, and time elements. In fact, the Fishbein and Ajzen model performed most effectively in the only domain for which intention was measured appropriately (i.e., attempts to quit smoking).

The second type of methodological problem occurs in the operational definition of a given variable. First, two variables labeled differently might amount to the same thing, and second, a given variable might not signify what the authors think it does. Dzewaltowski and co-workers (1990) concluded, for example, that self-efficacy is a better predictor of physical activity than intention. Nonetheless, the correlation between self-efficacy and intention was 0.81, and the two measures co-varied in parallel with all other variables measured. Did the two constructs measure the same thing, and if so, is one theory more effective than the other? Sallis et al. (1989) reported that perceived barriers strongly affect exercise behavior. They reported that among the most important perceived barriers to exercise were a lack of interest in and enjoyment of exercise. According to the social-cognitive theories of Fishbein and Ajzen and of Triandis, these perceived barriers correspond to affect, or the attitudinal dimension. Consequently, the conclusion of Sallis and co-workers (1989) that perceived barriers are important predictors of exercise would have to be re-interpreted as showing the importance of attitude (affect) in influencing exercise behavior.

Future research should be guided by a more rigorous application of social-cognitive theories. Researchers interested by and working in this area of research should carefully follow the recommendations and guidelines presented by the theories' authors for the development of their instruments. This would help researchers avoid reporting ambiguous conclusions regarding the relative efficiency of a given model or theoretical factor in predicting exercise behavior.

Another methodological concern is accurate documentation of the psychometric qualities of the variables and behavior. For example, Valois and Godin (1991) have shown that the internal consistency of an attitudinal scale was related to its ability to predict behavior—the lower the internal consistency of the scale, the lower the relation with behavior. Several researchers have also expressed concerns about the use of retrospective self-reports as a measure of exercise behavior in such analyses (Baranowski, 1988; Perkins & Epstein, 1988). Because this is a limitation in most social-cognitive studies, the quality of collected data remains an important problem.

Social-cognitive models admittedly account for no more than 35% of the variance in exercise behavior (Dishman, 1988). This fact is not surprising, however, given that the purpose of social-cognitive theory is to reveal the decision-making process that underlies and precedes an action. Numerous factors, both individual and environmental, moderate the prediction of behavior from intention (Ajzen, 1985); these include enabling and reinforcing factors (Green, Kreuter, Deeds, & Partridge, 1980). Predisposing factors initiate the behavior and involve variables such as those included in the social-cognitive models reviewed. Facilitating factors such as accessibility, availability of resources, and environmental temperature allow the behavioral intention to be realized. Reinforcing factors (such as rewards and incentives) follow behavior but contribute to the continuation or extinction of the behavior. The final behavior reflects the summed effect of all factors influencing the behavior since the beginning of observation, and all factors should be considered in program design. Social-cognitive models operate mainly in terms of predisposition and for this reason cannot explain more than a part of the variance in exercise behavior.

Since 1980 the average level of physical activity in the North American population has apparently plateaued (Shephard, 1986; Shephard, 1988; Stephens, 1987). The hope of further increasing the proportion of active individuals lies mainly in the development of new and more appropriately focused promotional programs, including encouraging regular physical activity without stressing its intensity. Over the past 10 years more women than men have adopted and sustained the habit of exercising regularly (Sallis et al., 1986; Stephens, 1987), possibly because they have elected a moderate rather than a strenuous pattern of exercise.

Promoting the habit of physical activity rather than fitness has the potential to yield to participants not only health but also rewards such as new experiences and social contacts. Moreover, such factors are significant motivators for some people (Dishman et al., 1985). A moderate exercise program is also likely to be perceived as enjoyable by those individuals who are sedentary but who manifest interest in becoming more active. Generating a positive attitude should in turn positively influence the intention to undertake further bouts of exercise.

Barriers to exercise seem to have a negative effect upon intention. Perceived barriers may exert a negative influence as strong as or stronger than true barriers because much of exercise behavior is under volitional control. Again, promoting the habit of moderate physical activity rather than vigorous fitness-seeking exercise should lower perceived barriers among a sedentary population.

An alternative approach to exercise promotion would be to explore the factors that sustain sedentary behavior in the majority of the North American population. Ajzen and Fishbein (1980) suggested considering attitudes toward alternative courses of action (including inaction) when predicting behavior. In agreement with this concept, Kendzierski and Davis Lamastro (1988) have documented that weight-lifting behavior was associated with positive and negative attitudes about weight lifting.

Future investigators should also explore differences in exercise behavior among subgroups of the population. For instance, women's intentions to exercise seem to be explained by different variables than their spouses' intentions (Godin & Shephard, 1985). Such subgroup effects have important practical implications, whether one is developing national or specifically targeted promotions of exercise behavior.

Although various empirical approaches have achieved some success in promoting exercise behavior, the choice of an optimal tactic must ultimately be based on an understanding of the factors underlying exercise behavior in each situation. To this end, we have need of further studies based on a sound and established theoretical framework, such as those reviewed in this chapter. An examination of the psychosocial determinants of exercise has practical value in defining the optimum content of any form of exercise promotion, whether it is an educational program, a social-marketing strategy, or persuasive communications.

References

Ajzen, I. (1985). From intention to actions: A theory of planned behavior. In J. Kuhl and J. Beckmann (Eds.), *Action-control: From cognition to behavior* (pp. 11-39). Heidelberg: Springer.

Ajzen, I. (1988). *Attitudes, personality, and behavior*. Chicago: Dorsey Press.

Ajzen, I. (1991). The theory of planned behavior. *Organizational Behavior and Human Decision Processes*, **50**, 179-211.

Ajzen, I., & Fishbein, M. (1980). *Understanding attitudes and predicting social behavior*. Englewood Cliffs, NJ: Prentice Hall.

Ajzen, I., & Madden, T.J. (1986). Prediction of goal-directed behavior: Attitudes, intentions, and perceived behavioral control. *Journal of Experimental Social Psychology*, **22**, 453-474.

Bandura, A. (1977). Self-efficacy: Toward a unifying theory of behavior change. *Psychological Review*, **84**, 191-215.

Bandura, A. (1982). Self-efficacy mechanism in human agency. *American Psychologist*, **37**, 122-147.

Baranowski, T. (1988). Validity and reliability of self-report measures of physical activity: An information-processing perspective. *Research Quarterly for Exercise and Sport*, **59**, 314-327.

Becker, M.H., & Maiman, L.A. (1975). Sociobehavioral determinants of compliance with health care and medical care recommendations. *Medical Care*, **13**, 10-24.

Bentler, P.M., & Speckart, G. (1981). Attitudes "cause" behaviors: A structural equation analysis. *Journal of Personality and Social Behavior*, **40**, 226-238.

Cooper, J., & Croyle, R.T. (1984). Attitudes and attitude change. *Annual Review of Psychology*, **35**, 395-426.

Desharnais, R., Bouillon, J., & Godin, G. (1986). Self-efficacy and outcome expectations as determinants of exercise adherence. *Psychological Reports*, **59**, 1155-1159.

Desharnais, R., Godin, G., & Jobin, J. (1987). Motivational characteristics of Evalu*Life and the Canadian Home Fitness Test. *Canadian Journal of Public Health*, **78**, 161-164.

Dishman, R.K. (1982). Compliance/adherence in health-related exercise. *Health Psychology*, **1**, 237-267.

Dishman, R.K. (1988). *Exercise adherence: Its impact on public health*. Champaign, IL: Human Kinetics.

Dishman, R.K., & Gettman, L.R. (1980). Psychobiologic influences on exercise adherence. *Journal of Sport Psychology*, **2**, 295-310.

Dishman, R.K., Ickes, W., & Morgan, W.P. (1980). Self-motivation and adherence to habitual physical activity. *Journal of Applied Social Psychology*, **10**, 115-132.

Dishman, R.K., Sallis, J.F., & Orenstein, D.R. (1985). The determinants of physical activity and exercise. *Public Health Reports*, **100**, 158-171.

Dzewaltowski, D.A. (1989). Toward a model of exercise motivation. *Journal of Sport and Exercise Psychology*, **11**, 251-269.

Dzewaltowski, D.A., Noble, J.M., & Shaw, J.M. (1990). Physical activity participation: Social-cognitive theory versus the theories of reasoned action and planned behavior. *Journal of Sport and Exercise Psychology*, **12**, 388-405.

Fishbein, M., & Ajzen, I. (1975). *Belief, attitude, intention and behavior*. Don Mills, NY: Addison-Wesley.

Gatch, C.L., & Kendzierski, D. (1990). Predicting exercise intentions: The theory of planned behavoir. *Research Quarterly for Exercise and Sport*, **61**, 100-102.

Godin, G. (1987). Importance of the emotional aspect of attitude to predict intention. *Psychological Reports*, **61**, 719-723.

Godin, G., Colantonio, A., Davis, G.M., Shephard, R.J., & Simard, C. (1986). Prediction of leisure time exercise behavior among a group of lower-limb disabled adults. *Journal of Clinical Psychology*, **42**, 272-279.

Godin, G., Cox, M., & Shephard, R.J. (1983). The impact of physical fitness evaluation on the behavioral intentions toward regular exercise. *Canadian Journal of Applied Sport Science*, **8**, 240-245.

Godin, G., & Desharnais, R. (1987). Knowledge that objectively measured fitness level differs from one's self-perception: The impact upon exercise behavior. In L.A. Miller (Ed.), *Proceedings of the 22nd Annual Meeting of the Society of Prospective Medicine* (pp. 95-97). Bethesda, MD: Society of Prospective Medicine.

Godin, G., Desharnais, R., Jobin, J., & Cook, J. (1987). The impact of physical fitness and health-age appraisal upon exercise intentions and behavior. *Journal of Behavioral Medicine*, **10**, 241-250.

Godin, G., & Gionet, N.J. (1991). Determinants of an intention to exercise of an electric power commission's employees. *Ergonomics*, **34**, 1221-1230.

Godin, G., & Shephard, R.J. (1983). Physical fitness promotion programs: Effectiveness in modifying exercise behavior. *Canadian Journal of Applied Sport Sciences*, **8**, 104-113.

Godin, G., & Shephard, R.J. (1985). Psycho-social predictors of exercise intentions among spouses. *Canadian Journal of Applied Sport Sciences*, **10**, 36-43.

Godin, G., & Shephard, R.J. (1986). Importance of type of attitude to the study of exercise-behavior. *Psychological Reports*, **58**, 991-1000.

Godin, G., & Shephard, R.J. (1990). Use of attitude-behavior models in exercise promotion. *Sports Medicine*, **10**, 103-121.

Godin, G., Valois, P., Jobin, J., & Ross, A. (1991). Prediction of intention to exercise of individuals who have suffered from coronary heart disease. *Journal of Clinical Psychology*, **47**, 762-772.

Godin, G., Valois, P., & Lepage, L. (1993). The pattern of influence of perceived behavioral control upon exercising behavior: An application of Ajzen's theory of planned behavior. *Journal of Behavioral Medicine*, **16**, 81-102.

Godin, G., Valois, P., Shephard, R.J., & Desharnais, R. (1987). Prediction of leisure-time exercise behavior: A path analysis (LISREL V) model. *Journal of Behavioral Medicine*, **10**, 145-158.

Godin, G., Vézina, L., & Leclerc, O. (1989). Factors influencing the intention of pregnant women to exercise after birth. *Public Health Reports*, **104**, 185-195.

Green, L.W., Kreuter, M.W., Deeds, S.G., & Partridge, K.B. (1980). *Health education planning: A diagnostic approach*. Palo Alto, CA: Mayfield.

Heinzelmann, P., & Bagley, R.W. (1970). Response to physical activity programs and their effects on health behavior. *Public Health Reports*, **85**, 905-911.

Holm, K., Fink, N., Christman, N.J., Reitz, N., & Ashley, W. (1985). The cardiac patient and exercise: A sociobehavioral analysis. *Heart and Lung*, **14**, 586-593.

Kendzierski, D., & Davis Lamastro, V. (1988). Reconsidering the role of attitudes in exercise behavior: A decision theoretical approach. *Journal of Applied Social Psychology*, **18**, 737-759.

Kenyon, G.S. (1968a). A conceptual model for characterizing physical activity. *Research Quarterly*, **39**, 96-105.

Kenyon, G.S. (1968b). Six scales for assessing attitude toward physical activity. *Research Quarterly*, **39**, 566-574.

Lindsay-Reid, E., & Osborn, R.W. (1980). Readiness for exercise adoption. *Social Sciences and Medicine*, **14A**, 139-146.

Maddux, J.E., & Rogers, R.W. (1983). Protection motivation and self-efficacy: A revised theory of fear appeals and attitude change. *Journal of Experimental Social Psychology*, **19**, 469-479.

McAuley, E., & Jacobson, L. (1991). Self-efficacy and exercise participation in sedentary adult females. *American Journal of Health Promotion*, **5**, 185-207.

McAuley, E., Wraith, S., & Duncan, T.E. (1991). Self-efficacy, perceptions of success, and intrinsic motivation for exercise. *Journal of Applied Social Psychology*, **21**, 139-155.

Miniard, P.W., & Cohen, J.B. (1981). An examination of the Fishbein-Ajzen behavioral-intention model's concepts and measures. *Journal of Experimental Social Psychology*, **17**, 309-339.

Mirotznik, J., Speedling, E., Stein, R., & Bronz, C. (1985). Cardiovascular fitness program: Factors associated with participation and adherence. *Public Health Reports*, **100**, 13-18.

Morgan, P.P., Shephard, R.J., Finucane, R., Schimmelfing, L., & Jazmaji, V. (1984). Health beliefs and exercise habits in an employee fitness program. *Canadian Journal of Applied Sport Sciences*, **9**, 87-93.

Muench, J. (1987). Health beliefs of patients with coronary heart disease enrolled in a cardiac exercise program. *Journal of Cardiopulmonary Rehabilitation*, **7**, 130-135.

Mullen, P.D., Hersey, J.C., & Iverson, D.C. (1987). Health behavior models compared. *Social Sciences and Medicine*, **24**, 973-981.

O'Connell, J.K., Price, J.H., Roberts, S.M., Jurs, S.G., & McKinley, R. (1985). Utilizing the health belief model to predict dieting and exercising behavior of obese and nonobese adolescents. *Health Education Quarterly*, **12**, 343-351.

Oldridge, N.B., & Streiner, D.L. (1990). The health belief model: Predicting compliance and dropout in cardiac rehabilitation. *Medicine and Science in Sports and Exercise*, **22**, 678-683.

Perkins, K.A., & Epstein, L.H. (1988). Methodology in exercise adherence research. In R.K. Dishman (Ed.), *Exercise adherence: Its impact on public health* (pp. 399-416). Champaign, IL: Human Kinetics.

Riddle, P.K. (1980). Attitudes, beliefs, behavioral intentions, and behaviors of women and men toward regular jogging. *Research Quarterly for Exercise and Sport*, **51**, 663-674.

Rogers, R.W. (1975). A protection motivation theory of fear appeals and attitude change. *Journal of Psychology*, **91**, 93-114.

Rogers, R.W. (1983). Cognitive and physiological processes in fear appeals and attitude change: A revised theory of protection motivation. In J.R. Cacioppo & R.E. Petty (Eds.), *Social psychology: A sourcebook* (pp. 153-176). New York: Guilford.

Rosenstock, I.M., Strecher, V.J., & Becker, M.H. (1988). Social learning theory and the health belief theory. *Health Education Quarterly*, **15**, 175-183.

Sallis, J.F., Haskell, W.L., Fortmann, S.P., Vranizan, K.M., Taylor, C.B., & Solomon, D.S. (1986). Predictors of adoption and maintenance of physical activity in a community sample. *Preventive Medicine*, **15**, 331-341.

Sallis, J.F., Hovell, M.F., Hofstetter, C.R., Faucher, P., Elder, J.P., Blanchard, J., Casperson, C.J., Powell, K.E., & Christenson, G.H. (1989). A multivariate study of determinants of vigorous exercise in a community sample. *Preventive Medicine*, **18**, 20-34.

Shephard, R.J. (1986). *Fitness of a nation: Lessons from the Canada Fitness Survey*. Basel, Switzerland: Karger.

Shephard, R.J. (1988). Fitness: Boom or bust? A Canadian perspective. *Research Quarterly for Exercise and Sport*, **59**, 265-269.

Shephard, R.J., Morgan, P.P., Finucane, R., & Schimmelfing, L. (1980). Factors influencing recruitment to an occupational fitness program. *Journal of Occupational Medicine*, **22**, 389-398.

Sheppard, B.H., Hartwick, J., & Warshaw, P.R. (1988). The theory of reasoned action: A meta-analysis of past research with recommendations for modification and future research. *Journal of Consumer Research*, **15**, 325-343.

Slenker, S.E., Price, J.H., Roberts, S.M., & Jurs, S.G. (1984). Joggers versus nonexercisers: An analysis of knowledge, attitudes and beliefs about jogging. *Research Quarterly for Exercise and Sport*, **55**, 371-378.

Sonstroem, R.J. (1974). Attitude testing examining certain psychosocial correlates of physical activity. *Research Quarterly*, **45**, 93-103.

Sonstroem, R.J. (1982). Attitudes and beliefs in the prediction of exercise participation. In R.C. Cantu and W.P. Gillepsie (Eds.), *Sports medicine, sports science: Bridging the' gap* (pp. 3-16). Toronto: Callemore Press.

Stanley, M.A., & Maddux, J.E. (1986). Cognitive processes in health enhancement: Investigation of a combined protection motivation and self-efficacy model. *Basic and Applied Social Psychology*, **7**, 101-113.

Stephens, T. (1987). Secular trends in adult physical activity: Exercise boom or bust? *Research Quarterly for Exercise and Sport*, **58**, 94-105.

Tappe, M.K., Duda, J.L., & Ehrnwald, P.M. (1989). Perceived barriers to exercise among adolescents. *Journal of School Health*, **59**, 153-155.

Tirrell, B.E., & Hart, L.K. (1980). The relationship of health beliefs and knowledge to exercise compliance in patients after coronary bypass. *Heart and Lung*, **9**, 487-493.

Triandis, H.C. (1977). *Interpersonal behavior*. Monterey, CA: Brooks/Cole.

Valois, P., Desharnais, R., & Godin, G. (1988). A comparison of the Fishbein and Ajzen and the Triandis attitudinal models for the prediction of exercise intention and behavior. *Journal of Behavioral Medicine*, **11**, 459-472.

Valois, P., & Godin, G. (1991). The importance of selecting appropriate adjective pairs for measuring attitude based on the semantic differential method. *Quality and Quantity*, **25**, 57-68.

Wankel, L.M. (1985). Personal and situational factors affecting exercise involvement: The importance of enjoyment. *Research Quarterly for Exercise and Sport*, **56**, 275-282.

Wankel, L.M., & Beatty, B.D. (1975). Behavior intentions and attendance of an exercise program: A field test of Fishbein's model. Actes du 7ᵉ symposium en apprentissage moteur et psychologie du sport. *Mouvement*, 381-386.

Wurtele, S.K., & Maddux, J.E. (1987). Relative contributions of protection motivation theory components in predicting exercise intentions and behavior. *Health Psychology*, **6**, 453-466.

CHAPTER 5

Schema Theory: An Information Processing Focus

Deborah Kendzierski

Decision theory has proved useful for studying the effects of exercise interventions. One line of research, based on Lewin's (1947) classic research on group decision, demonstrated that interventions that include a small-group discussion component have a positive effect on recruitment to exercise programs (Faulkner & Stewart, 1978; Heinzelmann, 1973). A second line of research was based on Janis and Mann's (1968, 1977) conflict theory. According to this theory, the more relevant information individuals consider before making decisions, the more committed they will be to implementing their decisions. Studies have shown that use of a decisional balance sheet (designed to help individuals systematically consider the pros and cons associated with each course of action) increases exercise-program attendance (Hoyt & Janis, 1975; Wankel, 1984; Wankel & Graham, 1980; Wankel & Thompson, 1977; Wankel, Yardley, & Graham, 1985).

Given the success of decision theory as a theoretical framework for exercise interventions, it seemed reasonable to examine its usefulness in regard to exercise behavior. Within a decision-theory framework, exercise behavior can be viewed as involving a series of decisions. First, someone must decide that he or she is interested in a particular type of exercise. Second, the person must decide whether to begin such an exercise program. Finally, once the person has begun an exercise program, he or she must decide whether to continue it, switch to another program, or stop exercising.

Subjective Expected Utility Theory

Many theories fall under the rubric of decision theory, with subjective expected utility (SEU) theory probably the best known (Edwards, 1961). According to

SEU theory, choice among a set of alternatives depends on one's evaluation of the utility or worth (Ui) of each outcome associated with an alternative and the subjective probability that each outcome will occur if the alternative is chosen (Pi). These two estimates are multiplied, and their products are summed over all the outcomes to yield the SEU for a given alternative. The alternative with the greatest SEU is predicted to be the chosen alternative. An advantage of this theory is that it provides a framework within which to study the role of attitudes in exercise behavior, because one conceptualization of attitude is an expectancy-value model (Feather, 1982; Fishbein & Ajzen, 1975). Essentially, an SEU is an attitude toward a course of action.

In a set of studies, Kendzierski and LaMastro (1988) examined the usefulness of SEU theory in regard to interest in weight lifting and adherence to a weight-lifting exercise program among a college student population. The main findings: SEU theory predicted interest but not adherence. Furthermore, there was no relationship between attitudes toward weight lifting and the number of days subjects lifted, but there was a significant negative relationship between attitudes toward *not* weight lifting and the number of days that experienced (but not inexperienced) subjects lifted. In a subsequent study (Kendzierski, 1990a, Study 1) SEU theory successfully predicted college students' intentions to adopt an exercise program but not whether they actually did so within 2 months.

These studies appeared to indicate that SEU theory could predict decision-making (forming an intention to exercise) but not decision implementation (following through on one's intention to start or continue an exercise program). This early work, then, led to redefining the key problem as understanding decision implementation, or what it takes to get people to act on intentions to exercise.

The Self and Exercise Behavior

Many people intend to exercise. However, implementing a decision to exercise regularly may prove difficult in light of the time and effort required and the fact that anticipated benefits (e.g., weight loss, feelings of well-being, increased endurance) do not occur immediately.

What might motivate people to devote the time and effort needed to exercise regularly (or to engage in any other complex decision implementation)? One possibility is their self-image. To the extent that people consider themselves to be exercisers, they should be motivated to engage in behavior, such as exercise, that verifies their self-image (Swann, 1983, 1985). Moreover, once they begin to exercise, they gain the immediate benefit of knowing that they are acting in accordance with their self-image. That immediate benefit could help maintain the behavior until exercisers begin to physically adapt to their activity and the other anticipated benefits of exercising start to accrue.

A self-schema approach (Markus, 1977) was chosen as a framework for conceptualizing an exerciser's self-image. This approach, borrowed from the social cognition literature, focuses on an individual's self-image in regard to a particular attribute or dimension, such as exercising. It is an information processing approach because the self-schema is viewed as a type of schema, a cognitive structure that guides the processing of information.

Schema Theory and the Self

Although cognitive psychologists differ in their use of the term, there is general agreement that a *schema* is an organized body of knowledge (Fiske & Taylor, 1984). A schema may include both general abstract knowledge regarding some domain and specific instances of the domain, as well as information about relationships among domain attributes (Taylor & Crocker, 1981). Schemata are thought to guide information processing in that they provide a basis for selecting and organizing incoming information as well as retrieving information stored in memory; they affect perception, inference, and memory (Bartlett, 1932; Brewer & Nakamura, 1984; Neisser, 1976; Rumelhart & Ortony, 1977; Taylor & Crocker, 1981).

Self-schemata are cognitive structures involving generalizations about the self that are derived from experience and focused on those aspects of the self that are regarded by the individual as important (Markus, 1977). Research has demonstrated that self-schemata affect the processing of information about the self and others (Fiske & Taylor, 1984; Markus & Smith, 1981). For example, self-schemata influence the speed and content of judgments about oneself, predictions about one's future behavior, and resistance to schema-inconsistent information, as well as memory for schema-related behavior (Markus, 1977). In addition, self-schemata influence the traits people notice in others and the inferences they make about others (Catrambone & Markus, 1987; Markus & Smith, 1981; Markus, Smith, & Moreland, 1985). This research has involved such diverse domains as independence (Markus, 1977), body weight (Markus, Hamill, & Sentis, 1987), sex roles (Markus, Crane, Bernstein, & Siladi, 1982), creativity (Markus & Smith, 1981), Type A and Type B behavior patterns (Strube et al., 1986), clothing (Pines & Kuczkowski, 1987), and dieting (Parisi & Kendzierski, 1991).

Although there is a dearth of research on the effect of self-schemata on behavior, the original theoretical formulation held that self-schemata "can be viewed as implicit theories used by individuals to make sense of their own past behavior and to direct the course of future behavior" (Markus, 1977, p. 78). The suggestion that the self plays an important role in regulating behavior has been echoed in the context of more recent theorizing as well (Cantor, Markus, Niedenthal, & Nurius, 1986; Markus & Wurf, 1987).

Exercise Self-Schema Measure

Using methodology devised by Markus (1977; Catrambone & Markus, 1987; Markus et al., 1985), an exercise self-schema measure was developed (Kendzierski, 1988). The measure was designed to identify exerciser schematics (those who are schematic for exercising), aschematics (those who are not schematic for exercising), and nonexerciser schematics (those who are schematic for *not* exercising). As defined by Markus (1977), individuals are schematic in regard to a particular attribute when

- they consider that attribute to be extremely self-descriptive (as do exerciser schematics) or extremely nondescriptive (as do nonexerciser schematics), and
- they consider that attribute extremely important to their self-image.

Likewise, individuals are aschematic when

- they consider the attribute only moderately descriptive or nondescriptive, and
- they do not consider the attribute important to their self-image.

In summary, schematicity requires both that people view their behavior as very reflective of the attribute in question and that they consider the attribute an important part of their self-image.

This definition, then, suggests that unless people categorize relevant physical activity as exercise behavior, they may fail to develop an exerciser self-schema even though it might be warranted by their behavior. Consider, for example, the Cape Cod octogenarian who walks 3 or more miles each day ''to see what's new in the neighborhood and how high the tide is.'' Behaviorally, this person is an exerciser, even though he does not view himself as such. Conversely, some individuals persist in thinking of themselves as exercisers or athletic when they might more objectively be described as occasional weekend warriors. Presumably, physical activity is important to them, and they construe their infrequent bouts of activity as evidence supportive of their self-image. The definition also suggests that engagement in exercise behavior, even when it is thus categorized by the individual, will not lead to the development of an exerciser schema unless the individual comes to view being an exerciser as important to his or her self-image. Such would be the prediction in the case of a young woman who spends 18 months in physical therapy as the result of an automobile accident: She faithfully does her prescribed home exercises but disdains physical activity and prefers to reflect on her other activities. In order to adopt the identity of an exerciser, this woman would require a change in values.

The exercise self-schema measure requires that subjects indicate on 11-point scales whether each of three key phrases describes them: ''someone who exercises regularly,'' ''someone who keeps in shape,'' and ''physically active.'' These phrases are included among a set of filler items such as ''spontaneous'' and ''friendly.'' Each scale ranges from 1 (does not describe me) to 11 (describes me). Subjects are also asked to indicate on 11-point scales (for which 1 = *not at all important* and 11 = *very important*) how important each descriptor phrase is ''to the image you have of yourself, regardless of whether or not the trait describes you.'' To be classified as an exerciser schematic, an individual must

- rate at least two of the three exercise descriptors as extremely self-descriptive (points 8-11) and
- rate at least two of the three exercise descriptors as attributes that are extremely important (points 8-11) to his or her self-image.

To be classified as a nonexerciser schematic, an individual must

- rate at least two of the three exercise descriptors as extremely nondescriptive (points 1-4) and
- rate at least two of the three exercise descriptors as attributes that are extremely important (points 8-11) to his or her self-image.

Lastly, to be classified as aschematic, an individual must

- rate at least two of the three exercise descriptors in the middle range (points 5-7) and
- rate at least two of the three exercise descriptors as attributes that are not extremely important (points 1-7) to his or her self-image.

Initial Validation Study

A crucial early step was to determine whether individuals identified as having exercise self-schemata process exercise-related information the same way that individuals identified as having self-schemata in other domains have been shown to process information relevant to those domains. If the standard self-schema findings were replicated, initial evidence of the exercise self-schema measure's construct validity would be provided.

The study (Kendzierski, 1990b, Study 1) involved three tasks developed by Markus (1977). In the first the content and latency of subjects' self-descriptions were assessed. Subjects viewed a series of words and phrases on a computer monitor and indicated whether each stimulus was or was not self-descriptive by pressing a key labeled *me* or one labeled *not me*. The computer recorded subjects' responses and reaction times. In the second task subjects were asked to supply behavioral evidence for their self-descriptions. Specifically, subjects were given a booklet containing both exercise-related and filler words and phrases and were asked to circle each word or phrase that described them, then list the reasons they felt the word or phrase was self-descriptive, giving specific evidence from their own past behavior. In the third task subjects were asked to predict their future behavior. Subjects were given a booklet containing pairs of behavioral alternatives; one alternative in each pair reflected a pro-exercise orientation (for example, "If I were at the mall and did not have a lot to carry, I would (a) use the stairs instead of taking the escalator or (b) take the escalator instead of the stairs"). Subjects indicated the likelihood that they would behave in the way described by assigning a number from 0 to 100 to each alternative so that the total for the pair equaled 100.

Based on self-schema theory, it was predicted that, relative to nonexerciser schematics, exerciser schematics would

- endorse as self-descriptive more words and phrases related to exercising and fewer related to not exercising (because of the composition of their self-image),
- take less time to make schema-consistent judgments (because having a schema facilitates the processing of schema-congruent information),
- recall more specific instances of exercise behavior (because having a schema facilitates retrieval of information in the domain), and
- predict that they would be more likely to engage in future pro-exercise behavior (because schematics, having reflected more on their behavior in the domain, should be more aware of how they would behave in domain-relevant situations and thus should be more confident in predicting their behavior in such situations).

Furthermore, it was predicted that aschematics' scores on these variables would fall between those of the other groups.

A clear, consistent, and theoretically meaningful pattern of data was obtained on all variables. Exerciser schematics judged more words and phrases self-descriptive than did aschematics or nonexerciser schematics, and aschematics judged more exerciser stimuli self-descriptive than did nonexerciser schematics. The reverse was found with regard to nonexerciser stimuli, although the difference between aschematics and nonexerciser schematics was not statistically significant. As can be seen in Figure 5.1, the latency data also showed the predicted pattern. For example, exerciser schematics were quicker at responding *me* to exerciser stimuli and *not me* to nonexerciser stimuli than were nonexerciser schematics. Mean reaction times for aschematics were between those of the other groups for both types of responses and differed significantly from those of the nonexerciser schematics, although not from those of the exerciser schematics. The data for the mean reaction time to respond *not me* to exerciser stimuli also showed the predicted pattern. Exerciser schematics were slower to respond *not me* to exerciser stimuli than were either aschematics or nonexerciser schematics; the latter two groups, however, did not differ in their mean reaction time. Finally, the data for the mean reaction time to respond *me* to the nonexerciser stimuli showed the predicted pattern, but none of the groups differed significantly; interpretation of these results is complicated by the fact that fewer exerciser schematics and aschematics were included because many did not make this type of response even once (see the published article for further details).

The predicted pattern of data was also obtained for the final two tasks. Exerciser schematics provided more behavioral examples for exerciser stimuli than did aschematics or nonexerciser schematics, and aschematics provided more than did nonexerciser schematics. Moreover, exerciser schematics thought it more likely that they would choose the exercise-oriented alternatives than did either aschematics or nonexerciser schematics, whereas aschematics thought it more likely than did nonexerciser schematics.

The results of this study suggest that individuals identified as having exercise self-schemata (i.e., both exerciser and nonexerciser schematics) process exercise-related information in the same way that individuals identified as having self-schemata in other domains have been shown to process information relevant to

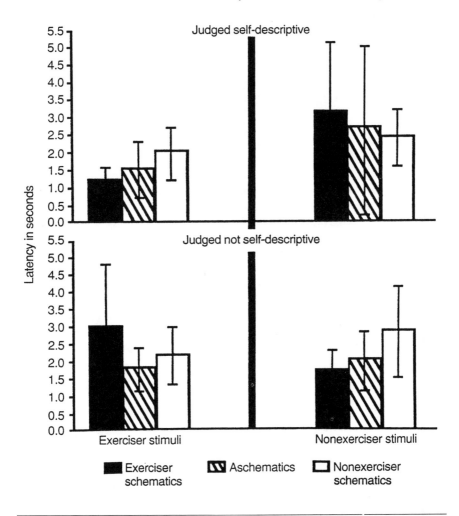

Figure 5.1   Mean response latency for exerciser and nonexerciser stimuli judged self-descriptive and not self-descriptive.
Reprinted from Kendzierski (1990b).

those domains. These findings thus provide initial evidence of the exercise self-schema measure's construct validity.

Self-Schemata and Exercise Behavior

As a first step toward determining whether any relationship exists between an individual's self-schema status and his or her exercise behavior, a concurrent study was conducted (Kendzierski, 1988). Two hundred twenty Villanova University undergraduates enrolled in a general psychology class completed the exercise self-schema measure and answered a series of questions about their exercise behavior as part of a considerably larger questionnaire study. Of the 220 participants, 116 were classified as exerciser schematics, 14 as nonexerciser schematics, and 19 as aschematics; the remaining 71 did not fit the criteria for inclusion in these groups. Because of the considerable discrepancy in sample sizes for the three groups, a subset of 20 exerciser schematics was selected for inclusion in the analyses.

The analyses revealed that exerciser schematics exercised more frequently, performed more exercise activities, and were more likely to report having exercised at least 3 times a week on average than aschematics or nonexerciser schematics (see Table 5.1). In addition, exerciser schematics were more likely than nonexerciser schematics to report having exercised at least 2 times a week the previous semester and having already begun to exercise regularly after returning to college from Christmas vacation. On these latter two variables, exerciser schematics were not significantly different from aschematics, although the pattern of data was in the predicted direction. Moreover, aschematics differed significantly from nonexerciser schematics on all variables except the number of activities done for exercise (differences were in the predicted direction).

Although these data were very encouraging, it was not possible to determine whether self-schema status has any predictive value, given that self-schemata and exercise behavior were assessed concurrently. Individuals who had exercised more in the recent past may simply be more likely to develop an exerciser

Table 5.1   Reported Exercise Behavior as a Function of Self-Schema Status

	Self-schema status		
	Exerciser schematics	Aschematics	Nonexerciser schematics
Mean number of days/week	5.10_a	3.11_b	1.36_c
Mean number of exercise activities	3.20_a	2.21_b	1.79_b
Percent who had already begun to exercise after returning from Christmas vacation	85.0_a	68.4_a	28.6_b
Percent who reported having exercised 3 times/week during the last semester	90.0_a	47.4_b	7.1_c
Percent who reported having exercised 2 times/week during the last semester	95.0_a	84.2_a	14.3_b

Note. Within each row, numbers with different subscripts differ significantly; for all, $p < .05$.

self-schema. It cannot be concluded that having an exerciser self-schema made individuals more likely to exercise.

The next step was a prospective study (Kendzierski, 1990b, Study 2) designed to determine whether individuals with an exerciser self-schema were more likely to start an exercise program than individuals without such a self-image (i.e., aschematics and nonexerciser schematics). Ninety-five Villanova University undergraduates who participated in a survey conducted at the beginning of the semester, reported that they had not already started an exercise program that semester, and were identified as exerciser schematics ($n = 43$), aschematics ($n = 22$), or nonexerciser schematics ($n = 30$) were contacted by mail in the 11th or 12th week of the semester and invited to participate in an exercise-behavior survey.

Questionnaire return rates were comparable for the three groups of participants. A relatively large proportion of subjects (19.7% overall; the groups did not differ significantly) reported suffering an illness or injury that prevented them from starting an exercise program, raising the possibility that some individuals may have cited illness or injury as an excuse for not starting an exercise program or may have misread the question as asking whether they had suffered an illness or injury that semester. Consequently, two sets of analyses were conducted: one including subjects who did not report suffering an illness or injury that would have prevented them from exercising and one including all subjects. As can be seen in Table 5.2, in both sets of analyses the proportion of exerciser schematics who reported starting an exercise program was greater than that of either aschematics or nonexerciser schematics; the proportion of aschematics and nonexerciser schematics who reported starting an exercise program did not differ. It should be noted that this study speaks only to the issue of exercise adoption. The extent to which individuals adhered to their exercise program is unknown, as is whether the adopted exercise programs were adequate for increasing physical fitness.

The exercise-behavior studies described in this section have definite limitations (e.g., reliance on self-report data, relatively short time frame, and lack of detail concerning subjects' exercise programs). Despite their limitations, however, these studies are valuable because they provide initial evidence that exercise self-schema status is associated with exercise behavior. It now seems reasonable to invest the necessary time, effort, and resources in better, more detailed studies of the association between exercise self-schemata and exercise behavior. Future research should definitely use more objective and more detailed measures of exercise behavior in long-term prospective designs with large samples. Although other studies of exercise adoption are needed, studies of exercise adherence should be given priority because adherence is the more difficult problem—it is much easier to start an exercise program than to adhere to one.

These initial studies have also raised an important question: If self-schemata guide behavior, how do they do so? Such a question focuses on the process involved in producing exercise behavior. As will be seen, it is possible to provide a more complex analysis of the problem than the one that led to this point in the research.

Table 5.2   Proportion of Exerciser Schematics, Aschematics, and Nonexerciser Schematics Who Reported Starting an Exercise Program

	Exerciser schematics	Aschematics	Nonexerciser schematics
Subjects not reporting an illness/injury			
Proportion who reported that they had started an exercise program	.520$_a$	.200$_b$	.167$_b$
n	25	10	18
All Subjects			
Proportion who reported that they had started an exercise program	.467$_a$	.200$_b$	.190$_b$
n	30	15	21

Note. Within each row, proportions with different subscripts differ significantly; for all, $p < .05$.
Reprinted from Kendzierski (1990b).

Linking Intentions and Behavior: A Self-Schema Process Model

It has been suggested that having an exerciser self-image provides the motivation to expend the time and effort necessary to follow through on exercise intentions. This reasoning led to the prediction that individuals who see themselves as exercisers (i.e., exerciser schematics) will engage in more exercise behavior than individuals who do not have such a self-image (i.e., aschematics and nonexerciser schematics). It should be noted, however, that this assumes that exerciser schematics tend to have favorable intentions toward exercising. Such was found to be the case in the Kendzierski (1988) study, in which exerciser schematics reported both being interested in ($M = 9.70$ on a 10-point scale) and committed to ($M = 8.60$ on a 10-point scale) exercising regularly during the current semester.[1]

Whereas exerciser schematics (and others) may generally intend to exercise, they will not always intend to exercise. Work demands, family obligations, or other personal priorities may cause individuals to decide to put exercise on hold for a while. Likewise, individuals may be aware that an illness or injury contraindicates exercise for some period of time. In such cases, one would not expect individuals—even exerciser schematics—to intend to exercise. And, to the extent that individuals do not intend to exercise, one would not expect them to engage in exercise behavior.

The basic model being proposed, then, is that both favorable exercise intentions and some motivation to implement them are required for exercise behavior to occur. It is suggested that, in addition to whatever other motivations individuals may have for exercising, exerciser schematics should be motivated to exercise as a means of verifying their self-image as exercisers. Aschematics would not have this motivation because they have no such self-image. The situation is more complicated with regard to nonexerciser schematics. Self-verification theory predicts that nonexerciser schematics would be inclined not to exercise in order to maintain their self-image as nonexercisers. This presupposes, however, that individuals have a vested interest in maintaining that self-image. If individuals disdain the self-image and seek to change it, acting in a manner consistent with the self-image should not be a source of satisfaction. There is reason to think that at least some nonexerciser schematics may be in this position.

Nonexerciser schematics are an interesting group: individuals who say that being "someone who exercises regularly," "someone who keeps in shape," and "physically active" is important to their self-image yet who also claim that these attributes do not describe them. It seems likely that two very different types of individuals may be among those classified as nonexerciser schematics. Some nonexerciser schematics may be proud couch potatoes. Such individuals should derive satisfaction (via self-verification) from not exercising. Other nonexerciser schematics, however, may possess what Elissa Wurf and Hazel Markus have described as negative self-schemata, which develop when individuals view themselves either as not possessing a desired positive attribute, or as possessing a negative attribute (Markus, Cross, & Wurf, 1990; Wurf & Markus, 1983). Research by Wurf (1987) suggests that negative self-schemata are markers of anticipated self-concept change. That is, an individual with a negative self-schema may have developed the schema as a result of thinking about his or her self-image in preparation for doing something to change it. Thus, some nonexerciser schematics may be in the process of attempting to become exercisers. Such individuals should derive no satisfaction from acting in accordance with their current but not desired self-image by not exercising.[2] Because two distinct subgroups of nonexerciser schematics may exist, any predictions about the type of motivation such individuals should have as a group in regard to acting on their nonexerciser self-images would be unsound from a theoretical perspective. It would be far better to devise a method for identifying members of the two subgroups; only then would it make sense to discuss nonexercisers' motivation to act in accordance with their self-image.

An additional factor should be considered as one enumerates the conditions necessary for producing exercise behavior. Even if individuals have an intention to exercise and a self-image that motivates implementing that intention, they would not be expected to exercise unless their intentions were brought to mind. Consider the case of an individual who intends to exercise but is kept so busy on a particular day that he or she never thinks of the intention to exercise. The idea that a behavioral guide must be accessed from memory in order to direct behavior is not new. In the literature on attitude-behavior consistency, Fazio

(1986) and Snyder and Kendzierski (1982) suggest that attitudes must be accessed from memory if they are to guide behavior. Likewise, Kuhl's (1985) model of action control holds that in order for intentions to be enacted, they must be accessed from long-term memory and enter working memory.

If it is true that in order to act on their intentions people must access those intentions from memory and be motivated to implement them, exerciser self-schema status should moderate the relationship between intentions and behavior. One reason for this is that, as discussed earlier, exerciser schematics should be motivated to act on their intentions in order to verify their self-image. A second reason, however, is that the intentions of schematics should be more accessible than those of aschematics, assuming that behavioral intentions are stored in memory as part of an individual's self-schema. Research from cognitive psychology provides indirect support for this assumption. Rosch and Mervis (1975) found that behavioral information is encoded along with other attributes of categories (which can be conceptualized as schemata). For example, one attribute of "bicycle" may be "something you ride." Based on this and other research, Carver and Scheier (1981) have argued that a schema can include "behavior-specifying information" and that "when a schema that includes such information is accessed and used in the classification of a stimulus input, the response-specifying information may also be accessed as part of a schema" (p. 121). Consider, for example, the individual who is driving and sees someone bicycling along the side of the road. An exerciser schematic should be more likely to interpret the situation as an exercise situation, and, consequently, to bring to mind his or her own exercise intentions. An aschematic, on the other hand, might be more likely to interpret the situation in another way, for example, as a "road hazard situation." To the extent that individuals repeatedly use schemata to interpret incoming information and that intentions are part of an individual's self-schema, schematics should more frequently access their intentions in that domain than aschematics. Since frequency of activation affects accessibility (Higgins & King, 1981; Wyer & Srull, 1980), the intentions of schematics should be more accessible than those of aschematics. To the extent that schematics' intentions are more accessible, schematics should be in a better position to use their intentions as behavioral guides.

Self-Schemata: Moderator of Exercise Intention–Behavior Consistency?

As a rough first test of the hypothesis that individuals with exerciser self-schemata will show a higher correlation between their exercise intentions and their behavior, a two-part questionnaire survey was conducted (Kendzierski, 1991) through recruitment of Villanova University undergraduates enrolled in a general psychology course. At the beginning of the semester subjects completed a questionnaire as part of a considerably larger screening survey.

This questionnaire included both the self-schema measure and five semantic differential scales designed to measure subjects' intentions about exercising regularly that semester (e.g., "I intend to exercise regularly" and "I will try my best to exercise regularly," both with endpoints of *extremely likely/ extremely unlikely*). In the 11th or 12th week of the semester subjects completed a second questionnaire, which focused on their physical activity over the past week. Subjects were asked to specify the number of days on which they had exercised during the past week, and complete the Stanford 7-Day Recall (a measure of physical activity over the past week that has been shown to have construct validity; see Blair, 1984, and Dishman & Steinhardt, 1988). In order to recruit enough subjects, this study was conducted over three semesters. During the last two semesters the study was conducted, the measure of exercise intentions was added to the second questionnaire in order to determine whether exerciser schematics, aschematics, and nonexerciser schematics showed similar consistency in their exercise intentions over time.

As can be seen in Table 5.3, exerciser schematics showed moderate but significant correlations between their intentions and behavior, whereas aschematics and nonexerciser schematics did not. In addition, the correlation between subjects' exercise intentions and the number of days on which they reported exercising during the past week was significantly greater for exerciser schematics than for aschematics or nonexerciser schematics; the correlations for the latter two groups

Table 5.3   Correlation Between Exercise Intentions and Exercise Behavior as a Function of Self-Schema Status

	Self-schema status		
	Exerciser schematics	Aschematics	Nonexerciser schematics
Correlation of exercise intentions with number of days subjects exercised	$.31_a$	$.02_b$	$.01_b$
n	330	53	50
p	<.01	.892	.932
Correlation of exercise intentions with Stanford 7-Day Recall scores	$.21_a$	$.09_a$	$.11_a$
n	333	54	51
p	<.01	.506	.446

Note. Within each row, correlations with different subscripts differ significantly; for all, $p < .05$.

were almost identical. A similar but weaker pattern was found in the correlation between subjects' exercise intentions and their Stanford 7-Day Recall scores; none of the correlations, however, were significantly different. It should be noted that the Stanford 7-Day Recall measure assesses physical activity in general—including, but not limited to, exercise. For this reason it is not an ideal measure of exercise behavior over the past week. Consequently, the fact that a similar pattern of data was found is encouraging.

These data have two noteworthy features: the lack of correlation between intention and behavior for nonexerciser schematics and the relatively low magnitude of the correlation for exerciser schematics. In regard to the first point, the data make sense if indeed there are two distinct subgroups of nonexerciser schematics, one of which has no motivation to act in accordance with the nonexerciser self-image. For this subgroup, whose negative self-schemata may have developed as part of their efforts to change their behavior and identity, a mismatch should exist between intentions and self-image. To the extent that a self-verification motivation fuels intention–behavior consistency, a lack of such motivation on the part of these nonexerciser schematics could lead to lack of intention–behavior consistency for the whole group.

The pattern of correlations for exerciser schematics, aschematics, and nonexerciser schematics cannot be explained by differences between the three groups on variables known to affect the size of correlations, such as the variances or ranges of either the intention or primary behavioral measures. Moreover, analysis of data collected from subjects tested in the latter two semesters of the study revealed no significant differences between the three groups of subjects in the stability of their intentions over time. This analysis ruled out the possibility that the lower intention–behavior correlation of nonexerciser schematics might have been due to their having been more prone than exerciser schematics to change their exercise intentions during the study.

The second point that deserves discussion is the magnitude of the exerciser schematics' correlation between exercise intentions and the number of days on which they exercised during the key week. Although the correlation is significant, it is only moderate in magnitude. In their theory of reasoned action, Ajzen and Fishbein (1980) claimed that intention should predict behavior if three conditions are met:

1. Intention and behavior are measured at corresponding levels of specificity.
2. Intentions have not changed in the time between their measurement and the measurement of behavior.
3. The behavior is under volitional control.

In the present situation, all three factors seem likely to have been operating to produce a lower intention–behavior correlation. First, subjects were asked about their intention to exercise regularly, defined as "exercising at least 3 times a week this semester." The behavioral measure, on the other hand, involved a count of the number of days during the key week on which subjects had exercised.

Although using this global measure of intention made it possible also to consider the correlation between intention and scores on the Stanford 7-Day Recall measure, it did not result in a high degree of correspondence between the intention measure and either measure of behavior. Second, it appears that exerciser schematics (as well as aschematics and nonexerciser schematics) may have changed their exercise intentions from the beginning of the semester to the 11th or 12th week. The correlation between exerciser schematics' intentions at the beginning of the semester and at the 11th or 12th week of the semester was .55 ($n = 227$, $p<.001$), despite the intention measure having a high internal-consistency reliability (alpha = .95).[3] Such instability may have been a function of the approaching end of the semester: Some students may have responded to an expected increase in workload by decreasing their exercise intentions in an effort to free more time, whereas others may have responded by maintaining or increasing their exercise intentions in an effort to use exercise to combat stress. As for the final requirement, that the behavior be under volitional control, the increased academic workload at the end of the semester should make it more difficult for students to implement their exercise intentions. For all of these reasons the moderate magnitude of the correlation between exerciser schematics' intentions and behavior seems reasonable.

This research needs to be replicated under optimal circumstances for obtaining strong intention–behavior correlations, and the replication should overcome the present study's limitation of reliance on self-report data. A focus on intention to engage in a particular exercise program for which objective behavioral data could be collected, over a period of time during which exercise intentions are unlikely to change because of situational pressures, would be ideal.

Self-Schemata and Accessibility of Intentions

The research provides initial evidence that having an exerciser self-schema facilitates intention–behavior consistency. The big question is why this should be so. It was suggested earlier that exerciser schematics meet all three conditions necessary for exercise behavior to occur:

1. They intend to exercise.
2. They are motivated to act on their intentions (for self-verification).
3. They possess exercise intentions that are relatively accessible in memory.

Clearly, testing this model will require a number of studies.

As a start Kendzierski and Shannon (1992) tested the general hypothesis that the intentions of schematics should be more accessible than those of aschematics. Ninety-five Villanova University students identified as either exerciser schematics ($n = 48$) or aschematics ($n = 47$) by a screening study participated in a self-description study. Subjects viewed on a computer monitor a series of 30 statements concerning intentions toward everyday activities. The first 6 statements served as practice stimuli; the remaining 24 appeared in random order. Of these, 4 referred to exercise intentions (i.e., "I intend to exercise regularly," "I am determined to exercise regularly," "I will try my best to exercise regularly," and "I am aiming at exercising regularly"). The other 20 statements consisted of the same four stems (e.g., "I intend to . . ."), each paired with five other everyday activities (i.e., "attend class regularly," "balance my checkbook regularly," "clean my room regularly," "read the newspaper regularly," and "attend church regularly").

Subjects were instructed to read each statement and respond as quickly as possible by pressing a key labeled *yes* or a key labeled *no* with the appropriate index finger (the *yes* key was always positioned for use by the dominant hand). Both the subject's response and his or her reaction time were automatically recorded by the computer. Analyses indicated that exerciser schematics responded "yes" to more of the exercise intention items than did aschematics (there were no differences in the mean number of "yes" responses to the other intention items). Because individuals used their dominant hand when making such judgments (and thus could be expected to make them more quickly), any analysis of reaction times for the exercise intention items that ignored the type of judgment would be biased in favor of the hypothesis (i.e., exerciser schematics could have faster reaction times simply because they used their dominant hand more when responding). To avoid this problem, an analysis of variance was performed only on mean reaction times for "yes" responses to exercise versus other intention items. The analysis yielded a significant main effect for item type, such that subjects responded more quickly to the exercise intention items, as well as for the predicted significant interaction between self-schema status and item type. As seen in Table 5.4, exerciser schematics were significantly faster than aschematics to respond "yes" to the exercise intention items but not to the other intention items. Also, while there was no difference in aschematics' reaction times for the exercise versus other intention items, exerciser schematics made significantly faster judgments

Table 5.4   Mean Response Latencies for Exercise and Other Intention Items as a Function of Self-Schema Status

| | Self-schema status | |
	Exercise schematics	Aschematics
Exercise intention items	1.26_a	1.48_b
Other intention items	1.61_b	1.47_b

Note. Within each row, means with different subscripts differ significantly ($p < .05$); within each column, means with different subscripts differ significantly ($p < .01$).

about exercise intention items—a finding consistent with previous research showing an advantage in processing schema-relevant information.

How generalizable are these findings? To determine the extent to which self-schema findings are generalizable across health-behavior domains, a measure was developed to assess diet-related self-schema status (Parisi & Kendzierski, 1991). In a subsequent study there was evidence that dieter schematics made significantly faster affirmative judgments about dieting intentions than did aschematics (Langer, 1992; Langer & Kendzierski, 1992). This study suggests that the finding is generalizable across at least two health-behavior domains and provides additional support for the model.

Self-Regulatory Correlates of an Exerciser Self-Schema

Focusing on the problem of decision implementation and trying to understand the processes involved in linking exercise intentions to behavior have led to other interesting findings concerning exerciser schematics. Both theorists and clinicians have suggested the importance of people's making specific plans to perform the behavior and of developing tricks or strategies to enable them to perform the behavior (Cantor et al., 1986). Do exerciser schematics differ from aschematics and nonexercisers on these supposedly important self-regulatory variables? Research suggests that they do. In the concurrent study mentioned earlier (Kendzierski, 1988), exerciser schematics reported having made significantly more plans to help them exercise regularly both during that semester and within the past 2 years; aschematics and nonexerciser schematics did not differ on either variable. Moreover, exerciser schematics reported having marginally significantly more ($p < .10$) strategies for getting themselves to exercise on days when they did not feel like exercising (e.g., "imagining myself looking like a beached whale" or "calling a friend to go running"); again, aschematics and nonexerciser schematics did not differ.

Given the correlational nature of these findings, it is unclear whether possession of an exerciser self-schema leads in some way to the development of plans and strategies for exercising or whether possession of plans and strategies leads in some way to the development of an exerciser self-schema. This is an important question if we are to gain a full understanding of the development and conse-quences of exerciser self-schemata. An equally important question concerns the possible role that the plans and strategies of exerciser schematics play in regard to their exercise behavior.

Self-Schema Versus Experience

As noted earlier, self-schemata involve generalizations about the self that are based on experience and focused on those aspects of the self that are regarded by the individual as important. Given this, it might be argued that an exercise self-schema measure simply reflects exercise experience and that any effects associated with possession of an exerciser self-schema (e.g., increased exercise behavior) may simply be due to exercise experience. Although this is certainly a possibility, both conceptual and empirical arguments may be made against it. Conceptually, experience is considered necessary but not sufficient for the development of a self-schema (Markus, 1977). The dimension must also be perceived as self-relevant by the individual. Two people could have identical exercise experience (e.g., both be doing exercise for rehabilitative purposes) but differ in the importance they place on exercising as regards their self-image; only the individual who considered (or came to consider) exercising important to his or her self-image would be classified as an exerciser schematic and expected to behave as one. Likewise, two people could have identical exercise experience (e.g., formerly sedentary neighbors who begin regularly walking through the neighborhood together as part of a Neighborhood Watch unit) but differ in whether they construe their common experience as getting exercise in addition to protecting the neighborhood. Only the individual who construes the activity in both ways would be in a position to begin developing an exerciser self-schema.

From an empirical perspective, exercise experience does not appear to be consistently related to exercise adherence. As noted by Dishman, Sallis, and Orenstein (1985), although past participation in supervised exercise programs relates to current participation, there are conflicting findings concerning the relationship between past experience in unsupervised settings and participation in supervised exercise programs. Moreover, although sports experience was found to correlate with exercise adherence in one cross-sectional study, no correlation has been found in any prospective study. If future research shows that exerciser schematics are more likely to adhere to both supervised and unsupervised exercise programs, the exercise self-schema concept would provide the more powerful approach. By emphasizing both experience and the importance of such experience to the individual, the exercise self-schema concept has the potential to resolve the conflicting findings on the role of exercise experience in subsequent exercise behavior.

The research program began with an attempt to understand the process of complex decision implementation as it relates to exercise behavior. Self-schema theory has proven useful from a heuristic standpoint, leading us to examine variables as diverse as response latencies and self-reports of exercise behavior. These initial studies have been promising; now it is time to collect better behavioral data on the role of exercise self-schemata in exercise and in linking exercise intentions and exercise behavior. It is also time to examine the complicated issue of the relationships between the constructs of exercise self-schema, its various correlates (e.g., accessibility of exercise intentions, possession of plans and strategies for exercising, and exercise experience), and exercise behavior. And it is time to test the model of exercise behavior outlined earlier, a model suggesting that such behavior results from having favorable intentions to exercise that are activated in memory, as well as motivation to act on those intentions that may derive in part from a desire to affirm one's self-image as an exerciser. These components are viewed as necessary conditions for exercise behavior, provided that exercising is under the individual's behavioral control (i.e., is possible given the individual's physical ability and situation).

A picture of an exerciser is emerging from this program of research. Whether or not self-schema theory will provide the most parsimonious explanation for the exercise self-schema findings remains to be determined. All that is certain is that the approach has led researchers to consider exercise behavior and decision implementation from previously unexamined angles. To the extent that the resulting findings contribute to the development of a good theory of exercise behavior, the approach will have been worth taking.

Notes

[1]Exerciser schematics reported being more interested in and committed to exercising regularly during the current semester than either aschematics (Ms = 7.16 and 5.79, respectively) or nonexerciser schematics (Ms = 7.93 and 4.29, respectively). Aschematics and nonexerciser schematics did not differ in their interest in exercising regularly, but aschematics were significantly more committed to exercising regularly than were nonexerciser schematics. Among the college students studied, interest in exercising was fairly high regardless of self-schema status.

[2]Data concerning nonexerciser schematics' intentions are consistent with the idea that two distinct subgroups of nonexerciser schematics may exist. Scores on the intention measure ranged from 9 to 35 out of a possible range of 5 to 35, with a mean of 23.90 and a standard deviation of 6.72. Clearly, some nonexerciser schematics have favorable intentions regarding exercise, whereas others have unfavorable intentions. If all nonexerciser schematics were either proud couch potatoes or would-be exercisers, one would expect less variability in their intention scores.

[3]The corresponding correlation was .44 (n = 39, p < .01) for aschematics and .48 (n = 41, p < .01) for nonexerciser schematics.

References

Ajzen, I., & Fishbein, M. (1980). *Understanding attitudes and predicting social behavior*. Englewood Cliffs, NJ: Prentice Hall.

Bartlett, F.C. (1932). *Remembering*. Cambridge, England: Cambridge University Press.

Blair, S.N. (1984). How to assess exercise habits and physical fitness. In J.D. Matarazzo, J.A. Herd, N.E. Miller, & S.M. Weiss (Eds.), *Behavioral health: A handbook for health enhancement and disease prevention* (pp. 424-447). New York: Wiley.

Brewer, W.F., & Nakamura, G.V. (1984). The nature and functions of schemas. In R.A. Wyer & T.K. Srull (Eds.), *Handbook of social cognition: Vol. 1* (pp. 119-160). Hillsdale, NJ: Erlbaum.

Cantor, N., Markus, H., Niedenthal, P., & Nurius, P. (1986). On motivation and the self-concept. In R.M. Sorrentino & E.T. Higgins (Eds.), *Handbook of motivation and cognition: Foundations of social behavior* (pp. 96-121). New York: Guilford Press.

Carver, C.S., & Scheier, M.F. (1981). *Attention and self-regulation: A control-theory approach to human behavior.* New York: Springer-Verlag.

Catrambone, R., & Markus, H. (1987). The role of self-schemas in going beyond the information given. *Social Cognition,* **5**, 349-368.

Dishman, R.K., Sallis, J.F., & Orenstein, D.R. (1985). The determinants of physical activity and exercise. *Public Health Reports,* **100**, 158-171.

Dishman, R.K., & Steinhardt, M. (1988). Reliability and concurrent validity for a 7-day recall of physical activity in college students. *Medicine and Science in Sports and Exercise,* **20**, 14-25.

Edwards, W. (1961). Behavioral decision theory. *Annual Review of Psychology,* **12**, 473-498.

Faulkner, R.A., & Stewart, G.W. (1978). Exercise programs—Recruitment/retention of participants. *Recreation Canada,* **36**, 21-27.

Fazio, R.H. (1986). How do attitudes guide behavior? In R.M. Sorrentino & E.T. Higgins (Eds.), *The handbook of motivation and cognition: Foundations of social behavior* (pp. 204-243). New York: Guilford Press.

Feather, N.T. (1982). *Expectations and actions: Expectancy-value models in psychology.* Hillsdale, NJ: Erlbaum.

Fishbein, M., & Ajzen, I. (1975). *Belief, attitude, intention and behavior: An introduction to theory and research.* Reading, MA: Addison-Wesley.

Fiske, S., & Taylor, S.E. (1984). *Social cognition.* Reading, MA: Addison-Wesley.

Heinzelmann, F. (1973). Social and psychological factors that influence the effectiveness of exercise programs. In J. Naughton & H.K. Hellerstein (Eds.), *Exercise testing and exercise training in coronary heart disease* (pp. 275-287). New York: Academic Press.

Higgins, E.T., & King, G. (1981). Accessibility of social constructs: Information-processing consequences of individual and contextual variability. In N. Cantor & J.F. Kihlstrom (Eds.), *Personality, cognition, and social interaction* (pp. 69-121). Hillsdale, NJ: Erlbaum.

Hoyt, M.F., & Janis, I.L. (1975). Increasing adherence to a stressful decision via a motivational balance-sheet procedure: A field experiment. *Journal of Personality and Social Psychology,* **31**, 833-839.

Janis, I.L., & Mann, L. (1968). A conflict-theory approach to attitude change and decision making. In A. Greenwald, T. Brock, & T. Ostrom (Eds.), *Psychological foundations of attitudes* (pp. 327-360). New York: Academic Press.

Janis, I.L., & Mann, L. (1977). *Decision making: A psychological analysis of conflict, choice, and commitment.* New York: Free Press.

Kendzierski, D. (1988). Self-schemata and exercise. *Basic and Applied Social Psychology,* **9**, 45-59.

Kendzierski, D. (1990a). Decision making versus decision implementation: An action control approach to exercise adoption and adherence. *Journal of Applied Social Psychology*, **20**, 27-45.

Kendzierski, D. (1990b). Exercise self-schemata: Cognitive and behavioral correlates. *Health Psychology*, **9**, 69-82.

Kendzierski, D. (1991). [*Self-schema as a moderator of intention-behavior consistency*]. Unpublished raw data.

Kendzierski, D., & LaMastro, V. (1988). Reconsidering the role of attitudes in exercise behavior: A decision theoretic approach. *Journal of Applied Social Psychology*, **18**, 737-759.

Kendzierski, D., & Shannon, D. (1992, August). *Exerciser self-schemata and the accessibility of exercise intentions*. Paper presented at the meeting of the American Psychological Association, Washington, DC.

Kuhl, J. (1985). Volitional mediators of cognition-behavior consistency: Self-regulatory processes and action versus state orientation. In J. Kuhl & J. Beckmann (Eds.), *Action control: From cognition to behavior* (pp. 101-128). New York: Springer-Verlag.

Langer, S. (1992). *Self-schemata and the accessibility of judgments about dieting intentions*. Unpublished master's thesis, Villanova University, Villanova, PA.

Langer, S., & Kendzierski, D. (1992, April). *Self-schemata and the accessibility of judgments about dieting intentions*. Paper presented at the meeting of the Eastern Psychological Association, Boston.

Lewin, K. (1947). Group decision and social change. In T.M. Newcomb & E.L. Hartley (Eds.), *Readings in social psychology* (pp. 330-344). New York: Holt.

Markus, H. (1977). Self-schemata and processing information about the self. *Journal of Personality and Social Psychology*, **35**, 63-78.

Markus, H., Crane, M., Bernstein, S., & Siladi, M. (1982). Self-schemas and gender. *Journal of Personality and Social Psychology*, **42**, 38-50.

Markus, H., Cross, S., & Wurf, E. (1990). The role of the self-system in competence. In R.J. Sternberg & J. Kolligian, Jr. (Eds.), *Competence considered* (pp. 205-225). New Haven, CT: Yale University Press.

Markus, H., Hamill, R., & Sentis, K.P. (1987). Thinking fat: Self-schemas for body weight and the processing of weight relevant information. *Journal of Applied Social Psychology*, **17**, 50-71.

Markus, H., & Smith, J. (1981). The influence of self-schemata on the perception of others. In N. Cantor & J. Kihlstrom (Eds.), *Personality, cognition, and social interaction* (pp. 233-262). Hillsdale, NJ: Erlbaum.

Markus, H., Smith, J., & Moreland, R.L. (1985). Role of the self-concept in the perception of others. *Journal of Personality and Social Psychology*, **49**, 1494-1512.

Markus, H., & Wurf, E. (1987). The dynamic self-concept: A social psychological perspective. *Annual Review of Psychology*, **38**, 299-337.

Neisser, V. (1976). *Cognition and reality: Principles and implications of cognitive psychology*. San Francisco: W.H. Freeman and Co.

Parisi, M., & Kendzierski, D. (1991, April). *Dieting self-schemata.* Paper presented at the meeting of the Eastern Psychological Association, New York.

Pines, H., & Kuczkowski, R. (1987, August). *A self-schema for clothing.* Paper presented at the meeting of the American Psychological Association, New York.

Rosch, E., & Mervis, C.B. (1975). Family resemblances: Studies in the internal structure of categories. *Cognitive Psychology*, **7**, 573-605.

Rumelhart, D.E., & Ortony, A. (1977). The representation of knowledge in memory. In R.C. Anderson, R.J. Spiro, & W.E. Montague (Eds.), *Schooling and the acquisition of knowledge* (pp. 99-136). Hillsdale, NJ: Erlbaum.

Snyder, M., & Kendzierski, D. (1982). Acting on one's attitudes: Procedures for linking attitudes and behavior. *Journal of Experimental Social Psychology*, **18**, 165-183.

Strube, M.J., Berry, J.M., Lott, C.L., Fogelman, R., Steinhart, G., Moergen, S., & Davison, L. (1986). Self-schematic representation of the Type A and B behavior patterns. *Journal of Personality and Social Psychology*, **51**, 170-180.

Swann, W.B., Jr. (1983). Self-verification: Bringing social reality into harmony with the self. In J. Suls & A.G. Greenwald (Eds.), *Social psychological perspectives on the self: Vol. 2* (pp. 33-66). Hillsdale, NJ: Erlbaum.

Swann, W.B., Jr. (1985). The self as architect of social reality. In B. Schlenker (Ed.), *The self and social life* (pp. 100-125). New York: McGraw-Hill.

Taylor, S.E., & Crocker, J. (1981). Schematic bases of social information processing. In E.T. Higgins, C.P. Herman, & M.P. Zanna, *Social cognition: The Ontario Symposium: Vol. 1* (pp. 89-134). Hillsdale, NJ: Erlbaum.

Wankel, L.M. (1984). Decision-making and social support strategies for increasing exercise adherence. *Journal of Cardiac Rehabilitation*, **4**, 124-135.

Wankel, L.M., & Graham, J. (1980). *The effects of a decision balance-sheet intervention upon exercise adherence of high and low self-motivated females.* Paper presented at the Canadian Psycho-motor Learning and Sport Psychology Symposium, Vancouver, BC.

Wankel, L.M., & Thompson, C.E. (1977). Motivating people to be physically active: Self-persuasion versus balanced decision-making. *Journal of Applied Social Psychology*, **7**, 332-340.

Wankel, L.M., Yardley, J.K., & Graham, J. (1985). The effects of motivational interventions upon the exercise adherence of high and low self-motivated adults. *Canadian Journal of Applied Sport Sciences*, **10**, 147-155.

Wurf, E. (1987). *Structure and functioning of regularity in the self-concept.* Unpublished doctoral dissertation, University of Michigan, Ann Arbor.

Wurf, E., & Markus, H. (1983). *Cognitive consequences of the negative self.* Paper presented at the meeting of the American Psychological Association, Anaheim, CA.

Wyer, R.S., Jr., & Srull, T.K. (1980). The processing of social stimulus information: A conceptual integration. In R. Hastie, T.M. Ostrom, E.B. Ebbesen, R.S. Wyer, D. Hamilton, & D.E. Carlston (Eds.), *Person memory: The cognitive basis of social perception* (pp. 227-300). Hillsdale, NJ: Erlbaum.

Research reported in this chapter was supported in part by National Institute of Mental Health Grant No. 1 R03 MH41690-01 and by a Villanova University Faculty Summer Research Grant. Portions of this chapter were written while the author was supported by National Science Foundation Grant No. BNS-9021105.

CHAPTER 6

The Transtheoretical Model: Applications to Exercise

James O. Prochaska
Bess H. Marcus

In the first half of this chapter we examine stages and processes as core constructs of the transtheoretical model of behavior change. We explore how core constructs from other theories, such as self-efficacy and decisional balance, can be integrated within a transtheoretical approach. Next we consider key concerns for behavioral interventions, comparing transtheoretical and more traditional approaches to such issues as recruitment, retention, resistance, relapse, and recovery. A sixth *R* for intervention is the relevance of a particular model to the behavior targeted for change. In the second half of the chapter we investigate the relevance of the transtheoretical model to the acquisition and maintenance of exercise behavior. We review current research applying core constructs of the transtheoretical model to individuals struggling to adopt and maintain exercise as an integral part of a healthier lifestyle.

Most of the research we cite focuses on extinction of negative behaviors, particularly smoking, rather than on acquisition of positive behaviors, such as exercise. As we discuss core constructs of the transtheoretical model, we raise questions about how certain constructs might differ for exercise acquisition. Then we explain similarities and differences in data and constructs when the transtheoretical model is applied to the acquisition and maintenance of exercise.

Our initial approach to understanding how individuals change was to study smokers attempting to change their behavior without professional intervention. What the individuals taught us was not available in any of the 300 systems of psychotherapy (Prochaska, 1979). Self-changers taught us that they progress through specific stages as they struggle to reduce or remove high-risk behaviors.

Stages of Change

The concept of stages is important for understanding change, in part because it reflects the temporal dimension in which change unfolds. Such constructs as self-efficacy, locus of control, decisional balance, barriers and facilitators, reinforcers and punishers, cues and consequences, cognitions, and norms lack a temporal dimension or a sense of directionality. Stages may represent an appropriate level of abstraction for understanding chronic behavioral risk factors such as smoking, obesity, high-fat diets, and sedentary lifestyles. The concept of stages falls somewhere between traits and states. Traits are typically construed as stable and not open to change. States, on the other hand, are readily changed and typically lack stability. Stages can be both stable and dynamic in nature. That is, although stages may last for considerable periods of time, they are open to change. This is the nature of most high risk behaviors—stable over time yet open to change.

The stages have been labeled

- precontemplation,
- contemplation,
- preparation,
- action,
- maintenance, and
- termination.

In the precontemplation stage, individuals do not intend to change their high-risk behaviors in the foreseeable future—usually within the next 6 months, as that period is about as far in the future as people anticipate making behavior changes. Individuals may be in this stage because

- they are uninformed about the long-term consequences of their behavior,
- they are demoralized about their ability to change and don't want to think about it, or
- they are defensive, in part because of social pressures to change.

With smokers, precontemplation is a very stable stage, with the majority of precontemplators remaining in it for the entire 2 years we have followed them. Precontemplation may not be as stable a stage for exercise behavior if people alternate between active and sedentary phases. As a group, precontemplators evaluate the pros of their risk behavior as greater than the cons (Velicer, DiClemente, Prochaska, & Brandenburg, 1985).

Contemplation is the stage in which people seriously intend to change in the next 6 months. Despite their intentions, we estimate that, on the average, individuals stay in this relatively stable stage for at least 2 years, telling themselves that someday they will change but putting off change. We refer to individuals who substitute thinking for acting as chronic contemplators. Contemplators see the pros and cons of their risk behavior as about equal. Consequently, they are ambivalent about changing.

Preparation is the stage in which individuals intend to take action in the near future, usually the next month. They typically have a plan of action and have taken action in the past year or made some behavior changes, such as reducing the number of cigarettes they smoke or increasing their activity levels, without reaching a criterion, such as exercising 3 times a week. This stage has both intentional and behavioral criteria. In it the downside of the risk behavior is evaluated as greater than the pros. Preparation is not a stable stage, and people in it are more likely than precontemplators or contemplators to progress over the next 6 months.

Action is the stage in which overt behavioral changes have occurred within the past 6 months. This is the busiest stage, in which the most processes of change are being used. It is also the least stable stage and tends to correspond with the highest risk for relapse. We originally compared 0 to 3 months and 3 to 6 months and found no significant differences in the number of processes of change used. Consequently, 0 to 6 months is the usual time criteria for the action stage (Prochaska & DiClemente, 1983). The behavioral-change criterion we try to apply is the one health professionals agree places the person at low risk for a particular behavior. Smokers, for example, are not in the action stage if they have reduced their smoking by 50% or 75% or have switched to cigarettes low in tar and nicotine: The action criterion is having quit smoking. Obviously, problems exist in areas for which there are no agreed-upon criteria. A research rule of thumb is, when in doubt, use a stricter criterion in order to obtain clearer results about how people change.

Maintenance is the period from 6 months after the criterion has been reached until such time as the risk of returning to the old behavior has terminated. Maintenance is a period of continued change, though fewer processes are typically needed to prevent relapse. When we use a time criterion, we consider 5 years of continuous maintenance as likely to result in termination. Researchers in the field used to assume that 12 months of continuous abstinence put smokers at minimal risk for relapse. Recent research now reveals that even after 12 months of continuous abstinence, 37% of individuals will return to regular smoking. After 5 years of continuous abstinence, the risk for relapse falls to 7% (U.S. Department of Health and Human Services, 1990).

Termination is the stage in which there is no temptation to engage in the old behavior and 100% self-efficacy in all previously tempting situations. With samples of maintainers for both smoking and alcohol abuse, we found only 15% and 17% of the individuals, respectively, had terminated their problem. There is reason to question whether formerly sedentary individuals can reach termination or whether they remain at risk for relapse and must continue to work to maintain regular exercise.

Processes of Change

In a number of retrospective, cross-sectional, longitudinal, and intervention studies, we have found that different change processes are emphasized at the various stages of change (DiClemente & Prochaska, 1982; DiClemente et al., 1991; Prochaska & DiClemente, 1983, 1984; Prochaska, DiClemente, Velicer, Ginpil, & Norcross, 1985; Prochaska, Velicer, DiClemente, Guadagnoli, & Rossi, 1991). Processes of change are covert or overt activities that individuals use to modify their experiences and environments in order to modify behavior. The 10 processes we have studied the most are

- consciousness raising,
- dramatic relief,
- self-reevaluation,
- social reevaluation,
- social liberation,
- environmental reevaluation,
- relationship fostering,
- counterconditioning,
- contingency management, and
- stimulus control.

Theoretically, these processes have their heritage in diverse therapy systems, including behavioral, cognitive, existential, experiential, gestalt, humanistic, interpersonal, psychodynamic, and radical therapies.

The 10 processes can be organized in a hierarchical manner consisting of two higher-order constructs, experiential and behavioral (Prochaska, Velicer, DiClemente, & Fava, 1988). The experiential construct includes the first five processes listed, and the behavioral incorporates the second five.

Experiential processes are much more important than behavioral processes for understanding and predicting progress in the early stages of change (DiClemente et al., 1991; Prochaska & DiClemente, 1983; Prochaska et al., 1988). Behavioral processes are much more important for understanding and predicting transitions from preparation to action and from action to maintenance.

Researchers' discovery of an integration of stages and processes of change has provided a useful guide for interventions. Once an individual's stage has been assessed, interventionists have a better idea of which processes to emphasize in order to help him or her progress to the next stage.

Decisional Balance

Decision-making theories help deepen our understanding of behavior change. In our research we have drawn upon the model of Janis and Mann (1977). In their model, decision-making involves balancing eight central constructs:

- instrumental benefits to self,
- instrumental benefits to others,
- instrumental costs to self,
- instrumental costs to others,

- approval from self,
- approval from others,
- disapproval from self, and
- disapproval from others.

In developing decisional balance measures for problem behaviors, we have consistently included items representing each of these constructs. We have developed a much simpler two-factor structure for our instruments, namely, the pros and cons or benefits and costs of specific behaviors (O'Connell & Velicer, 1988; Velicer et al., 1985).

The pros and cons are clearly relevant for understanding and predicting transitions between the first three stages of change (DiClemente et al., 1991; Prochaska et al., 1985; Velicer et al., 1985). During the action and maintenance stages, however, these decisional balance measures are much less important as predictors of progress.

The pattern of the pros and cons across stages is revealing. In studies of 12 problem behaviors, cons of changing always outweigh pros during the precontemplation stage (Prochaska, Velicer, et al., 1994). The opposite is true in the action and maintenance stages, the cross-over in relative importance of the pros and cons taking place during the contemplation or preparation stage, depending on the problem being studied. These studies suggest that a core construct such as decisional balance can be borrowed from other theories of behavior change and integrated into the stage dimension of the transtheoretical model.

Self-Efficacy

Self-efficacy has become a central concept within social learning theory (Bandura, 1977, 1982). Self-efficacy evaluations are assumed to influence choice, effort expenditure, thoughts, emotional reactions, and behavioral performance (Bandura, 1977, 1982). Self-efficacy involves people's degree of confidence that they can abstain from engaging in a problem behavior in a broad range of situations. Besides assessing confidence levels, we also assess the salience of specific situations. To do so, we assess how much individuals are tempted to engage in problem behaviors when in specific situations, such as when depressed, anxious, or socializing.

Across the stages, self-efficacy scores increase linearly, and temptation scores decrease linearly from precontemplation to maintenance. In the precontemplation stage self-efficacy is very low and temptations are very high. The gap between the two narrows somewhat in the contemplation and preparation stages.

Individuals in the action stage strike a precarious balance between efficacy and temptation, which reflects their high risks of relapse. In the maintenance stage the precontemplation period is reversed, with low temptation and high self-efficacy. The termination stage involves maximum self-efficacy and minimal temptation.

Self-efficacy is an important predictor of progress, but only in the action and maintenance stages. It is particularly striking that during the early stages, the higher people's self-efficacy, the more they apply the relevant processes of change. The opposite is true in later stages; the higher people's self-efficacy, the less they apply relevant processes of change. These findings indicate how a core construct from an alternative model of change can be further elucidated when integrated into the transtheoretical model.

Intervention Issues

Comparing a transtheoretical approach to intervention research with more traditional approaches reveals intervention mistakes that have been made with common risk factors. First, the vast majority of behavior-change research and behavior-change interventions are designed for individuals who are prepared for action. The available research indicates, however, that only a small percentage of people at risk are in the preparation stage. With smoking, for example, our best estimates are that only 10% to 20% of people at risk are prepared to take action, 30% to 40% are in the contemplation stage, and the majority are in the precontemplation stage (Abrams, Follick, & Biener, 1988; Gottlieb, Galvotti, McCuan, & McAlister, 1990; Pallonen, Fava, Salonen, & Prochaska, 1991).

If we try to help sedentary populations with action-oriented interventions, we risk serving many of them badly. We must survey what stage of change such populations are in so we can match their needs rather than expect them to match our action-oriented interventions. We shall examine five Rs of intervention to see how we have fared with action-oriented research and how we might fare with a stage-matched approach.

Recruitment

Tracy Orleans et al. (1988) surveyed a representative sample of smokers at the largest health maintenance organization (HMO) in Seattle, and 70% to 80% said they would take advantage of home-based self-help programs if offered for free through their HMO. After considerable publicity about this action-oriented program and a year of recruitment, 4% signed up. David Abrams and his colleagues (1988) surveyed a representative sample of employees at a work site, and 70% to 80% said they would take advantage of self-help programs if offered for free at work. Knowing the recruitment rates in Seattle, Abrams offered incentives for those who signed up. Chances to win VCRs, TVs, days off from work, and a weekend in Newport, Rhode Island, did increase recruitment rates—to 7%. Researchers at the Minnesota Heart Health program randomly assigned individuals to one of three recruitment strategies, including personalized letters announcing home-based programs for smoking cessation and weight loss. They found that recruitment rates for their action-oriented smoking cessation programs ranged from 1% to 5%; for their weight-loss programs the rates were 3% to 12% (Schmid, Jeffrey, & Hellerstedt, 1989).

When we ran small ads for home-based self-help programs for smokers who were prepared to take action on their smoking, about 100 people signed up in Rhode Island and 100 in Houston. We then ran ads of the same size for smokers who did not want to quit and recruited about 200 in Rhode Island and 200 in Houston. These results are not surprising when we consider that many more smokers are in the precontemplation stage than the preparation stage.

Traditionally, action-oriented interventions rely on reactive recruitment strategies: Advertise or announce your program, and let potential participants react. The act of calling or writing for a program may be a bigger action step than we can expect from most contemplators and precontemplators. From a stage perspective, we recommend proactive recruitment strategies. In our current random digit dialing study of 5,000 smokers in Rhode Island, proactive recruitment has enabled us to recruit 75% to 80% of the eligible smokers to our stage-matched self-help programs.

Retention

In three separate studies of work site–based weight-control programs, 80% of the participants dropped out. In a prediction study, we found that the best predictors of dropout were the stages clients were in and the processes they used early in treatment. These predictor variables outperformed the best predictors available in the literature, including demographics, problem history and severity, goals and expectations, self-esteem, and self-efficacy (Prochaska, Norcross, Fowler, Follick, & Abrams, 1992).

In the mental-health area 40% to 60% of individuals drop out of therapy prematurely and before their third session. In another prediction study we were not able to predict premature dropouts although we used the best predictors in the literature, including demographics, problem history, and severity and type of problem. Using our stage-related measures, assessed at the start of therapy, we were able to correctly predict 93% of the dropouts (Medeiros & Prochaska, 1993). We can now predict—if only we could control. In our current random digit dialing study of 5,000 smokers, we have been able to retain 75% of the participants after 3 months in our stage-matched programs, which is comparable to our retention rates with reactively recruited smokers.

Resistance

It is not uncommon for the administrator of self-help programs to find that about 50% of the people who call or send for materials do not read them, let alone use them. In self-help programs for smokers, we have found that among contemplators who report that they seriously intend to quit in the next 6 months, less than 50% quit for even 24 hr over the next 12 months. Our telephone counselors had the strong impression that the more we prodded contemplators to make a 24-hr quit attempt, the more resistance we encountered. We now believe that to help contemplators move to the preparation stage, we may need to help them take smaller behavioral steps such as reducing the number of cigarettes smoked daily by 4 or delaying the first cigarette of the day by an extra 30 min. Those, at least, are the main behavioral differences we have found between smokers in the contemplation stage and those in the preparation stage (DiClemente et al., 1991).

Relapse

This used to be thought of as the major challenge for behavior change, especially for addictive problems (Marlatt & Gordon, 1985). Relapse is a major problem, especially for those in the action stage. But helping individuals think about changing is a major challenge for those in the precontemplation stage. Helping individuals to take action is more of a problem for those in the contemplation stage.

Relapse prevention is a continuing concern for many researchers. One of our approaches is trying to help individuals become well prepared before taking action. We assume that the more effectively individuals have progressed through the stages before taking action, the more successful their attempts will be. We have found that the more individuals in the action stage continue to use change processes that are more appropriate to earlier stages, the more likely they are to relapse.

Given the current stage of our knowledge, however, we are convinced that no matter what we do, the majority of people will relapse after any single attempt to overcome most chronic behavior problems. Our strategy is to recycle relapsers to help them take action more effectively on their next attempt. We provide systematic feedback from our expert system, explaining what they did right and wrong and what they failed to do on their most recent attempt.

Recovery

This is our ultimate goal for behavior change. But as our stage model suggests, recovery is a process rather than an immediate outcome. The amount of progress individuals make toward recovery following intervention is usually a function of the stage they are in before intervention. We assessed the percentage of individuals now smoking at four points in the 18 months following intervention, as a function of their pretreatment stage of change. Precontemplators made the least progress, contemplators made considerably more, and individuals in the preparation stage made the most. Furthermore, the rate of progress appeared to plateau after 18 months for precontemplators but seemed to accelerate for those who began in the preparation stage.

Judith Ockene, Ira Ockene, and colleagues (1992) found clear stage relationships in smokers who entered the hospital for cardiovascular disease. At 12-month follow-up about 22% of their precontemplators, 44% of their contemplators, and about 80% of those in the preparation or action stage were not smoking. With Mexican-Americans in small towns in Texas, Nell Gottlieb and colleagues (1990) replicated most of what we have found in majority populations in terms of stages and processes of change. At follow-ups ranging from 12 to 18 months, however, they found that about four times as many contemplators as precontemplators had quit smoking.

Treatment Matching

One strategy to help people progress is to match treatment with their current stage and help them progress one stage in 1 month. With our self-help programs for smokers, we found a doubling in quit rates at 6 months for smokers who progressed one stage in 1 month. Among contemplators who progressed to preparation in 1 month, for example, 41% were not smoking at 6 months, compared with 20% who were still in the contemplation stage after the 1st month.

In a recent study we compared three interventions we have developed for smokers based on our stage model (Prochaska, DiClemente, et al., 1993). The treatment protocol involved randomly assigning 870 Rhode Island subjects by stage to one of four treatment conditions: standardized, individualized, interactive, or personalized. Standardized treatment involved the best self-help program currently available, namely, the action and maintenance manuals developed and tested by the American Lung Association. These manuals were supplemented by the best available materials for smokers not prepared for action. The standardized condition was used instead of a no-treatment condition. If new approaches cannot outperform the best available programs, there is no reason for the field to adopt them.

The self-help manuals were individualized to each participant's stage of change. Rather than assume that participants were prepared for action, we assessed their stages of change and started them on the appropriate manual.

The interactive condition involved the use of computer generated progress reports, which were based on participants' responses to questionnaires. These were scored and interpreted by expert computer systems that generated a unique report for each respondent. The reports included information on the participant's stage of change, decisional balance measures regarding the pros and cons of quitting smoking (Velicer et al., 1985), up to six processes of change that were being underused, overused, or used appropriately (Prochaska et al., 1988), temptations and self-efficacy in the most important smoking situations (Velicer, DiClemente, Rossi, & Prochaska, 1990), and techniques for coping with specific situations. The reports also referred participants to the stage-based manuals. Reports were mailed to participants as promptly as possible.

The personalized condition included stage-based manuals, computer reports, and personalized calls initiated by the counselors. A reactive hotline was offered to participants, and scarcely any used it. The calls were delivered at the start of treatment and at 1-, 3-, and 6-month follow-ups. Except for the month 3 call, counselors had copies of the computer reports to help them counsel clients about their progress on key process variables.

The two manual conditions replicated each other through the 12-month follow-up. At the 18-month follow-up, however, the individualized transtheoretical manuals (18.5% abstained) appeared to be performing better than the standardized American Lung Association (ALA) manuals (11% abstained).

The interactive (ITT) computer reports outperformed both manual conditions at each of the four follow-ups. The computer reports produced more than twice as much quitting at each follow-up than did the gold standard ALA manuals (e.g., 25.2% versus 11% at 18 months).

The personalized counselor call condition about doubled the quit rates of the two manual conditions up to the 12-month follow-up. Up to the 12-month follow-up the personalized and interactive (PITT) condition appeared to be producing a somewhat weaker replication of the interactive computer condition. By the 18-month follow-up, however, effects from the PITT condition appeared to have plateaued (at 18%). At 18 months the PITT condition outperformed only the ALA manuals, whereas the transtheoretical manual condition seemed to have caught up with the counselor call condition.

It is not clear why the counselor condition did not perform as well as the computer condition. Our counselors felt that we may have pushed participants, particularly contemplators, too vigorously toward action. This approach may have produced resistance. It is also possible that participants in this condition became more dependent on the proactive counselor calls. Once the counselors had completed their four calls, some participants may have had a sense of being abandoned in their efforts to change.

The results suggest that interactive computer feedback on stage-related variables has the potential to outperform the best self-help program currently available. Confidence in these results is enhanced by several findings: First, the two manual conditions replicated each other over the first 12 months of follow-up, which suggests that the outcomes were not due to chance; second, results for the two conditions that included interactive reports (ITT and PITT) paralleled each other for the first 12 months, although the personalized counselor condition consistently produced somewhat weaker results. Nevertheless, enough replication occurred across the two conditions to suggest the outcomes can be replicated and did not result from chance. Finally, stage by treatment comparisons indicate that the interactive computer condition outperformed the standardized manuals for smokers in each stage of change.

These results suggest that for the first time the field may have self-help programs that are appropriate and effective for the vast majority of smokers who are not prepared to take action on their smoking. Providing smokers interactive feedback about their stages of change, decisional balance, processes of change, self-efficacy, and temptation levels in critical smoking situations can produce greater success than providing only the best available self-help manuals.

That the interactive computer condition at least equaled and somewhat outperformed trained counselors suggests that our computer system can deliver expert help more cost-effectively than trained counselors. This expert system could be used by physicians and other health professionals to intervene with individuals who smoke. It could also be used as a freestanding service delivered by health promotion agencies such as the American Cancer Society and the American Lung Association.

We are now testing our expert system on a representative sample of 4,200 smokers in Rhode Island and an entire population of 5,000 smokers in an HMO in Massachusetts. In the latter study we are examining methods to enhance and simplify the system. As reported, we have been able to proactively recruit 75% to 80% of eligible smokers to our programs.

Although these results are encouraging, we must remember that the majority of individuals in our programs were still smoking at 18-month follow-up. Given the state of our science, we are convinced that we cannot help most people reach the maintenance stage with one trial of a brief intervention. We believe we can accelerate the process of change, and our initial data with stage-matched interventions are promising. A computer system providing expert feedback about stages, processes, decisional balance, self-efficacy, and other key variables could have considerable impact on helping people acquire and maintain the habit of exercise. But we should not make the same mistake with exercise that has been made with smoking—that is, to expect one trial of brief interventions to move most people. Such a strategy is likely to disappoint us and, more important, discourage the people we hope to help.

We want our models, measures, and intervention modalities to be relevant to as many problems and populations as possible. For example, many of the people we hope to serve have multiple risk factors. Using entirely new models, measures, and modalities with each problem or person could be overwhelming for them and for us. When we work with health professionals and those who deliver preventive medicine, it would help if they could learn models, measures, and modalities relevant to multiple risks rather than learn new approaches for each risk factor.

One of our research missions is to develop more relevant models of change. The stages of change model appears to be potentially relevant to a relatively broad range of problems. We have mentioned studies on 12 problem areas with data integrating the stages of change and decisional balance measures of the pros and cons of a behavior. The data revealed striking similarities among the following behaviors: smoking cessation, exercise acquisition, weight control, high-fat diets, quitting cocaine, delinquent behavior, condom use, safer sex, radon exposure, sun exposure, mammography screening, and physicians' preventive practices with smoking. A more in-depth analysis of studies can reveal the relevance of the transtheoretical model to understanding and intervening in exercise behavior.

Applications to Physical Exercise

Participation in physical exercise provides numerous benefits for both physical and mental health. Regular exercise can help prevent and treat diseases and conditions such as coronary heart disease, osteoporosis, hypertension, diabetes, and depression (Harris, Caspersen, DeFriese, & Estes, 1989). Although the benefits of exercise are well-established, getting inactive individuals to start exercising and active individuals to keep exercising remains somewhat mysterious.

Little is known about population-based interventions aimed at increasing the proportion of people interested in initiating physical activity. Media-based and other campaigns to reach large numbers of people have met with poor results. These results may be due to the educational rather than behavioral and motivational focus of such campaigns (Knapp, 1988). They may also be due to the campaigns' positioning to individuals who are already seriously considering participation in physical activity or are already exercising.

Across a variety of populations approximately 50% of individuals who join an exercise program will drop out in the first 3 to 6 months (Carmody, Senner, Manilow, & Mattarazzo, 1980; Dishman, 1988b). Although numerous investigations have been conducted to study the problem of exercise relapse, and some have shown positive effects on short-term adherence to relatively brief exercise programs, little success has been attained in improving long-term maintenance of exercise behavior (Dishman, 1982, 1988a, 1988b; Martin & Dubbert, 1982, 1984). This may be because most exercise programs are designed for people who have decided to begin or continue in an exercise program, yet a large portion of the North American population participates in virtually no exercise and likely has little interest in starting to exercise. This mismatch between current offerings (action-oriented programs) and the condition of the population (not exercising and probably not interested in exercise) indicates that successful interventions must be tailored to the needs of the population of interest (i.e., the very sedentary). The transtheoretical model has been successfully applied to tailoring interventions for such precontemplators in the domain of addictive behaviors and may be useful in guiding the design of successful exercise interventions (Prochaska, DiClemente, et al., 1993).

The pattern of exercise relapse is similar to the negatively accelerated relapse curve often seen in the study of addictions (Hunt, Barnett, & Branch, 1971). This similarity suggests that theoretical models, such as the transtheoretical model, that have guided research in the addictions may be useful for guiding exercise research. Adequate data on whether common processes are involved in the acquisition of positive behaviors such as exercise and the cessation of negative behaviors such as smoking, however, are unavailable (Sonstroem, 1987).

A particular strength of applying the transtheoretical model to the study of exercise behavior is its dynamic nature. Exercise researchers have recommended dynamic models that focus on the transitions that occur in adoption and maintenance of a behavior (Dishman, 1982; Sallis & Hovell, 1990; Sonstroem, 1988). In accordance with its dynamic focus, the transtheoretical model suggests that behavior change is not an all-or-none phenomenon and that individuals who stop performing a behavior may intend to start again.

The initial application of the transtheoretical model to exercise was conducted at the University of Rhode Island (Sonstroem, 1988; Sonstroem & Amaral, 1986).

Two hundred and twenty males over age 30 were classified into four stages of change:

- precontemplators,
- contemplators,
- recruits (initiated a program of vigorous exercise for at least 20 min at least 3 times a week within the past 2 years), and
- adherers (exercising at the recruit level for 2 or more years)

based on self-reported exercise history over the previous 4 years. Sixty-nine belief statements about the outcome of regular participation in a program of exercise, based on the Fishbein and Ajzen model (1975), were administered. A major discriminant function composed of 9 belief statements produced a canonical r of .75 with stage of exercise adoption, along with a correct overall classification of 67.9%. Furthermore, accuracy was consistent across stages, with a range from 28.1% above baseline for recruits to 47.2% above baseline for adherents. Interestingly, when 48 subjects who reported previous attrition from exercise were included in the analyses, classification accuracy dropped to 50.9% across the five categories of subjects. Group centroids for dropouts were not significantly different from those of contemplators. Because 37 dropouts were considering joining another exercise program, they were recategorized as contemplators, thereby increasing the overall accuracy to 60.3% across five categories and providing significant differences between the centroids of contemplators and dropouts. Thus, it appears that dropouts include both people who intend to resume participation in exercise and those who do not.

A second investigation was conducted by Barke and Nicholas (1990), who measured the stages of change in a group of older adults and compared the stages between an active and an inactive subgroup. Fifty-nine subjects aged 59 to 80 completed a 32-item stages of change scale for physical activity. Eighteen subjects were exercise-program participants, 20 were a matched group of retirees, and 21 were participants in an elderhostel program. Action and maintenance subscale scores were significantly higher than those of precontemplation, indicating that a large number of older adults are not sedentary. Analyses between groups revealed that exercise and elderhostel groups scored significantly higher on action and maintenance subscales than retirees, who scored significantly higher on the precontemplation subscale. These findings demonstrate that the stages of change scale does effectively distinguish groups of older adults who differ in level of physical activity.

Another group of investigators has been working on measurement development and model testing in the area of exercise adoption and maintenance. Marcus, Selby, Niaura, and Rossi (1992) developed scales to measure stages of change for exercise and self-efficacy for exercise. For the five-item self-efficacy measure, internal consistency was .76. Test-retest reliability for the self-efficacy scale over a 2-week period was .90. The Kappa index of reliability for the stages of change instrument over a 2-week period was .78. Two work-site samples ($n1 = 1,063$,

$n2 = 429$) were used to determine prevalence information on stage of adoption and the relationship between stage of adoption and self-efficacy. In the samples 34% to 39% of employees were regularly participating in physical activity (action or maintenance). Scores on efficacy items significantly differentiated employees at most stages, with proportions of variance accounted for (*eta* ^{2}) at .23 ($n1$) and .28 ($n2$). These results indicate that employees who had not yet begun to exercise, in contrast with those who exercised regularly, had little confidence in their ability to exercise. These findings support the smoking-related work of DiClemente, Prochaska, and Gilbertini (1985).

Marcus, Rossi, Selby, Niaura, and Abrams (1992) developed stages and processes of change questionnaires and administered them to a sample of 1,172 participants in a work-site health promotion project. This sample was randomly split into halves for initial model development and testing and confirmatory measurement model testing. Further model confirmation was obtained by examining the hierarchical structure of the processes of change and conducting stage by process analyses. Subjects used all 10 processes of change hypothesized by the transtheoretical model (Prochaska et al., 1988). The processes were organized in a hierarchical manner, using two hypothesized higher-order constructs, experiential and behavioral. Subjects in different stages of change used the processes of change in significantly different ways. Precontemplators used all 10 processes significantly less than individuals in the other stages. Subjects in preparation (exercising some but not regularly) used behavioral processes more than those in contemplation, whereas the two groups used experiential processes to a similar degree. Subjects in action used both experiential and behavioral processes more than those in preparation. Individuals in maintenance used the experiential processes less and the behavioral processes about the same amount as those in action. Although there are many similarities between these findings and those for smoking cessation, important differences were also revealed. In smoking cessation, the use of experiential processes peaks in preparation and declines in action and maintenance, whereas in exercise adoption its use peaks in action. Second, in smoking cessation the use of behavioral processes declines from action to maintenance; this is not the case in exercise adoption. These differences may or may not be due to the differences between acquisition and cessation behaviors.

Selby and DiLorenzo (1991) also developed stages and processes of change questionnaires and administered them to 443 college students. A series of factor analyses was conducted on the 65 process items, generating a 7-factor 32-item solution. Next, an analysis of variance was conducted to determine differential use of the change processes by current exercise stage. A multivariate analysis of variance and all but one univariate analysis of variance were significant, indicating increased use of the experiential processes in the early stages and of the behavioral processes in the late stages. Whereas this study resulted in a 7-factor 32-item solution and the Marcus, Rossi, et al. (1992) study resulted in a 10-factor 39-item solution, the pattern of process use by subjects in the different stages is consistent.

In another study, Marcus, Rakowski, and Rossi (1992) developed a decisional balance measure for exercise similar to that used for smoking cessation (Velicer et al., 1985). A sample of 778 men and women recruited from five work sites answered a 40-item questionnaire composed of items reflecting positive and negative aspects of exercise. Principal components analysis identified two factors, one a 6-item component representing avoidance of exercise (Cons), the other a 10-item component representing positive perceptions of exercise (Pros). Analysis of variance showed that the Pros, Cons, and a decisional balance measure (pros minus cons) were significantly associated with stage of exercise adoption, consistent with the application of these constructs to smoking cessation (Velicer et al., 1985), weight control (O'Connell & Velicer, 1988), and mammography (Rakowski et al., 1992).

In a cross-sectional study Marcus and Owen (1992) examined the prevalence of stages of readiness to exercise and their relationship to self-efficacy and the costs and benefits of exercising in samples of 1,093 U.S. employees and 801 Australian employees. In both samples 41% of the subjects were in precontemplation and contemplation, and 59% were in preparation, action, and maintenance. Scores on the five-item self-efficacy measure were significantly related to stage of change in both samples. Self-efficacy reliably differentiated most stages in a manner consistent with the findings of DiClemente et al. (1985). In both samples scores on the decisional balance scales were also significantly related to stage. These measures reliably differentiated subjects at most stages, supporting the smoking-related work of Velicer et al. (1985) and the weight-loss-related work of O'Connell and Velicer (1988). Although there were some differences in demographics and response rates between the two samples, a pattern emerged. These findings may be helpful for those designing community exercise programs.

Marcus and Simkin (1993) examined the validity of the stages of exercise adoption instrument by comparing it with the Seven Day Physical Activity Recall Questionnaire (Blair, 1984). A stages of exercise behavior questionnaire and the Seven Day Physical Activity Recall Questionnaire were given to a sample of 235 employees. Results revealed that 51% of employees were participating in no exercise (precontemplation and contemplation), and 49% were participating in occasional or regular exercise (preparation, action, and maintenance). Scores on physical-activity behavior items significantly differentiated employees among the stages, demonstrating that the stage instrument has concurrent validity with a well-accepted activity instrument. Continued work to integrate this model with self-report and objective measures of physical activity is important.

Marcus, Eaton, Rossi, and Harlow (in press) conducted a study on 698 employees to examine the relationships among stage of exercise behavior, self-reported level of physical activity, self-efficacy for exercise, and decision-making for exercise. Exploratory analyses revealed three independent components: pros, cons, and self-efficacy for exercise. Confirmatory analyses revealed an excellent fit between the hypothesized model and the data, that much of the variance in the stage of exercise construct was explained by the independent constructs, and that much of the variance in physical activity was explained by stage. Prediction analyses also revealed that the model did a good job of predicting exercise behavior 6 months later. Thus, these findings demonstrated that subjects' level of physical activity could be largely predicted by knowing their stage of exercise behavior, their perceptions of the costs and benefits of exercise, and their self-efficacy for exercise.

In the only intervention study conducted to date, Marcus, Banspach, et al. (1992) used the transtheoretical model to design an intervention to increase the adoption of physical activity among 610 community volunteers. At baseline 39% of subjects were in contemplation, 37% were in preparation, and 24% were in action. A 6-week stage-matched intervention consisting of three sets of self-help materials, a resource manual describing activity options, and weekly fun walks and activity nights was delivered. A random sample of participants ($n = 236$) stratified by baseline stage was telephoned postintervention. At that time 17% of subjects were in contemplation, 24% were in preparation, and 59% were in action, demonstrating that they had become significantly more active during the intervention. Although future work will need to include a proper control group and to assess maintenance of behavior change, it appears that using subjects' stage of exercise adoption to design and conduct an activity intervention enhances exercise adoption.

Researchers at San Diego University are involved in a Centers for Disease Control–funded research study called Project PACE (Physician-Based Assessment and Counseling for Exercise). The project's goal is to develop standardized assessment and counseling protocols that will help increase the frequency and adequacy of physician counseling about exercise. The PACE protocols are designed to stratify patients into three groups, based on their level of physical activity and their interest in it. The approach for stratification is based on the stages of change model and the stages in the natural history of exercise model (Sallis & Hovell, 1990). Patients will be stratified into precontemplation, contemplation, or action/maintenance groups. Each protocol is designed to help patients move closer to adopting or maintaining an active lifestyle.

Interest in applying the transtheoretical model to the study of exercise behavior appears to have accelerated in recent years. To date, a number of cross-sectional studies, one longitudinal study, and one intervention study have been conducted. Instrument development studies have been conducted, and it is probable that valid, reliable instruments for measuring all of the key transtheoretical model constructs will soon exist. It is likely that this model that has been so helpful in guiding research in the cessation of addictive behavior will also successfully guide research in the acquisition of exercise behavior. This is not surprising, in that the process of initiating physical activity can also be conceptualized as the cessation of a sedentary lifestyle.

A number of limitations are present in existing studies, and we hope that future studies will be able to rectify them. First, all of the studies have relied on self-reports of physical activity. Validity studies using objective measures of physical activity are needed. Second, more longitudinal studies are needed, as this model deals with behavior change and only some aspects of change can be studied with a cross-sectional design. Third, more intervention studies are needed to determine whether matching treatment to stage makes intervention more effective. Finally, the use of more representative and diverse samples is desirable.

References

Abrams, D.B., Follick, M.J., & Biener, L. (1988, November). Individual versus group self-help smoking cessation at the workplace: Initial impact and twelve month outcomes. In T. Glynn (Chair), *Four National Cancer Institute–funded self-help smoking cessation trials: Interim results and emerging patterns.* Symposium conducted at the meeting of the Association for the Advancement of Behavior Therapy, New York.

Bandura, A. (1977). Self-efficacy: Toward a unifying theory of behavioral change. *Psychological Review*, **84**, 191-215.

Bandura, A. (1982). Self-efficacy mechanism in human agency. *American Psychologist*, **87**, 122-147.

Barke, C.R., & Nicholas, D.R. (1990). Physical activity in older adults: The stages of change. *Journal of Applied Gerontology*, **9**(2), 216-223.

Blair, S.N. (1984). How to assess exercise habits and physical fitness. In J. Matarazzo, S. Weiss, J. Herd, & N. Miller (Eds.), *Behavioral health: A handbook of health enhancement and disease prevention* (pp. 424-447). New York: Wiley.

Carmody, T.P., Senner, J.W., Manilow, M.R., & Mattarazzo, J.D. (1980). Physical exercise rehabilitation: Long-term dropout rate in cardiac patients. *Journal of Behavioral Medicine*, **3**, 163-168.

DiClemente, C.C., & Prochaska, J.O. (1982). Self-change and therapy change of smoking behavior: A comparison of processes of cessation and maintenance. *Addictive Behaviors*, **7**, 133-142.

DiClemente, C.C., Prochaska, J.O., & Gilbertini, M. (1985). Self-efficacy and the stages of self-change of smoking. *Cognitive Therapy and Research*, **9**(1), 181-200.

DiClemente, C.C., Prochaska, J.O., Velicer, W.F., Fairhurst, S., Rossi, J.S., & Velasquez, M. (1991). The process of smoking cessation: An analysis of precontemplation, contemplation and preparation stages of change. *Journal of Consulting and Clinical Psychology*, **9**, 295-304.

Dishman, R.K. (1982). Compliance/adherence in health-related exercise. *Health Psychology*, **1**, 237-267.

Dishman, R.K. (1988a). Exercise adherence research: Future directions. *American Journal of Health Promotion*, **3**, 52-56.

Dishman, R.K. (1988b). Overview. In R.K. Dishman (Ed.), *Exercise adherence* (pp. 1-9). Champaign, IL: Human Kinetics.

Fishbein, M., & Ajzen, I. (1975). *Belief, attitude, intention, and behavior: An introduction to theory and research.* Reading, MA: Addison-Wesley.

Gottlieb, N.H., Galavotti, C., McCuan, R.S., & McAlister, A.L. (1990). Specification of a social cognitive model predicting smoking cessation in a Mexican-American population: A prospective study. *Cognitive Therapy and Research*, **14**, 529-542.

Harris, S.S., Caspersen, C.J., DeFriese, G.N., & Estes, E.H., Jr. (1989). Physical activity counseling for healthy adults as a primary preventive intervention in the clinical setting: Report of the U.S. Preventive Services Task Force. *Journal of the American Medical Association, 261,* 3590-3598.

Hunt, W.A., Barnett, L.W., & Branch, L.G. (1971). Relapse rates in addictions programs. *Journal of Clinical Psychology, 27,* 455-456.

Janis, I.L., & Mann, L. (1977). *Decision making.* New York: Macmillan.

Knapp, D.N. (1988). Behavioral management techniques and exercise promotion. In R.K. Dishman (Ed.), *Exercise adherence* (pp. 203-235). Champaign, IL: Human Kinetics.

Marcus, B.H., Banspach, S.W., Lefebvre, R.L., Rossi, J.S., Carleton, R.A., & Abrams, D.B. (1992). Using the stages of change model to increase the adoption of physical activity among community participants. *American Journal of Health Promotion, 6,* 424-429.

Marcus, B.H., Eaton, C.A., Rossi, J.S., & Harlow, L.L. (in press). Self-efficacy, decision-making and stages of change: A model of physical exercise. *Journal of Applied Social Psychology.*

Marcus, B.H., & Owen, N. (1992). Motivational readiness, self-efficacy and decision-making for exercise. *Journal of Applied Social Psychology, 22,* 3-16.

Marcus, B.H., Rakowski, W., & Rossi, J.S. (1992). Assessing motivational readiness and decision-making for exercise. *Health Psychology, 11,* 257-261.

Marcus, B.H., Rossi, J.S., Selby, V.C., Niaura, R.S., & Abrams, D.B. (1992). The stages and processes of exercise adoption and maintenance in a worksite sample. *Health Psychology, 11,* 386-395.

Marcus, B.H., Selby, V.C., Niaura, R.S., & Rossi, J.S. (1992). Self-efficacy and the stages of exercise behavior change. *Research Quarterly for Exercise and Sport, 63,* 60-66.

Marcus, B.H., & Simkin, L.R. (1993). The stages of exercise behavior. *Journal of Sports Medicine and Physical Fitness, 33,* 83-88.

Marlatt, G.A., & Gordon, J.R. (Eds.) (1985). *Relapse prevention: Maintenance strategies in the treatment of addictive behaviors.* New York: Guilford Press.

Martin, J.E., & Dubbert, P.M. (1982). Exercise applications and promotion in behavioral medicine: Current status and future directions. *Journal of Consulting and Clinical Psychology, 50,* 1004-1007.

Martin, J.E., & Dubbert, P.M. (1984). Behavioral management strategies for improving health and fitness. *Journal of Cardiac Rehabilitation, 4,* 200-208.

Medeiros, M., & Prochaska, J.O. (1993). *Predicting premature termination from psychotherapy.* Manuscript submitted for publication.

Ockene, J., Kristeller, J., Goldberg, R., Ockene, I., Merriam, P., Barrett, S., Pekow, P., Hosmer, D., & Gianelly, R. (1992). Smoking cessation and severity of disease: The Coronary Artery Smoking Intervention Study. *Health Psychology, 11,* 119-126.

O'Connell, D., & Velicer, W.F. (1988). A decisional balance measure for weight loss. *The International Journal of Addictions, 23,* 729-750.

Orleans, C.T., Schoenbach, V.J., Salmon, M.A., Wagner, E.A., Pearson, D.C., Fiedler, J., Quade, D., Porter, C.Q., & Kaplan, B.A. (1988, November).

Effectiveness of self-help quit smoking strategies. In T. Glynn (Chair), *Four National Cancer Institute–funded self-help smoking cessation trials: Interim results and emerging patterns*. Symposium conducted at the meeting of the Association for the Advancement of Behavior Therapy, New York.

Pallonen, U.E., Fava, J.L., Salonen, J.T., & Prochaska, J.O. (1991). *Readiness for smoking change among middle-aged Finnish men: The KUOPIO CVD risk factor trial*. Manuscript submitted for publication.

Prochaska, J.O. (1979). *Systems of psychotherapy: A transtheoretical analysis*. Homewood, IL: Dorsey Press.

Prochaska, J.O., & DiClemente, C.C. (1983). Stages and processes of self-change of smoking: Toward an integrative model of change. *Journal of Consulting and Clinical Psychology*, **51**, 390-395.

Prochaska, J.O., & DiClemente, C.C. (1984). *The transtheoretical approach: Crossing traditional boundaries of therapy*. Pacific Grove, CA: Brooks/Cole.

Prochaska, J.O., DiClemente, C.C., Velicer, W.F., Ginpil, S., & Norcross, J.C. (1985). Predicting change in smoking status for self-changers. *Addictive Behaviors*, **10**, 395-406.

Prochaska, J.O., DiClemente, C.C., Velicer, W.F., & Rossi, J.S. (1993). Standardized, individualized, interactive and personalized self-help programs for smoking cessation. *Health Psychology*, **12**, 399-405.

Prochaska, J.O., Norcross, J.C., Fowler, J., Follick, M., & Abrams, D.B. (1992). Attendance and outcome in a work-site weight control program: Processes and stages of change as process and predictor variables. *Addictive Behaviors*, **17**, 35-45.

Prochaska, J.O., Velicer, W.F., DiClemente, C.C., & Fava, J.L. (1988). Measuring processes of change: Applications to the cessation of smoking. *Journal of Consulting and Clinical Psychology*, **56**, 520-528.

Prochaska, J.O., Velicer, W.F., DiClemente, C.C., Guadagnoli, E., & Rossi, J.S. (1991). Patterns of change: Dynamic typology applied to smoking cessation. *Multivariate Behavioral Research*, **26**, 83-107.

Prochaska, J.O., Velicer, W.F., Rossi, J.S., Goldstein, M., Marcus, B., O'Connell, D., Rakowski, W., Fiore, C., Harlow, L., Redding, C., Rosenbloom, D., & Rossi, S. (1994). Stages of change and decisional balance for twelve problem behaviors. *Health Psychology*, **13**, 39-46.

Rakowski, W., Dubé, C., Marcus, B.H., Prochaska, J.O., Velicer, W.F., & Abrams, D.B. (1992). Assessing elements of women's decision-making about mammography. *Health Psychology*, **11**, 111-118.

Sallis, J.F., & Hovell, M.F. (1990). Determinants of exercise behavior. In J.O. Holloszy & K.B. Pandolf (Eds.), *Exercise and sport sciences review*, **18**. Baltimore: Williams & Wilkins.

Schmid, T.L., Jeffrey, R.W., & Hellerstedt, W.L. (1989). Direct mail recruitment to house-based smoking and weight control programs: A comparison of strengths. *Preventive Medicine*, **18**, 503-517.

Selby, V.C., & DiLorenzo, T.M. (1991). *Processes of change in the acquisition and maintenance of exercise*. Manuscript submitted for publication.

Sonstroem, R.J. (1987, August). *Stage model of exercise adoption.* Paper presented at the meeting of the American Psychological Association, New York.

Sonstroem, R.J. (1988). Psychological models. In R.K. Dishman (Ed.), *Exercise adherence* (pp. 125-154). Champaign, IL: Human Kinetics.

Sonstroem, R.J., & Amaral, L. (1986, April). *Beliefs and stages in exercise adoption.* Paper presented at the meeting of the American Alliance for Health, Physical Education, Recreation and Dance, Cincinnati.

U.S. Department of Health and Human Services. (1990). *The health benefits of smoking cessation* (DHHS Publication No. CDC 90-8416). Office on Smoking and Health. Washington, DC: Government Printing Office.

Velicer, W.F., DiClemente, C.C., Prochaska, J., & Brandenburg, N. (1985). A decisional balance measure for assessing and predicting smoking status. *Journal of Personality and Social Psychology*, **48**, 1279-1289.

Velicer, W.F., DiClemente, C.C., Rossi, J.S., & Prochaska, J.O. (1990). Relapse situations and self-efficacy: An integrative model. *Addictive Behaviors*, **15**, 271-283.

PART III

Interventions for Adoption and Maintenance

CHAPTER 7

Clinical and Community Interventions to Promote and Support Physical Activity Participation

Abby C. King

During the past several decades a tremendous amount of attention from both public and private sectors has been placed on physical exercise and fitness. Such attention notwithstanding, we remain an underactive and generally unfit society. As noted in Part I of this book, exercise participation rates rarely reach 50% even in the more affluent and younger sectors of the population and tend to diminish with age. What's more, a sizeable proportion of the U.S. population remains completely sedentary (Caspersen, Christenson, & Pollard, 1986).

The size and scope of the exercise adherence problem in the U.S. and a number of other Western nations demand a multilevel, multidisciplinary approach combining knowledge and expertise from behavioral science, exercise science, and public health. Such an approach emphasizes all levels of interventions, including personal and interpersonal strategies that target individuals or small groups and organizational, environmental, and societal strategies that influence the broader milieu (Winett, King, & Altman, 1989). Examples of strategies for promoting regular exercise at each of these levels are shown in Table 7.1.

Although a growing number of studies on exercise behavior have been conducted over the past several decades, much of the work remains focused on personal and interpersonal interventions that specifically target the individual. Although gains in knowledge have been made, it is clear that to achieve a significant impact on the whole population, strategies that target the environmental and social forces influencing exercise behavior will require far greater attention.

Table 7.1 Examples of Physical-Activity Programs, by Level of Intervention, Channel, Target, and Strategy

Level of intervention	Channel	Target	Strategy
Personal	Face-to-face: physician's office, health clinic, health spas and clubs	Patients, clients	Information on risk and health benefits, counselor support, personal monitoring and feedback, problem-solving (relapse prevention)
	Mediated/Not face-to-face: telephone, mail (feedback systems, correspondence courses, self-help kits and booklets)		Same as above
Interpersonal	Classes, telephone/mail systems, health spas and clubs, peer-led groups	Patients, healthy individuals, families, peers	Information; peer, family, & counselor support; group affiliation; personal or public monitoring and feedback; group problem-solving

Organizational/Environmental	Schools, worksites, neighborhoods, community facilities (e.g., par courses, walk/bike paths), churches, community organizations, sites for activities of daily living (public stairs, shopping malls, parking lots)	Student body, all employees, local residents, social norms or milieu	Curricula, point-of-choice education and prompts, organizational support, public feedback, incentives
Institutional/Legislative	Policies, laws, regulations	Broad spectrum of the community or population	Standardization of exercise-related curricula, insurance incentives for regular exercisers, flexible work time to permit exercise, monetary incentives for the development of adequate public facilities for exercise, Surgeon General's report on physical activity and health

Reprinted from King (1991).

This chapter provides a review of the intervention strategies that promote exercise participation in clinical and community settings and that have received scientific support. The review is not exhaustive but highlights particularly promising strategies as well as areas requiring further scientific attention. Before reviewing the literature several important issues relevant to the topic are discussed. Given that other chapters in this book focus specifically on children, the focus of this chapter is primarily on adults.

Exercise Adoption Versus Adherence

The term *adherence* generally refers to the level of participation achieved in a behavioral regimen once the individual has agreed to undertake it. This definition of exercise change has led researchers to focus their attention on increasing exercise participation in those individuals who are already somewhat active or are in the stages of becoming more active (Marcus & Owen, in press). As noted, however, a significant portion of the U.S. population is completely sedentary. It is this segment of the population that has the most to gain in disease prevention and health promotion through even modest increases in activity levels (Leon, Connett, Jacobs, & Rauramaa, 1987). Thus, a more relevant focus for this high-risk group is methods for increasing initial attempts to become more active (i.e., exercise adoption).

Despite the clear importance of developing strategies to encourage exercise adoption in sedentary individuals, controlled research in this area has been sparse for several reasons. As is the case in most health behavior areas, exercise researchers have tended to use a clinical approach in defining and measuring exercise behavior. That is, research and programming efforts have focused on those individuals who seek formal exercise programs that take place at a setting and time and in a format designated by the health professional. Such efforts usually attract individuals who are reasonably motivated or have a history of participation in formal exercise rather than the more typical sedentary individual in the community (King, Harris, & Haskell, 1988).

An alternative to the clinical model is a public health approach, whereby the scientist or health professional seeks out the sedentary members of a population rather than waiting for such individuals to present themselves. Epidemiological methodologies are applied in defining the population of interest (e.g., a community, a work site) and identifying sedentary individuals for further intervention. In one such study a community sample of approximately 600 sedentary or intermittently active women were recruited through community-wide promotion under the auspices of the Pawtucket Heart Health Program (Marcus, 1991). Using the stages of change approach described by Prochaska and DiClemente (1986), the researchers evaluated each individual's stage of exercise readiness at baseline, implemented a 6-week stage-matched intervention, and evaluated the stage of readiness again postintervention. Although the use of a quasi-experimental design limits the strength of the results, the investigators found that 30% of individuals identified as contemplators at baseline and more than 60% of those who reported being prepared to begin exercise but were not currently doing so had advanced to beginning an exercise regimen at 6 weeks.

In a Northern California community a random digit dialing telephone survey was used to identify sedentary individuals aged 50 to 65 years (King, Haskell, Taylor, Kraemer, & DeBusk, 1991). Those sedentary individuals who met other study criteria were invited to participate in a clinical trial evaluating the effects of different formats and intensities of endurance exercise on fitness levels and cardiovascular risk factors. They were compared with a group of individuals recruited by the more typical avenues of media promotion and physician referral. It was found that individuals recruited through the random digit dialing telephone survey had a greater number of risk factors for cardiovascular disease, including higher smoking rates and poorer plasma cholesterol profiles, than those recruited through the media promotion and physician referrals (King, Harris, & Haskell, 1988). The former group of individuals resembled the larger community more closely than did the latter group.

Such studies suggest that the application of epidemiological methods may indeed result in identifying sedentary individuals not typically reached by more clinically oriented approaches. Such strategies are more costly and complicated to use than other methods, however, especially when applied across an entire community. An alternative to using the community at large is to focus such public health approaches on a specific setting, such as a school or work site. In one extremely successful public health effort, the Johnson & Johnson Live for Live program, interventions to increase physical activity levels among all employees were evaluated in four Johnson & Johnson companies (Blair, Piserchia, Wilbur, & Crowder, 1986). The intervention consisted of a number of components, including an annual health assessment, a multifaceted health education campaign, and a series of health promotion seminars and exercise classes. The purpose of the program was to reach more than the small number of highly motivated employees who typically participate in the supervised exercise classes held at many work sites. Three other companies that received only the annual health assessment served as controls.

The exercise participation rates reported at 24 months were notable. During that time the prevalence of participation in vigorous physical activity more than doubled in the intervention companies, compared with only a 33% increase among employees at the comparison companies (Blair, Piserchia, et al., 1986). These changes occurred across all levels of employees. The changes in physical-activity levels were corroborated using estimates of $\dot{V}O_2$max obtained from a submaximal bicycle ergometer test.

These results underscore the utility of public health strategies for increasing physical-activity levels among a greater number and broader spectrum of individuals than will typically be reached with clinical approaches. Scientists will increasingly be required to turn their attention to the continued development of such broad-based strategies if the nation's objectives for exercise and physical fitness are to be reached (U.S. Department of Health and Human Services, Public Health Service, 1991).

In addition to the need to investigate methods for increasing initial participation rates, more attention is required in developing strategies for maintaining increases in physical activity beyond the 3- to 6-month period that is the typical length of most studies in this field (Dishman, 1991; Dubbert, 1992).

Exercise Versus Physical Activity

Research on exercise adherence has typically focused on planned bouts of high-intensity exercise scheduled for specific times and days. The individual is usually supplied with a formal exercise prescription, and adherence levels are calculated based on that prescription. Increased energy expenditure, however, which has been associated with a number of positive health effects of physical activity (Paffenbarger, Hyde, Wing, & Hsieh, 1986), can be generated by activities other than scheduled sessions of high-intensity exercise. Increasing one's level of routine or daily activities is an alternative way of expending energy that, if undertaken regularly, can decrease risk for cardiovascular disease and other chronic diseases (Leon et al., 1987). Given this fact, evaluating an individual's energy expenditure throughout the week would likely provide a more sensitive measure with which to assess the effects of physical activity on health and function than would a narrow focus on scheduled exercise sessions.

A focus on energy-expenditure levels—and the more routine types of physical activities (e.g., brisk walking) that form an important part of energy expenditure—demands a reconceptualization of both definitions and measures of adherence. It has been noted that the accurate assessment of light and moderate physical activity is an important challenge facing scientists interested in further evaluation of physical-activity participation rates and activity-related health effects (King et al., 1992). Similarly, it has become clear that in order to continue to advance the field of exercise behavior, researchers must develop broader definitions of physical-activity participation that extend beyond the traditional definitions of program adherence. Few studies have applied a broader concept of physical-activity participation in evaluating specific programs or strategies.

Review of Interventions

Having discussed several caveats, I will now review the types of interventions that show promise at each of the four levels of analysis.

Personal Approaches

Personal approaches target the individual for change, focusing largely on biological, cognitive, and behavioral variables that may influence physical-activity patterns. Theories and models of behavior change applied at this level include social learning and social-cognitive theories, applied behavior analysis, biopsychology models, health-belief models, and relapse-prevention approaches (Dishman, 1991; King et al., in press).

Such theories, along with exercise prevalence data broken down by demographic categories such as gender, age, and education, have provided researchers with a better understanding of the types of individuals at risk for inactivity and the factors that might affect adoption and adherence (Sallis, Haskell, et al., 1986; Sallis et al., 1989). Some of the more frequently noted variables influencing exercise participation and adherence are presented in Table 7.2. The variables are divided into three categories—personal, program-based, and environmental factors—based on social learning theory and its derivatives (Bandura, 1977, 1986). These variables have been described in detail in other recent reviews (Dishman, 1991; Dubbert, 1992; King et al., 1992) and will be discussed only briefly here.

In the personal arena, a variety of demographic, health-related, and psychological variables have been associated with rates of both initial and ongoing exercise participation in clinical and healthy populations. Individuals at risk for inactivity include older people, women (particularly if vigorous activity is the target), the less educated, and those who smoke or are overweight (Dishman, 1991; Dubbert, 1992; King et al., 1992). Despite consistent identification of these population segments as at risk for underactivity, few interventions have been tailored to their preferences or needs. Similarly, although psychological variables such as self-motivation (Dishman & Ickes, 1981) and self-efficacy (Bandura, 1977) have been associated with increased exercise participation in a variety of clinical and

Table 7.2   Examples of Factors Associated With Physical Activity

	Factor type		
	Personal	Program-based	Environmental or social
Adoption	Age, gender	Convenience	Available facilities, locale
	Education	Intensity	Social support
	Occupation	Choices	Weather
	Smoking status	Costs (monetary,	Environmental prompts, cues
	Body weight	psychological)	
	Self-efficacy		
	Attitudes, beliefs		
Maintenance	Smoking	Convenience	Social support
	Body weight	Intensity	Incentives, rewards
	Time issues	Flexibility	Minimal disincentives or
	Self-reguatory skills	Skills training	environmental barriers
	Self-motivation		
	Self-efficacy		

healthy populations (Garcia & King, 1991; Knapp, 1988), the most effective methods for using or modifying such factors to promote physical activity remain unclear.

In contrast, several programs aimed at enhancing an individual's behavioral and cognitive skills for increasing and maintaining exercise despite barriers and challenges have had short-term success in both clinical (i.e., cardiac) and healthy populations. Among those cognitive-behavioral strategies that appear useful in promoting at least short-term exercise adherence are self-monitoring (Martin et al., 1984; Oldridge & Jones, 1983), goal-setting (Martin et al., 1984; Owen, Lee, Naccarella, & Haag, 1987), feedback (Martin et al., 1984; Owen, Lee, Naccarella, & Haag, 1987), decision balance sheets (Hoyt & Janis, 1975; Wankel, Yardley, & Graham, 1985), relapse-prevention training (Belisle, Roskies, & Levesque, 1987; King & Frederiksen, 1984; King, Taylor, Haskell, & DeBusk, 1988), written agreements and contracts (Oldridge & Jones, 1983), stimulus control strategies (Kau & Fischer, 1974; Owen, Lee, Naccarella, & Haag, 1987), and contingency management (Allen & Iwata, 1984; Kau & Fischer, 1974). Unfortunately, evaluation of the majority of these strategies has been limited to intervention periods lasting less than 6 months. Although several investigations have found such strategies useful in maintaining exercise participation levels for a longer time (Blair, Piserchia, et al., 1986; King, Haskell, et al., 1991), the strategies have typically been administered in combination, preventing conclusions about the utility of any one strategy. In addition, the evidence suggests that some level of ongoing monitoring on the part of a health professional or other interested party may be necessary to ensure that such strategies continue to be used (King, Frey-Hewitt, Dreon, & Wood, 1989).

One behavioral strategy for increasing physical activity that has typically involved feedback and other educational components is the use of health risk appraisal or physical-fitness testing. The impact of health risk appraisal or fitness assessment, alone or combined with general education, on subsequent levels of physical activity occurring outside of a structured program has been evaluated in both healthy and cardiac populations. The majority of controlled investigations in this area have reported little success in increasing physical activity with such methods regardless of the targeted population (Ewart, Taylor, Reese, & DeBusk, 1983; Godin, Desharnais, Jobin, & Cook, 1987). Although fitness testing, combined with knowledge of results and other educational information, has been found to increase intention to exercise in some populations (Godin et al., 1987), minimal increases in exercise levels were found 3 to 6 months later (Daltroy, 1985; Godin et al., 1987; Reid & Morgan, 1979). The results suggest that health risk appraisal and fitness testing, although potentially useful in enhancing motivation to become more active, must be combined with more powerful strategies to bring about behavior change.

With respect to the exercise regimen itself, factors such as the enjoyability, convenience, and intensity of the prescribed exercise can have a significant impact on participation and adherence (King, Taylor, Haskell, & DeBusk, 1990; Sallis et al., 1990). Although vigorous frequent exercise can result in injury and thus reduced adherence (Pollock, 1988), at least one study found little difference in

1-year adherence rates between moderate-intensity regimens undertaken 3 or 5 days a week (King, Haskell, et al., 1991). In addition, although a recent study has demonstrated that breaking a 30-min exercise bout into three 10-min bouts undertaken throughout the day can achieve fitness increases similar to those achieved with longer bouts (DeBusk, Stenestrand, Sheehan, & Haskell, 1990), the long-term effects on adherence of these more frequent "minibouts" are unclear.

Environmental strategies undertaken on a personal level often involve guidance and support from a health professional (e.g., a physician). Because this type of support is typically removed in time from the exercise bout, however, it is likely to be less potent than forms of support that occur during the higher levels of intervention (e.g., interpersonal, institutional) that will be discussed in this chapter. Investigations of such strategies clearly indicate that social support for physical activity is invaluable in obtaining initial participation as well as long-term adherence. It is less clear how such support might best be delivered if the convenience and flexibility of the individual's physical-activity regimen are to be preserved.

The cognitive-behavioral, regimen-based, and environmental variables I have discussed can be applied personally with several formats. I will now describe these channels of delivery.

Face-to-Face Counseling.   In most health behavior areas, face-to-face counseling has been considered the sine qua non for achieving behavior change. This approach offers intensive, individualized attention by a trained health professional and the opportunity for clients' behavioral prescriptions to be tailored to fit their needs. In the physical-activity arena, such counseling has often occurred in a clinical setting with patients who have suffered a cardiac event. Physician- or office-based behavioral counseling of cardiac patients has been shown to increase their physical-activity levels relative to those of controls (Fraser et al., 1988). As noted in this volume's chapter 8, however, many primary-care physicians lack confidence in their ability to counsel patients about exercise and do not typically provide patients with an exercise prescription or other exercise-related information (Rosen, Logsdon, & Demak, 1984; Wells, Ware, & Lewis, 1984). Consequently, physicians remain an untapped resource for promoting increased physical activity among sedentary people.

The health promotion counterpart to face-to-face individual counseling by health-care professionals is the service provided over the past several decades by personal trainers (American Council on Exercise, 1991). The clientele of such trainers typically consists of healthy, affluent individuals who aim to achieve high levels of physical conditioning. Although it seems logical that the ongoing attention, instruction, and support provided by a personal trainer would result in adherence to an exercise regimen, controlled evaluations of the effectiveness of such an approach relative to other strategies are scarce.

The advantages of face-to-face individual counseling notwithstanding, the time- and labor-intensiveness of this approach, for both health professionals and clients, precludes its ongoing use for all but a select few.

Mediated Approaches.   At the other end of the continuum from face-to-face counseling are personal approaches that are primarily or entirely mediated. Such strategies rely on broadcast or print media to provide people with instructions and guidance for initiating or maintaining a physical-activity program. They range from videotapes that provide information on increasing physical activity, viewed in a physician's office or work site, to booklets, self-help kits, and correspondence courses designed to guide people through the behavioral steps involved in becoming more active.

Although advances in the use of personal mediated approaches have been noted in health areas such as smoking cessation (Sallis, Hill, et al., 1986) and weight loss (Brownell, 1988), much less attention has been paid to physical activity. As part of the Stanford Five-City Project (Farquhar et al., 1990), walking and jogging self-help kits were developed and distributed to the experimental communities. The kits provided a step-by-step program for becoming more active that incorporated behavioral strategies such as self-monitoring, goal-setting, and shaping. Formative evaluation revealed a great deal of interest in the kits among community members. Because the kits were disseminated to the community as part of a multicomponent program for increasing physical activity, however, their effectiveness as a tool for influencing physical activity is difficult to gauge.

Efforts to evaluate the feasibility and effectiveness of mediated self-instructional training methods for increasing endurance exercise have been undertaken by Owen, Lee, and colleagues in Australia (Owen, Lee, Naccarella, & Haag, 1987). They evaluated the effects of both single mailings and correspondence courses in samples of healthy young to middle-aged adults. Using a quasi-experimental design, they found that the 10-month exercise participation rates from the single-mailing and multiple-mailing self-instructional programs were similar to those reported from a face-to-face exercise program conducted in the same locale, although rates for all three programs were fairly low (approximately 36% of participants met the study criteria for regular vigorous exercise; Owen, Lee, Naccarella, & Haag, 1987).

The results support the continued investigation of mediated methods for supplying instruction and support to groups of individuals who are not typically reached by face-to-face or class approaches to physical activity. Continued research is required to develop mediated programs that are flexible and interactive enough to meet individual needs and interest levels while maintaining their convenient format.

Telephone Plus Mediated Approaches.   In an attempt to broaden the applicability and flexibility of personal interventions and reduce their costs, researchers have recently developed and evaluated telephone-based interventions to increase physical-activity levels (Houston-Miller, 1993). The goal of such programs is to allow individuals greater flexibility and convenience in choosing when, where, and in what manner to be physically active but to retain contact with and support from a knowledgeable instructor or health professional. These supervised home-based programs, as they have been labeled, differ from earlier attempts to evaluate regular physical activity outside of a formal class or group in that they provide ongoing contact with the health professional rather than end with the fitness assessment or brief counseling (Daltroy, 1985; Godin et al., 1987; Heinzelman & Bagley, 1970; Reid & Morgan, 1979).

Supervised home-based regimens have incorporated a number of cognitive-behavioral strategies demonstrated to be useful in face-to-face contexts. These strategies include self-monitoring, goal-setting, written contracts, feedback, structured problem-solving, and relapse-prevention training (King, Taylor, et al., 1988). Participants typically receive one individual counseling session with a trained staff member, during which an individualized exercise program is outlined and questions are answered. Subsequent interactions with the staff member occur primarily by telephone and mail. Telephone contacts initially occur about once every week or two, diminishing to an average of once a month as the individual progresses. Simple exercise logs are completed and sent back to the staff person each month. The logs are used to provide the individual with feedback and to identify problem areas in adhering to the exercise regimen. Research on such programs indicates that logging one's exercise on a daily basis promotes better long-term exercise adherence than keeping a weekly log (King, Taylor, et al., 1988). A sample home-based exercise regimen is outlined in Table 7.3.

Supervised home-based exercise training was originally designed for patients who had experienced an uncomplicated myocardial infarction (MI) (DeBusk et al., 1985). DeBusk and colleagues found in their studies of exercise training that patients randomly assigned to the home-based supervised exercise rehabilitation program had essentially the same level of adherence as those assigned to the gymnasium-based program. Adherence levels remained similar throughout the 23-week program.

An innovative variation of such telephone-mediated approaches to exercise participation has recently been developed by DeBusk and colleagues for post-MI

Table 7.3   Sample Supervised Home-Based Exercise Program

Introductory session	Physical-activity prescription tailored to individual preferences and physical, behavioral, and psychosocial needs
	Discussion of initial expectations for change
	Information on potential barriers to adherence and solutions (relapse prevention)
	Realistic goal-setting
	Contracting for behavior change
	Instruction in simple logging procedures (mailed back monthly)
Weeks 1-3	Brief weekly staff-initiated telephone contacts to
	Discuss progress
	Provide feedback and support
	Identify problem areas and discuss alternatives, solutions
	Encourage regular logging of behavior
Weeks 4-8	Biweekly staff-initiated telephone contacts
Months 3-12	Monthly staff-initiated telephone contacts

patients in five health maintenance organizations (HMOs) in northern California (Thomas et al., 1991). The purpose of this large-scale randomized, controlled trial is to evaluate the effectiveness of a home-based nurse-managed exercise program relative to the usual care condition. Data have been collected from 455 patients thus far. A large proportion of the post-MI patients (71%) were deemed eligible for exercise training. Patient reports, validated by treadmill exercise testing, indicate high levels of patient adherence (91%) with their prescription of low-intensity walking following hospital discharge. The prescription appears to be reasonably well maintained 180 days post-MI.

Supervised home-based exercise training has also been evaluated in a variety of populations of healthy middle-aged and older adults of both sexes (Gossard et al., 1986; Juneau et al., 1987; King et al., 1989; King, Haskell, et al., 1991; King, Taylor, et al., 1988). Both women and men have shown significant increases in exercise participation and fitness levels for periods of up to 2 years (King, Taylor, & Haskell, 1991). In addition, long-term exercise adherence has been found to be significantly greater in those women and men randomly assigned to home-based rather than group-based exercise training (King, Haskell, et al., 1991). In the few studies that have compared telephone plus mediated strategies with mediated strategies alone, individuals receiving brief monthly telephone contacts achieved significantly better exercise adherence than those receiving mailings alone, both during the initial (King, Taylor, et al., 1988) and long-term (King et al., 1989) phases of exercise participation.

A distinct advantage of such home-based programs is that they make it easier for individuals to participate in frequent episodes of light and moderate-intensity activity. This allows them to achieve weekly energy expenditures similar to those achieved by people engaged in high-intensity activities in a class setting. A wider variety of activities can also be targeted in home-based programs relative to standard class-based programs. Whereas most individuals enrolled in the studies chose to complete their exercise episodes on their own, people who wished to exercise with others could also be accommodated.

The expense of face-to-face personal approaches argues against their use for solving our society's inactivity problem, although brief counseling by physicians and other health professionals can likely aid and reinforce other strategies for enhancing physical-activity levels. In contrast, telephone and mediated approaches offer promise for reaching a broader segment of the sedentary or intermittently active population in a more cost-effective manner. Telephone approaches in particular offer the incentive of personal contact and support, coupled with a convenience not typically afforded by face-to-face strategies. Identifying the most effective methods for delivering ongoing low-cost telephone contact represents the next task in the development of such programs for the community. Potential channels for delivering periodic telephone contact include work sites; public-health outreach programs; and volunteer organizations and other groups operating through city parks and recreation departments, senior centers, HMOs, clinics, community colleges, and nonprofit health organizations.

Research on personal interventions has provided the scientific community with a foundation of potentially influential variables and strategies with which to intervene in physical activity. Profitable next steps include developing a clearer understanding of how these variables interact in influencing exercise behavior at the stages of adoption, adherence, and long-term maintenance; designing a more comprehensive conceptual and theoretical framework for organizing the strategies that have proved useful and for investigating new ones; and continuing to explore methods for identifying broader channels and levels for population-based dissemination of effective strategies. In addition, it would behoove researchers to evaluate strategies for formally training this country's exercise instructors in methods of systematically applying the knowledge already available for promoting regular exercise. It is questionable whether even basic behavioral strategies, such as logging, feedback, and use of incentives, are systematically applied by the organizers of the myriad exercise classes and facilities in the United States.

Interpersonal Approaches

Interpersonal approaches have focused largely on group or class formats. Such formats remain the most popular method for delivering exercise programs in clinical settings and the community and for studying factors and interventions related to exercise adherence (Owen, Lee, & Sedgwick, 1987). Group formats have a number of potential advantages, including a larger professional-to-client ratio, making such formats potentially more cost-effective than individual approaches; on-site supervision; visual modeling by the instructor; a set structure with respect to location, exercise format, and time; face-to-face encouragement by the instructor; and potential peer support.

Despite the widespread use of group formats, most such exercise programs remain focused on the individual. Indeed, the majority of the studies summarized in the previous section used a group or class format. In general, however, there has been minimal formal or structured involvement of exercise peers or the other social factors, such as co-workers or families, that are typically the hallmark of interpersonal programs. A notable exception is the San Diego Family Health Project (Nader et al., 1989), which has targeted the family as a major focus of intervention for bringing about improvements in children's dietary and physical-activity behaviors. The data collected demonstrate the impact of parental physical-activity behaviors on a child's physical-activity patterns (Sallis, Patterson, Mc-Kenzie, & Nader, 1988). Such factors are discussed in more detail in chapter 12.

Social support from peers can take the form of buddy systems (Rich & King, 1986), which, if used appropriately, could reduce the high incidence of dropout that plagues most exercise programs. The use of public monitoring and feedback systems, competitions, and group problem-solving can also enhance feelings of group affiliation and thus promote continued participation (Dishman, 1991; King, Carl, Birkel, & Haskell, 1988; Martin et al., 1984). As noted previously, an important challenge is to find ways to promote the use of such social forces in the already available group programs offered in most communities. This may be a difficult task, particularly in the private sector of the exercise industry, where initial enrollment, not ongoing attendance, dictates profits. In these and other settings, rewarding instructors for obtaining good attendance rates would likely facilitate participant adherence. It may also be useful to develop methods for teaching individuals self-management techniques to use in conjunction with or following their participation in exercise courses (Owen, Lee, & Sedgwick, 1987).

An additional way to enhance the attractiveness and effectiveness of group programs is to employ exercise instructors who are culturally and demographically similar to the population segment being targeted. This may be particularly important in attracting members of minority groups. A good example can be found in the Zuni Indian Diabetes Project (Heath, Leonard, Wilson, Kendrick, & Powell, 1987). Offered at several sites throughout the Zuni community in New Mexico, the program evaluated exercise as a means of aiding control of non-insulin-dependent diabetes mellitus, which is alarmingly prevalent in this cultural group. Community ownership of the program was increased through using 48 Zuni Indians in its delivery. These individuals were trained by project staff in exercise leadership and played an active role in the program. Program-based weight loss and fasting blood glucose values have been encouraging. An important side effect of the program has been the apparent diffusion of the physical-activity message throughout the community; the researchers noted that 18% of inactive individuals who had chosen not to participate in the classes subsequently initiated home exercise during the course of the study.

The advantages of formal exercise classes notwithstanding, the class approach carries with it a number of disadvantages. These include

- the inconvenience of getting to class several times a week, along with constraints related to class schedules;
- a limited variety of activities, which, in contrast with many people's preferences, typically take place indoors (King et al., 1990);
- constraints on individualizing the regimen for the individual;
- the expense of fees, equipment, and special attire;
- social costs, such as embarrassment or discouragement, that may develop from the social comparisons that inevitably occur in groups; and
- group leader effects.

Leader effects may involve dislike of the leader's style or disruptions in the class or group that inevitably occur with leader absence or turnover.

These difficulties, coupled with an increased emphasis on moderate-intensity activity, have led to an increase in walking groups and other clubs that provide group exercise in locations convenient to participants' homes or jobs. These include mall walking programs, which have grown in popularity particularly among older adults, and neighborhood-based efforts such as the Heart and Sole Program that was part of the Stanford Five-City Project (Farquhar et al., 1990; King, 1991). Such programs hold promise for reaching untapped segments of the inactive population yet have been minimally studied.

Group exercise programs and facilities will likely remain popular for people who enjoy the social aspects of such programs and are able and willing to overcome barriers related to convenience. Surveys suggest that this segment constitutes a minority of the American public, however (Iverson, Fielding, Crow, & Christenson, 1985; King et al., 1990). The majority of Americans seem to prefer to engage in physical activity outside a formal setting or program. For instance, in a recent epidemiological survey of more than 1,800 adults aged 50 to 65 years residing in a midsize northern California community, more than two thirds stated a preference for activities that, following some instruction, could be undertaken alone (Haskell, King, & Evans, 1988).

By applying a waiting rather than a seeking mode, organized programs are unlikely to touch the most sedentary segments of the population, which could potentially benefit the most from even relatively small increases in physical activity (Leon et al., 1987). In addition, even if most Americans were willing to try group activities, the sheer size of the underactive population would overwhelm the ability of exercise professionals to provide the number of exercise classes required to meet the need.

Organizational or Environmental Approaches

Organizational or environmental approaches focus on changing aspects of a setting or environment in order to promote the targeted health behavior. Interventions may include changing organizational rules or policies, community norms, or the availability of facilities to increase the occurrence of a health behavior. Such interventions may also include removing or minimizing environmental barriers to undertaking the behavior. An excellent example of the latter is found in the Community Health Assessment and Promotion Project (CHAPP), which was supported by the Centers for Disease Control (CDC). The goal of CHAPP was to modify dietary and exercise behaviors in approximately 400 obese women from a predominantly black Atlanta community (Lasco et al., 1989). Among the environmentally relevant strategies applied in promoting physical activity were providing security escorts for groups of participants walking in dangerous neighborhoods, installing curtains on the windows in the exercise room to ensure privacy, and making free transportation and child care available to promote participation. A particularly important aspect of CHAPP was the formation of a community coalition, which has helped bring together a variety of community organizations (e.g., churches, the YMCA) that are working to maintain the program. The data collected 4 months into the program were encouraging, with participation rates of approximately 60% to 70%.

An example of how community norms can be influenced is provided by the Zuni Indian Diabetes Project. The information campaign that launched the project, coupled, most likely, with word of mouth from participants in the exercise classes, resulted in an increase in physical activity among a notable percentage of Zuni Indians who were not formally participating in the exercise classes.

Community Settings—Work Sites. A number of community organizations provide attractive settings for physical-activity programs. Work sites have become particularly popular outlets for physical activity and other health promotion activities (W.S. Cohen, 1985). Work sites offer, among other things, an accessible and diverse population base, convenience, potential avenues for group support and environmental and social influence, and existing communication and health-care delivery channels (Winett et al., 1989). Work-site health promotion programs are often attractive to both employees and employers, who forsee potential benefits in employee morale and productivity as well as reduced health insurance costs and absenteeism (Blair, Smith, et al., 1986; Shephard, 1986).

Such advantages notwithstanding, the vast majority of work-site exercise programs have been limited to small-group instruction reminiscent of the clinical model previously discussed (Shephard, 1986). Although the results from many work-site studies are promising with respect to short-term employee participation, a lack of public-health focus and the many methodological constraints that often face researchers in this setting have prevented the development of programs that reach the full potential work sites offer. As noted previously, the Johnson & Johnson Live for Life program is one of the few programs employing a multilevel public-health approach to enhancing physical-activity levels (Blair, Piserchia, et al., 1986). Other programs that have taken advantage of the social, organizational, and environmental aspects of this setting include the Team Health Program (Knadler & Rogers, 1987), the Stanford Coming Alive Program (Altman et al., 1986), and the Minnesota Shape Up Challenge (Blake et al., 1987). All three programs targeted the entire work force and used a contest that incorporated goal-setting, regular tracking of physical activity, feedback, and incentives to promote increases in physical-activity participation. The Stanford and Minnesota programs involved a competition among a number of work sites in the community, whereas the Team Health Program focused on one work site housed in a 50-story Dallas high-rise building. A unique aspect of this program was that it focused on a mundane but readily accessible form of routine activity: stair climbing.

Results from all three programs indicated significant increases in physical-activity participation during the contest period. Team Health staff have reported reasonable success in maintaining exercise participation after the initial contest through the development of stair-climbing clubs and the continued distribution of low-cost incentives based on exercise levels (Knadler & Rogers, 1987). In addition, an effort to extend such contests to a traditionally hard-to-reach segment of the employee population—blue-collar workers—resulted in a 25% increase in the number of employees engaged in physical activity vigorous enough to improve fitness during the 4-month contest period (King, Carl, et al., 1988).

These findings reinforce the potential of the work place as an avenue for reaching a broad cross section of Americans in a systematic and ongoing fashion. Future efforts are required to develop organizational, social, and environmental strategies not only for initiating such programs but also for maintaining participation. Additional work should be aimed at developing viable physical-activity programs in smaller work places (i.e., those with fewer than 50 employees), which employ the majority of Americans. Most programming efforts have targeted larger work sites (Felix, Stunkard, R.Y. Cohen, & Cooley, 1985). It also should be noted that a number of these efforts, such as the Staywell Program for CDC employees and their spouses (Naditch, 1984) and the Johnson & Johnson Live for Life program, have focused on multiple health behaviors. It remains unclear whether physical-activity interventions are more likely to be successful if targeted alone or in combination with several risk factors (King, 1991).

Other Community Settings.   Schools, places of worship, and to an increasing degree, senior centers and senior residential settings are increasingly being explored as sites for exercise-program delivery.

Programs in primary and secondary schools have typically focused on multiple risk factors, with classroom instruction as the primary means of delivery (Killen et al., 1988; Walter, 1989). In a few cases classroom instruction has been supplemented with organizational or environmental strategies such as modifying the school's physical-education curriculum to include more class time spent in moderate and vigorous physical activity (Parcel et al., 1987). In addition, several programs have attempted to involve the family in enhancing physical activity and other risk-factor changes in children (Coates, Jeffery, & Slinkard, 1981; Nader et al., 1989). Although all of these interventions have resulted in significant increases in knowledge and some indications of increased physical activity in elementary to high school children, questions remain concerning the long-term stability of the changes.

An alternate approach to classroom instruction has been adopted by the Institute for Aerobics Research in designing and implementing a Campbell Soup Company–sponsored program called FITNESSGRAM (Blair, Clark, Cureton, & Powell, 1989). FITNESSGRAM, a physical-fitness assessment and feedback program for youth, is designed to enhance awareness of and encourage greater participation in physical activity. It incorporates exercise logging, with feedback and participation rewards, and is being implemented in a number of community settings throughout the country (e.g., YMCAs, recreation centers) and in schools. Available data on the program suggest that it provides a useful standardized method for assessing children's fitness levels and for encouraging continued improvement.

Places of worship offer a means of targeting the family and have been suggested as particularly appropriate settings for reaching population segments that have traditionally been underserved in health promotion. For instance, the Fitness Through Churches Project has targeted African-American residents of North Carolina with a health promotion campaign that includes aerobic exercise (Hatch, Cunningham, Woods, & Snipes, 1986). This and other programs, such as the Health and Religion Project (HARP) in Rhode Island (Lasater, B.L. Wells, Carleton, & Elder, 1986), use both personal-interpersonal strategies (e.g., exercise classes) and organizational strategies (e.g., training church volunteers to disseminate information to other members). Early results support the feasibility and accessibility of places of worship for the promotion of physical activity (Hatch et al., 1986; Lasater et al., 1986), but the effectiveness of such programs in achieving sustained physical-activity participation remains to be determined.

A number of other community settings, such as senior centers, have become increasingly active in offering physical-activity programs for their constituents. Few such programs have been evaluated systematically, however, and most use approaches limited to personal and interpersonal levels of intervention.

Community Events.   In addition to offering setting-specific programs, a number of community organizations sponsor annual community-wide exercise events such as races and fun runs or walking events. Evaluations of such events, when they occur, have generally indicated that they are most effective at increasing community awareness concerning physical activity, whereas physical-activity participation has been found to be greater in setting-specific programs (Blake et al., 1987).

Mass-Media Approaches.   Although the use of mass media has been identified as a potentially powerful means of influencing health (Maccoby & Alexander, 1980), systematic evaluations of physical-activity media campaigns on the community, regional, or national level have been few. All four of the major community-wide heart disease prevention programs undertaken in the United States have developed some form of mass-media programming in the physical-activity area, but the fact that these interventions were concurrent with a number of other community interventions makes their impact difficult to discern (King, 1991).

Results from the few systematically evaluated national physical-activity media campaigns have been equivocal. Evaluation of a media campaign initiated by the U.S. Department of Health and Human Services in 1981, that targeted physical activity and five other health behaviors, produced questionable results as to whether the campaign significantly increased even awareness related to physical activity (David & Iverson, 1984). The best predictor of postcampaign exercise levels remained precampaign exercise levels. Similarly ambiguous results were found for a 1977 national Australian physical-activity campaign, Life—Be in It (Iverson et al., 1985). Given the few evaluations of this type, it is unclear whether such mass-media approaches are ineffective for physical activity or rather need to be structured, executed, or evaluated differently.

Although they offer many advantages in accessibility, communication, and incentives for behavior change, work sites and other community settings have not yet reached their potential for increasing participation in regular physical activity. As is the case for interpersonal approaches, future efforts to develop organizational or environmental physical-activity interventions require the incorporation of strategies that move beyond personal approaches and take advantage of the additional factors operating in the organization and the environment. The majority of organizational-level interventions have not done so.

This limitation notwithstanding, study results point to the utility of more systematic investigations of the best methods for integrating organizational or environmental strategies across the community at large. The major U.S. community-wide heart disease prevention programs undertaken in California, Minnesota, Rhode Island, and Pennsylvania have initiated physical-activity interventions that span the variety of organizational or environmental approaches I have described (King,

1991). The amount of resources used to develop and evaluate such physical-activity programs, however, was generally less than that applied in other risk-factor areas. Much remains to be learned about combining both setting-specific and more general organizational or environmental approaches to obtain the best and most cost-effective outcomes.

The use of "point of decision" informational prompts, coupled with incentives and other environmental strategies, also deserves greater attention. These simple approaches, which have been used to encourage individuals to walk, bicycle, or use stairs rather than choose motor vehicles or escalators, have received support in several carefully controlled investigations undertaken in the early 1980s (Brownell, Stunkard, & Albaum, 1980; Mayer & Geller, 1982). Unfortunately, they have received minimal attention since then. Additional examples of potentially influential environmental strategies include making safe and accessible pedestrian and bicycle lanes available throughout the community and providing public transportation that allows residents ready access to community exercise settings.

Institutional or Societal Approaches

Institutional or societal approaches focus primarily on public policy and legislation as well as on developing passive prevention strategies that do not require action on the part of the individual in order to be effective. Such approaches are often employed in other health promotion areas in which the use of a product or substance is at issue. Modifications of the production, content, or packaging of items such as cigarettes, alcohol, eggs, and processed foods have been made in an effort to diminish the negative impact of using these products. Similarly, taxes have been levied, and laws have increasingly been enacted or enforced to curtail or otherwise influence the advertising and use of such items, with at times notable success (Winett et al., 1989).

Despite clear avenues for intervention and evidence that indicates the potency of such programs on behaviors such as cigarette use, the multiple and often divergent interests of different social sectors in a free-market economy typically make such interventions difficult to carry out. The problem is compounded in the area of physical activity, where the focus is not on control of a product but on participation in a behavior. Passive prevention approaches are consequently difficult to devise. An example of such an approach—which has gained popularity in Scandinavia, though is less popular in the United States—is the development of urban shopping areas as pedestrian malls where motorized traffic is prohibited.

Other potentially effective societal strategies include

- policies governing the standardization and dissemination of exercise curricula in schools and other community institutions,
- the development of a standard set of policies for the training and certification of exercise instructors,

- the use of monetary incentives (e.g., tax breaks) to encourage communities to make public facilities available for exercise,
- incentives to encourage employers to use more flexible work scheduling that would permit exercise during the workday, and
- the implementation of insurance-based incentives to encourage regular exercise among the public.

These strategies have received minimal systematic attention.

The major focus of current government efforts has been the development of a scientific data base with which to more effectively investigate health outcomes in the physical-activity field and the dissemination of physical-activity information to the public. Government agencies actively involved in these activities include the National Institutes of Health (NIH), CDC, the President's Council on Physical Fitness and Sports, and the Office of Disease Prevention and Health Promotion (ODPHP). Although some have argued that physical activity has traditionally taken a back seat to other health promotion areas when it comes to federal attention and resources, recent federal initiatives suggest that this may be changing. For instance, the NIH's National Heart, Lung, and Blood Institute recently convened a special workshop to outline the top scientific needs and research priorities in the physical-activity area. In addition, physical activity appears at the head of the list of health promotion priorities outlined in the recently released ODPHP document *Healthy People 2000* (U.S. Department of Health and Human Services, Public Health Service, 1991). Whether such activities will result in more resources being directed toward solving this country's inactivity problem remains to be seen.

Future Directions

The gaps in knowledge I have outlined underscore the challenges facing scientists and practitioners committed to increasing physical-activity levels in the United States. A note of urgency is added by trends suggesting that the scope of the problem is likely to continue increasing unless a variety of forces can be brought to bear on it.

In addition to the research directions I have suggested for each of the four levels of intervention described, I present the following list of areas that merit further consideration.

Multilevel Approaches to Physical-Activity Programming

Although each of the four major levels of intervention has been discussed separately, the strongest course of action will likely involve program development including all levels. In particular, methods for expanding the ongoing delivery of powerful personal strategies such as social support to other channels, settings, and levels of programming could have a substantial impact on population physical-activity levels.

As pointed out by those scientific groups undertaking comprehensive community-wide intervention in the area of heart disease prevention (Farquhar et al., 1990), there is likely to be substantial overlap across the four levels that would reinforce the health message. Given the current political, financial, and logistical constraints involved in executing a comprehensive, integrated program for physical activity in many parts of the country, however, smaller-scale alternatives that allow multilevel programming should continue to be sought. The work place and other such settings remain outstanding choices for such efforts (Blair, Piserchia, et al., 1986).

Interventions Targeting Physical Activity in Combination With Other Health Behaviors

Most research in this area has targeted physical activity alone. Yet an increasing amount of scientific evidence emphasizes the potential physiological and behavioral synergy that may accompany interventions that combine physical activity and other important health behaviors (Paffenbarger et al., 1986). Notable among such health behaviors are dietary change and smoking cessation. Current evidence suggests that such behaviors do not often change naturally as a consequence of increased levels of physical activity (King, Haskell, et al., 1991). Systematic intervention in these areas as a complement to the physical-activity program, however, may yield a number of benefits. For instance, a combined program of dietary change and regular exercise is more effective at facilitating weight loss than either strategy alone (Wood et al., 1988; Wood, Stefanick, Williams, & Haskell, 1991). In turn, successful weight loss may serve as an incentive for maintaining exercise adherence. Similarly, several studies have suggested that a well-run physical-activity program, coupled with formal smoking cessation instruction, may result in improved quit rates (Marcus, Albrecht, Niaura, Abrams, & P.D. Thompson, 1991). Regular exercise may also help moderate the weight changes that many smokers fear following smoking cessation and thus enhance mood and other psychological outcomes during and after quitting. Much remains to be learned, however, about implementing such multiple-risk-factor programs effectively.

Application of a Life-Span (Developmental) Approach to Intervention

In addition to continuing their research on the cognitive, behavioral, and social processes that accompany the stages of exercise initiation and long-term maintenance, researchers should broaden their perspective to include the effects of life stages and transitions. It is likely that the developmental transitions that affect other aspects of our lives (Felner, Farber, & Primavera, 1983; Winett et al., 1989) have a similarly important effect on physical-activity levels. Notable transitions or milestones include puberty, the transition from school to the work force, parenthood, retirement, and widowhood or caregiving situations (King, 1991). Although an understanding of the effects of such milestones on physical-activity patterns could greatly aid efforts to tailor interventions to population segments, the knowledge base related to such developmental transitions remains meager. To maximize the disease prevention effects of regular physical activity, it would be particularly useful to target those transitional periods that take place before the seventh decade of life, when chronic illness and diminished functioning often occur.

Some of the features associated with several important developmental milestones and their potential effects on physical-activity programming are shown in Table 7.4.

Continued Development of Measures to Assess Mild- to Moderate-Intensity Activities

Advances in physical-activity programming and adherence are predicated at least in part on our ability to accurately measure the behavior we are attempting to change. In light of the increasing emphasis on the value of mild and moderate as well as vigorous activity, new approaches to physical-activity assessment are required. It is imperative that more resources and effort be put into developing assessment tools that can measure lighter forms of activity in an accurate, reliable, convenient, and cost-effective manner.

It would also be worthwhile to expand both assessment and adherence efforts to include other aspects of physical conditioning, such as strength and flexibility, that are known to influence physical functioning and health (Bouchard, Shephard, Stephens, Sutton, & McPherson, 1990). Such areas are of special importance for aging adults (Buchner & de Lateur, 1991).

The body of research on physical-activity intervention provides a good foundation for future work on the personal intervention level and suggests strategies that may have implications for higher levels of intervention. The challenge is to broaden our focus beyond the traditionally applied clinical model to include public-health perspectives and concerns. Such a shift, coupled with research that is multidisciplinary in nature and design, is imperative if we are to achieve the population-wide increases in physical activity that are so clearly required. Only by making this shift will we be able to fully realize the potential of active lifestyles to improve our nation's health, physical and psychological functioning, and quality of life.

Table 7.4 Features and Examples of Physical-Activity Programs for Several Major Developmental Milestones

Milestone (critical period)	Specific features	Goals or strategies
Adolescence	Rapid physical and emotional changes Increased concern with appearance and weight Need for independence Short-term perspective Increased peer influence	Exercise as part of a program of healthy weight regulation (both sexes) Noncompetitive activities that are fun, varied Emphasis on independence, choice Focus on proximal outcomes (e.g., body image, stress management) Peer involvement, support
Initial work entry	Increased time and scheduling constraints Short-term perspective Employer demands	Choice of activities that are convenient, enjoyable Focus on proximal outcomes Involvement of work site (environmental prompts, incentives) Realistic goal-setting injury prevention Coeducational noncompetitive activities
Parenting	Increased family demands and time constraints Family-directed focus Postpartum effects on weight, mood	Emphasis on benefits to self and family (e.g., stress management, weight control, well-being) Activities appropriate with children (e.g., walking) Flexible, convenient, personalized regimen Inclusion of activities of daily living Neighborhood involvement, focus Family-based public monitoring, goal setting Availability of child-related services (child care)

(continued)

Table 7.4   (*continued*)

Milestone (critical period)	Specific features	Goals or strategies
Retirement age	Increased time availability and flexibility Long-term perspective on health, increased health concerns, "readiness" Caregiving duties, responsibilities (parents, spouse, children, grandchildren)	Identification of current and previous enjoyable activities Matching of activities to current health status Emphasis on mild- and moderate-intensity activities, including activities of daily living Use of "life path point" information and prompts Emphasis on activities engendering independence Garnering support of family members, peers Availability of necessary services (e.g., caretaking services for significant other)

Reprinted from King (1991).

References

Allen, L.D., & Iwata, B.A. (1984). Reinforcing exercise maintenance. *Behavior Modification*, **4**, 337-354.

Altman, D.G., Evans, A.J., Flora, J.A., Benjamin, L., Albright, C.L., King, A.C., Blaskovich, L.G., Schneider, M., & Fortmann, S.P. (1986). A worksite exercise content. In *Proceedings of the Society of Behavioral Medicine's Seventh Annual Scientific Sessions* (p. 38). Washington, DC: Society of Behavioral Medicine.

American Council on Exercise. (1991). *Personal trainer manual*. San Diego: Author.

Bandura, A. (1977). *Social learning theory*. Englewood Cliffs, NJ: Prentice Hall.

Bandura, A. (1986). *Social foundations of thought and action: A social cognitive theory*. Englewood Cliffs, NJ: Prentice Hall.

Belisle, M., Roskies, E., & Levesque, J-M. (1987). Improving adherence to physical activity. *Health Psychology*, **6**, 159-172.

Blair, S.N., Clark, D.G., Cureton, K.J., & Powell, K.E. (1989). Exercise and fitness in childhood: Implications for a lifetime of health. In C.V. Gisolfi & D.R. Lamb (Eds.), *Perspectives in exercise science and sports medicine: Vol. 2. Youth, exercise, and sport* (pp. 401-430). Indianapolis: Benchmark Press.

Blair, S.N., Piserchia, P.V., Wilbur, C.S., & Crowder, J.H. (1986). A public health intervention model for worksite health promotion: Impact on exercise and physical fitness in a health promotion plan after 24 months. *Journal of the American Medical Association, 255*, 921-926.

Blair, S.N., Smith, M., Collingwood, T.R., Reynolds, R., Prentice, M.C., & Sterling, C.L. (1986). Health promotion for educators: Impact on absenteeism. *Preventive Medicine, 15*, 166-175.

Blake, S.M., Jeffery, R.W., Finnegan, J.R., Crow, R.S., Pirie, P.L., Ringhofer, K.R., Fruetel, J.R., Caspersen, C.J., & Mittelmark, M.B. (1987). Process evaluation of a community-based physical activity campaign: The Minnesota Heart Health Program experience. *Health Education Research, 2*, 115-121.

Bouchard, C., Shephard, R.J., Stephens, T., Sutton, J.R., & McPherson, B.D. (Eds.) (1990). *Exercise, fitness, and health: A consensus of current knowledge.* Champaign, IL: Human Kinetics.

Brownell, K.D. (1988). Weight management and body composition. In S.N. Blair, P. Painter, R.R. Pate, L.K. Smith, & C.B. Taylor (Eds.) in collaboration with the American College of Sports Medicine, *Resource manual for guidelines for exercise testing and prescription* (pp. 355-361). Philadelphia: Lea & Febiger.

Brownell, K.D., Stunkard, A.J., & Albaum, J.M. (1980). Evaluation and modification of exercise patterns in the natural environment. *American Journal of Psychiatry, 137*, 1540-1545.

Buchner, D.M., & de Lateur, B.J. (1991). The importance of skeletal muscle strength to physical function in older adults. *Annals of Behavioral Medicine, 13*, 91-98.

Caspersen, C.J., Christenson, G.M., & Pollard, R.A. (1986). Status of the 1990 physical fitness and exercise objectives—evidence from NHIS 1985. *Public Health Reports, 101*, 587-592.

Coates, T.J., Jeffery, R.W., & Slinkard, L.A. (1981). Heart healthy eating and exercise: Introducing and maintaining changes in health behaviors. *American Journal of Public Health, 71*, 15-23.

Cohen, W.S. (1985, February). Health promotion in the workplace: A prescription for good health. *American Psychologist*, pp. 213-216.

Daltroy, L.H. (1985). Improving cardiac patient adherence to exercise regimens: A clinical trial of health education. *Journal of Cardiopulmonary Rehabilitation, 9*, 846-853.

David, M.F., & Iverson, D.C. (1984). An overview and analysis of the Health Style campaign. *Health Education Quarterly, 11*, 253-272.

DeBusk, R.F., Haskell, W.L., Miller, N.H., Berra, K., Taylor, C.B., Berger, W.E., III, & Lew, H. (1985). Medically directed at-home rehabilitation soon after clinically uncomplicated acute myocardial infarction: A new model for patient care. *American Journal of Cardiology, 55*, 251-257.

DeBusk, R.F., Stenestrand, U., Sheehan, M., & Haskell, W.L.. (1990). Training effects of long versus short bouts of exercise in healthy subjects. *American Journal of Cardiology, 65*, 1010-1013.

Dishman, R.K. (1991). Increasing and maintaining exercise and physical activity. *Behavior Therapy*, **22**, 345-378.

Dishman, R.K., & Ickes, W.D. (1981). Self-motivation and adherence to therapeutic exercise. *Journal of Behavioral Medicine*, **4**, 421-438.

Dubbert, P.M. (1992). Exercise applications and promotion in behavioral medicine. *Journal of Consulting and Clinical Psychology*, **60**, 613-618.

Ewart, C.K., Taylor, C.B., Reese, L.B., & DeBusk, R.F. (1983). Effects of early postmyocardial infarction exercise testing on self-perception and subsequent physical activity. *American Journal of Cardiology*, **51**, 1076-1080.

Farquhar, J.W., Fortmann, S.P., Flora, J.A., Taylor, C.B., Haskell, W.L., Williams, P.T., Maccoby, N., & Wood, P.D. (1990). The Stanford Five-City Project: Effects of community-wide education on cardiovascular disease risk factors. *Journal of the American Medical Association*, **264**, 359-365.

Felix, M.R.J., Stunkard, A.J., Cohen, R.Y., & Cooley, N.B. (1985). Health promotion at the worksite: A process for establishing programs. *Preventive Medicine*, **14**, 99-108.

Felner, R.D., Farber, S.S., & Primavera, J. (1983). Transitions and stressful life events: A model of primary prevention. In R.D. Felner (Ed.), *Preventive psychology: Theory, research, and practice*. Elmsford, NY: Pergamon Press.

Fraser, G.E., Schneider, L.E., Mattison, S., Kubo, C., LaClair, L., Johnson, K., Lee, G.G., & Caldwell, L. (1988). Behavioral interventions from an office setting in patients with cardiac disease. *Journal of Cardiopulmonary Rehabilitation*, **8**, 50-57.

Garcia, A.W., & King, A.C. (1991). Predicting long-term adherence to aerobic exercise: A comparison of two models. *Journal of Sport and Exercise Psychology*, **13**, 394-410.

Godin, G., Desharnais, R., Jobin, J., & Cook, J. (1987). The impact of physical fitness and health-age appraisal upon exercise intentions and behavior. *Journal of Behavioral Medicine*, **10**, 241-250.

Gossard, D., Haskell, W.L., Taylor, C.B., Mueller, J.K., Rogers, F., Chandler, M., Ahn, D.K., Miller, N.H., & DeBusk, R.F. (1986). Effects of low- and high-intensity home-based exercise training on functional capacity in healthy middle-aged men. *American Journal of Cardiology*, **57**, 446-449.

Haskell, W.L., King, A.C., & Evans, A.J. (1988, winter). Factors influencing physical activity in older adults. *CVD Epidemiology Newsletter*, p. 43.

Hatch, J.W., Cunningham, A.C., Woods, W.W., & Snipes, F.C. (1986). The Fitness Through Churches Project: Description of a community-based cardiovascular health promotion intervention. *Hygie*, **5**, 9-12.

Heath, G.W., Leonard, B.E., Wilson, R.H., Kendrick, J.S., & Powell, K.E. (1987). Community-based exercise intervention: Zuni diabetes project. *Diabetes Care*, **10**, 579-583.

Heinzelmann, F., & Bagley, R.W. (1970). Response to physical activity programs and their effects on health behavior. *Public Health Reports*, **85**, 905-911.

Houston-Miller, N. (1993). Home-based approaches to exercise training. In American College of Sports Medicine (Ed.), *Resource manual for guidelines for exercise testing and prescription* (2nd ed.) (pp. 350-355). Philadelphia: Lea & Febiger.

Hoyt, M.F., & Janis, I.L. (1975). Increasing adherence to a stressful decision via a motivational balance-sheet procedure: A field experiment. *Journal of Personality and Social Psychology*, **31**, 833-839.

Iverson, D.C., Fielding, M.E., Crow, R.S., & Christenson, G.M. (1985). The promotion of physical activity in the United States population: The status of programs in medical, worksite, community, and school settings. *Public Health Reports*, **100**, 212-224.

Juneau, M., Rogers, F., DeSantos, V., Yee, M., Evans, A., Bohn, A., Haskell, W.L., Taylor, C.B., & DeBusk, R.F. (1987). Effectiveness of self-monitored, home-based moderate-intensity exercise training in middle-aged men and women. *American Journal of Cardiology*, **60**, 66-70.

Kau, M.L., & Fischer, J. (1974). Self-modification of exercise behavior. *Journal of Behavior Therapy and Experimental Psychiatry*, **5**, 213-214.

Killen, J.D., Telch, M., Robinson, T., Maccoby, N., Taylor, C.B., & Farquhar, J.W. (1988). Cardiovascular risk reduction for tenth graders: A multiple factor school-based approach. *Journal of the American Medical Association*, **260**, 1728-1733.

King, A.C. (1991). Community intervention for promotion of physical activity and fitness. *Exercise and Sport Science Review*, **19**, 211-259.

King, A.C., Blair, S.N., Dishman, R.K., Dubbert, P.M., Marcus, B.H., Oldridge, N.B., Paffenbarger, R.S., Jr., Powell, K.E., & Yeager, K.K. (1992). Determinants of physical activity and interventions in adults. *Medicine and Science in Sports and Exercise*, **24**, S221-S236.

King, A.C., Carl, F., Birkel, L., & Haskell, W.L. (1988). Increasing exercise among blue-collar employees: The tailoring of worksite programs to meet specific needs. *Preventive Medicine*, **17**, 357-365.

King, A.C., & Frederiksen, L.W. (1984). Low-cost strategies for increasing exercise behavior. *Behavior Modification*, **8**, 3-21.

King, A.C., Frey-Hewitt, B., Dreon, D., & Wood, P. (1989). Diet versus exercise in weight maintenance: The effects of minimal intervention strategies on long term outcomes in men. *Archives of Internal Medicine*, **149**, 2741-2746.

King, A.C., Harris, R.B., & Haskell, W.L. (1988, winter). Clinical trial recruitment: Study- vs. subject-contact. *CVD Epidemiology Newsletter*, p. 38.

King, A.C., Haskell, W.L., Taylor, C.B., Kraemer, H.C., & DeBusk, R.F. (1991). Group- versus home-based exercise training in healthy older men and women: A community-based clinical trial. *Journal of the American Medical Association*, **266**, 1535-1542.

King, A.C., Taylor, C.B., & Haskell, W.L. (1991). Exercise adherence in the aging adult: Two-year results from a community-based clinical trial. *Medicine and Science in Sports and Exercise*, **23**(Suppl. 4), 520. (Abstract)

King, A.C., Taylor, C.B., Haskell, W.L., & DeBusk, R.F. (1988). Strategies for increasing early adherence to and long-term maintenance of home-based exercise training in healthy middle-aged men and women. *American Journal of Cardiology*, **61**, 628-632.

King, A.C., Taylor, C.B., Haskell, W.L., & DeBusk, R.F. (1990). Identifying strategies for increasing employee physical activity levels: Findings from the Stanford/Lockheed exercise survey. *Health Education Quarterly*, **17**, 269-285.

Knadler, G.F., & Rogers, T. (1987, October). Mountain climb month program: A low-cost exercise intervention program at a hig-rise worksite. *Fitness in Business*, pp. 64-67.

Knapp, D.N. (1988). Behavioral management techniques and exercise promotion. In R.K. Dishman (Ed.), *Exercise adherence: Its impact on public health* (pp. 203-236). Champaign, IL: Human Kinetics.

Lasater, T.M., Wells, B.L., Carleton, R.A., & Elder, J.P. (1986). The role of churches in disease prevention research studies. *Public Health Reports*, **101**, 125-131.

Lasco, R.A., Curry, R.H., Dickson, V.J., Powers, J., Menes, S., & Merritt, R.K. (1989). Participation rates, weight loss, and blood pressure changes among obese women in a nutrition–exercise program. *Public Health Reports*, **104**, 640-646.

Leon, A.S., Connett, J., Jacobs, D.R., Jr., & Rauramaa, R. (1987). Leisure-time physical activity levels and risk of coronary heart disease and death: The Multiple Risk Factor Intervention Trial. *Journal of the American Medical Association*, **258**, 2388-2394.

Maccoby, N., & Alexander, J. (1980). Use of media in lifestyle programs. In P.O. Davidson & S.M. Davidson (Eds.), *Behavioral medicine: Changing health lifestyles* (pp. 351-370). New York: Brunner/Mazel.

Marcus, B.H. (1991, August). Women and exercise: Enhancing adoption among lower income community participants. In B.H. Marcus & A.C. King (Chairs), *Women and exercise: Community and special populations*. Symposium conducted at the meeting of the American Psychological Association, San Francisco.

Marcus, B.H., Albrecht, A.E., Niaura, R.S., Abrams, D.B., & Thompson, P.D. (1991). Usefulness of physical exercise for maintaining smoking cessation in women. *American Journal of Cardiology*, **68**, 406-407.

Marcus, B.H., & Owen, N. (in press). Motivational readiness, self-efficacy and decision-making for exercise. *Journal of Applied Social Psychology*.

Martin, J.E., Dubbert, P.M., Katell, A.D., Thompson, J.K., Raczynski, J.R., Lake, M., Smith, P.O., Webster, J.S., Sikora, T., & Cohen, R.E. (1984). Behavioral control of exercise in sedentary adults: Studies 1 through 6. *Journal of Consulting and Clinical Psychology*, **52**, 795-811.

Mayer, J., & Geller, E.S. (1982). Motivating energy efficient travel: A community-based intervention for encouraging biking. *Journal of Environmental Systems*, **12**, 99-112.

Nader, P.R., Sallis, J.R., Patterson, T.L., Abramson, I.S., Rupp, J.W., Senn, K.L., Atkins, C.J., Roppe, B.E., Morris, J.A., & Wallace, J.P. (1989). A family approach to cardiovascular risk reductions: Results from the San Diego Family Health Project. *Health Education Quarterly*, **16**, 229-244.

Naditch, P. (1984). The Staywell Program. In J.D. Matarazzo, S.M. Weiss, J.A. Herd, N.E. Miller, & S.M. Weiss (Eds.), *Behavioral health: A handbook of health enhancement and disease prevention* (pp. 1071-1078). New York: Wiley.

Oldridge, N.B., & Jones, N.L. (1983). Improving patient compliance in cardiac rehabilitation. Effects of written agreement and self-monitoring. *Journal of Cardiopulmonary Rehabilitation*, **3**, 257-262.

Owen, N., Lee, C., Naccarella, L., & Haag, K. (1987). Exercise by mail: A mediated behavior-change program for aerobic exercise. *Journal of Sport Psychology*, **9**, 346-357.

Owen, N., Lee, C., & Sedgwick, A.W. (1987, June). Exercise maintenance: Developing self-management guidelines for community fitness courses. *The Australian Journal of Science and Medicine in Sport*, pp. 8-12.

Paffenbarger, R.S., Jr., Hyde, R.T., Wing, A.L., & Hsieh, C.C. (1986). Physical activity, all-cause mortality, and longevity of college alumni. *New England Journal of Medicine*, **314**, 605-613.

Parcel, G.S., Simons-Morton, B.G., O'Hara, N.M., Baranowski, T., Kolbe, L.J., & Bee, D.E. (1987). School promotion of healthful diet and exercise behavior: An integration of organizational change and social learning theory interventions. *Journal of School Health*, **57**, 150-156.

Pollock, M.L. (1988). Prescribing exercise for fitness and adherence. In R.K. Dishman (Ed.), *Exercise adherence: Its impact on public health* (pp. 259-277). Champaign, IL: Human Kinetics.

Prochaska, J.O., & DiClemente, C.C. (1986). The transtheoretical approach: Towards a systematic eclectic framework. In J.C. Norcross (Ed.), *Handbook of eclectic psychotherapy* (pp. 163-299). New York: Brunner/Mazel.

Reid, E.L., & Morgan, R.W. (1979). Exercise prescription: A clinical trial. *American Journal of Public Health*, **69**, 591-595.

Rich, T., & King, A.C. (1986). College dormitory-based interventions to prevent cardiovascular disease: Does a buddy help? *Society of Behavioral Medicine Proceedings* (p. 39). San Francisco (Abstract).

Rosen, M.A., Logsdon, D.N., & Demak, M. (1984). Prevention and health promotion in primary care: Baseline results on physicians from the INSURE Project on Lifecycle Preventive Health Services. *Preventive Medicine*, **13**, 535-548.

Sallis, J.F., Haskell, W.L., Fortmann, S.P., Vranizan, K.M., Taylor, C.B., & Solomon, D.S. (1986). Predictors of adoption and maintenance of physical activity in a community sample. *Preventive Medicine*, **15**, 331-341.

Sallis, J.F., Hill, R.D., Killen, J.D., Telch, M.J., Flora, J.A., Girard, J., Taylor, C.B., & Fortmann, S.P. (1986). Helping smokers quit on their own: A controlled evaluation of the Stanford Quit Kit. *American Journal of Preventive Medicine*, **2**, 342-344.

Sallis, J.F., Hovell, M.F., Hofstetter, C.R., Elder, J.P., Hackley, M., Caspersen, C.J., & Powell, K.E. (1990). Distance between homes and exercise facilities related to frequency of exercise among San Diego residents. *Public Health Reports*, **105**, 179-185.

Sallis, J.F., Hovell, M., Hofstetter, C.R., Faucher, P., Elder, J.P., Blanchard, J., Caspersen, C.J., Powell, K.E., & Christenson, G.M. (1989). A multivariate study of determinants of vigorous exercise in a community sample. *Preventive Medicine*, **18**, 20-34.

Sallis, J.F., Patterson, T.L., McKenzie, T.L., & Nader, P.R. (1988). Family variables and physical activity in preschool children. *Journal of Developmental and Behavioral Pediatrics*, **9**, 57-61.

Shephard, R.J. (1986). *Fitness and health in industry*. Basel, Switzerland: Karger.

Thomas, R.J., Miller, N.H., Taylor, C.B., Ghandour, G., Fisher, L., & DeBusk, R.F. (1991). Nurse-managed home-based exercise training after acute myocardial infarction: Methods and effects on functional capacity. *Circulation*, **84**(Suppl. 2), 540.

U.S. Department of Health and Human Services, Public Health Service. (1991). *Healthy people 2000: National health promotion and disease prevention objectives* (DHHS Publication No.[PHS] 91-50212). Washington, DC: U.S. Government Printing Office.

Walter, H.J. (1989). Primary prevention of chronic disease among children: The school-based "Know Your Body" intervention trials. *Health Education Quarterly*, **16**, 201-214.

Wankel, L.M., Yardley, J.K., & Graham, J. (1985). The effects of motivational interventions upon the exercise adherence of high and low self-motivated adults. *Canadian Journal of Applied Sport Science*, **10**, 147-155.

Wells, K.B., Ware, J., & Lewis, C. (1984). Physician practices in counseling patients about health habits. *Medical Care*, **22**, 240-246.

Winett, R.A., King, A.C., & Altman, D.G. (1989). *Health psychology and public health: An integrative approach*. Elmsford, NY: Pergamon Press.

Wood, P.D., Stefanick, M.L., Dreon, D.M., Frey-Hewitt, B., Garay, S.C., Williams, P.T., Superko, H.R., Fortmann, S.P., Albers, J.J., & Vranizan, K.M. (1988). Changes in plasma lipids and lipoproteins in overweight men during weight loss through dieting as compared with exercise. *New England Journal of Medicine*, **319**, 1173-1179.

Wood, P.D., Stefanick, M.L., Williams, P.T., & Haskell, W.L. (1991). The effects on plasma lipoproteins of a prudent weight-reducing diet, with or without exercise, in overweight men and women. *New England Journal of Medicine*, **325**, 461-466.

The current work was supported in part by U.S. Public Health Service grant AG-00440 from the National Institute on Aging, Bethesda, MD.

CHAPTER 8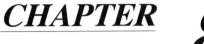

Health-Care Provider Counseling to Promote Physical Activity

Nola J. Pender
James F. Sallis
Barbara J. Long
Karen J. Calfas

> Increase to at least 50 percent the proportion of primary care providers who routinely assess and counsel their patients regarding the frequency, duration, type and intensity of each patient's physical activity practices. (From *Healthy People 2000*, U.S. Department of Health and Human Services, Public Health Service, 1991)

This health objective for the year 2000 indicates that the U.S. Public Health Service has judged primary health-care providers to be a significant resource for the promotion of regular physical activity in the American population. Primary-care providers have frequent and long-term personal contact with the public as well as a high degree of credibility. Thus, they have a unique opportunity to affect the lifestyle choices of their patients.

Promoting physical activity, a critical component of a healthy lifestyle, is a new focus for intervention in primary care. This chapter documents the rationale for primary-care interventions, presents an innovative and practical approach to physical-activity counseling, and focuses on the challenge of promoting physical activity among patients of all ages. Specific attention is given to health providers as role models of active lifestyles, determinants of physical-activity counseling, and future directions for research and counseling program design.

A major assumption underlying our collaboration as authors is that physical-activity counseling should be a team effort. At minimum the counseling team includes the physician and the nurse. Ideally, the team should also include a health educator, an exercise specialist, and a behavioral scientist with expertise in health-related behavior change. In the past much of the writing and research on preventive services has focused on physicians, so we seek to expand the discussion to include a larger team of health professionals.

The Promise of Physical-Activity Counseling by Health-Care Providers

The number of primary-care providers in the United States and their frequent contacts with patients underscore their potential impact on the physical-activity patterns of the population. According to the 1990 edition of *Physician Characteristics and Distribution in the U.S.* (Roback, Randolph, & Seidman, 1990) there are 240,420 active physicians in the primary-care specialities of family practice, general practice, internal medicine, pediatrics, and obstetrics-gynecology. This number represents 44% of the active physicians in the United States. Information from the National Health Interview Survey (National Center for Health Statistics [NCHS], 1990) shows that during 1989 nearly 80% of the population had contact with a physician. Approximately 63% of those contacts were with a primary-care physician (NCHS, 1990). In a 1978 Harris survey (Mutual Life Insurance Company, 1978) most respondents claimed they would be inclined to change their health habits if they were told to do so by a physician. This "white-coat" phenomenon is a result of physicians' being perceived as knowledgeable and trusted sources of health-care information.

Many patients also receive information and care from nurses during health-care encounters. According to 1990 data from the Division of Nursing, Bureau of Health Professions, 244,630 nurses work in primary-care settings. This represents approximately 15% of the number of active nurses in the United States. Of this group, 21,932 are nurse practitioners, and 3,375 are nurse midwives. Nurses employed in rural health centers and urban neighborhood clinics have the particularly challenging task of increasing health behaviors, including physical activity, among some of the nation's most vulnerable populations.

The combined number of physicians and nurses in primary care constitutes a force of almost half a million. Although the general public is frequently exposed to media messages on the benefits of healthy lifestyle choices such as stopping smoking, eating right, exercising regularly, and managing stress, people continue to look to health-care providers for knowledgeable guidance. Even a small increase in the frequency of effective health promotion messages by primary-care providers would affect millions of people and thereby have a substantial public-health impact.

Why Counsel About Physical Activity?

Though physical activity is a protective factor for a number of common diseases (Harris, Caspersen, DeFriese, & Estes, 1989), the greatest public-health benefit is likely to be gained from the prevention of cardiovascular disease (CVD). In their review of research, Powell, Thompson, Caspersen and Kendrick (1987) concluded that physical activity is inversely and causally related to the incidence of coronary heart disease, with a mean relative risk of 1.9. This is comparable with the relative risks for the other major risk factors for coronary heart disease. These relative risks are 2.1 for those with systolic blood pressure greater than 150 mmHg, 2.4 for men with cholesterol levels greater than 268 mg/dl, and 2.5 for those who smoke more than one pack per day. The prevalences of these risk factors within the general population are 10% hypertensive, 10% with elevated cholesterol, and 18% smokers. According to the 1988 Behavioral Risk Factor Surveillance Survey, the prevalence of physical inactivity is nearly 60% (Centers for Disease Control, 1990).

The relative risk of physical inactivity is comparable to the other major risk factors, but it is significantly more prevalent. Thus, the number of people at risk because of physical inactivity is higher than the number at risk for any other factor. This implies that promoting physical activity may be the single most effective method of lowering the risk of CVD in the population. In light of this information, health-care providers have underemphasized physical activity as a preventive measure. These recently published findings indicate that primary-care providers should work toward increasing their patients' regular physical activity.

The Provider as Role Model for Physical Activity

According to social-cognitive theory, most learning occurs through observation of others. Exposure to relevant models is thus one of the most powerful means of transmitting values, attitudes, and patterns of thought and behavior (Bandura, 1986). Role modeling an active lifestyle is an integral part of effective physical-activity counseling by health-care providers. Although only a few patients may observe their health-care providers engaging in exercise, patients are quick to recognize the extent to which providers value, enjoy, and participate in regular physical activity. The physical appearance of health-care providers also provides cues to the patient about whether health professionals advocating regular physical activity practice what they preach.

Wyshak, Lamb, Lawrence, and Curren (1980) conducted one of the earliest investigations of the health habits of physicians. Wyshak and her colleagues compared the health-promoting behaviors of 289 physicians and 316 lawyers practicing in the state of Massachusetts. Physicians were slightly less likely than lawyers to engage in vigorous physical activity such as jogging (31% versus

34%), calisthenics (24% versus 32%), and racquetball (24% versus 25%) but slightly more likely to bicycle (16% versus 14%). The health habits of 151 male physicians in California were surveyed by Wells, Lewis, Leake, and Ware (1984). An analysis of physical-fitness activity reported by the group revealed that only 27% spent more than 1 hr each week in vigorous exercise. Nonsurgeons reported being more physically active than surgeons and were also much more likely than surgeons to provide exercise counseling to their patients. In this study it appeared that physicians' physical-activity counseling patterns paralleled their own exercise habits. In client encounters, sedentary physicians were unlikely to address the health importance of regular physical exercise.

Holcomb and Mullen (1986) examined the personal health promotion and disease prevention behaviors of 250 randomly selected certified nurse midwives. Vigorous physical activity at least three times per week was reported by 48% of the respondents. Of those who reported exercising, 73% believed that exercise was very important to personal health. Only 25% of those who did not report exercising regularly held this belief. As a group the nurse midwives were less likely to ask patients about their level of physical activity than about smoking, weight, and alcohol intake.

Fasser, Mullen, and Holcomb (1988) examined the health beliefs and behaviors of 256 physician assistants (PA) practicing in Texas. Involvement in vigorous physical activity at least three times per week was reported by 58% of the sample. When PAs' history-taking practices were examined, however, information about exercise ranked 9th in frequency among 13 health promotion and disease prevention practices asked about. Approximately one third of the PAs reported having counseled some patients regarding regular exercise.

These studies have several limitations: All were retrospective rather than prospective, self-reports of health habits were not validated, and sample sizes were relatively small. The trend of the data in all of the studies indicates, however, that although the frequency of regular physical activity among health professionals is substantially higher than that of the general public, it could be increased. The data suggest that physically active providers are more likely to counsel patients regarding physical activity than providers with sedentary lifestyles.

Because the public looks to health professionals as role models of healthy lifestyles, intervention studies are needed that attempt to increase the extent to which health professionals engage in positive health habits, including regular exercise. The relationship between their exercise habits and the physical-activity counseling they give patients also needs further exploration.

Role modeling is a powerful educational approach. Health professionals who are active can better articulate the benefits of exercise, techniques for warming up and cooling down, ways of adapting exercise to personal needs, and injury prevention. Being in shape also adds to the health professional's attractiveness as a role model, increasing the patient's receptivity to education and counseling about physical activity. Programs that prepare health providers for physical-activity counseling are likely to be more effective if they initially focus on the exercise habits of health-care providers and various strategies for role modeling healthy lifestyles to patients.

Physical-Activity Counseling Practices of Health-Care Providers

Over the past decade researchers have attempted to describe health-care providers' knowledge, attitudes, beliefs, and clinical practices relevant to health promotion and prevention. Most of these studies are cross-sectional surveys of physicians. Survey limitations include small samples, self-report, and lack of information regarding how patients were assessed and what, if any, type of exercise prescription was provided. Investigations focused on physical-activity counseling practices have been hindered by a lack of operational definitions of counseling strategies and of reliable, valid measures of counseling behavior.

Wells, Ware, and Lewis (1984) conducted one of the earliest studies of physicians' practices in counseling patients about health habits. In a study of 151 male physicians in California, two dimensions of health counseling were explored: indications physicians used for routine counseling on health habits and the aggressiveness of counseling. Of physicians studied, 27% said they counseled all patients about exercise, 20% counseled only those who exhibited a cardiovascular or pulmonary disorder linked to inactivity, and 40% did not counsel patients about exercise. Physicians counseled less aggressively about exercise than about weight control and smoking. Only 13% of the physicians participating in the study spent more than 5 min during patient visits counseling about exercise. Given the complexity of maintaining regular physical activity, this is not enough time to assess activity patterns, provide an exercise prescription, counsel on relapse prevention, and answer any questions the patient may have.

Mullen and Tabak (1989) conducted a national study of the patterns of counseling and the techniques used by family practice physicians for smoking, weight, exercise, and stress. The sample of 903 physicians was predominantly male (90.8%). The data revealed that counseling about exercise occurred less frequently than counseling about cigarette smoking and weight control. The counseling techniques most frequently used for exercise and other health behaviors were

- suggesting specific steps to take,
- bringing up the subject again at a later visit, and
- referring patients to other office personnel for counseling.

Internal referral of patients by family practice physicians to nurses or nurse practitioners for physical-activity counseling appropriately uses important professional resources for patient education.

The majority of physicians surveyed believe that promotion of physical activity by the physician is important, but this attitude does not always translate into behavior. Depending on how counseling is defined, between 15% and 84% of primary-care physicians say they counsel their patients about physical activity. The quality of that counseling must be questioned, however, as few physicians spend more than 3 to 5 min in physical-activity counseling (Lewis, Clancy, Leake, & Schwartz, 1991; Wells, Lewis, et al., 1984).

Early studies of nurse practitioners showed that activities they frequently performed included teaching and counseling for health promotion and disease prevention in conjunction with disease management (Draye & Peznecker, 1980; Repicky, Mendenhall, & Neville, 1980; Wirth, Kahn, & Storm, 1977). Brown and Waybrant (1988) examined the health promotion counseling practices of nurse practitioners. Responses to a health promotion inventory by 110 nurse practitioners in primary-care settings were analyzed. When asked whether they had provided physical-activity counseling to at least one client on the previous day, 76.4% said they had. Physical-activity counseling was the third most frequently reported health promotion activity, surpassed in frequency only by screening activities and the provision of nutrition information. The content of physical-activity counseling and the strategies used were not ascertained. Sullivan (1982), in evaluating nurse practitioner research, concluded that the significant amount of health-oriented educational services nurse practitioners offered contributed to their successful patient encounters.

No studies of the efficacy of primary-care team approaches to physical-activity counseling were found in the literature. This area is ripe for innovation and further research. One empirical study has shown that primary-care providers can be effective counselors. The INSURE (Industrywide Network for Social, Urban and Rural Efforts) project (Logsdon, Lazaro, & Meir, 1989) found that the patients of physicians who received brief training in prevention counseling reported more physical activity than those of untrained physicians.

Reported Barriers to Physical-Activity Counseling

If health-care providers believe that physical-activity counseling is important, why do they not routinely provide it? Several studies cited such barriers as a lack of time, of reimbursement, of standard protocols, of perceived effectiveness as counselors, and of appropriate training.

Time Constraints

This appeared to be the most common barrier. Family and general practitioners average less than 15 min a patient visit (NCHS, 1990). Most of this time can easily be consumed by other tasks that are part of the traditional physician-patient encounter, such as history taking, physical exams, diagnosis, and record keeping. Such time pressures make it unlikely that primary-care physicians will spend more than a very few minutes counseling patients about physical activity. Time constraints that affect nurses and other providers need to be studied.

Lack of Reimbursement

This has been a major obstacle for primary-care providers (Johns, Hovell, Ganiats, Peddecord, & Agras, 1987; Orleans, George, Houpt, & Brodie, 1985; Rosen,

Logsdon, & Demak, 1984). Third-party payers reimburse for diagnostic tests, procedures, and hospitalization, but the activities of primary prevention, such as screening and counseling, are reimbursed inadequately if at all. Thus, time spent on prevention counseling reduces the time physicians can spend on income-generating activities. This situation may soon undergo a significant change, however, as the major providers of health insurance are beginning to recognize the economic advantages of preventive care. As appropriate reimbursement becomes available, physicians, nurses, and other health-care providers will become more involved in primary prevention.

Lack of Standard Protocols

This barrier to exercise counseling is frequently mentioned (Gemson & Elinson, 1986; Johns et al., 1987; Orleans et al., 1985). When standard protocols are available, as for hypertension control (National Heart, Lung, and Blood Institute, 1988b) and hyperlipidemia (National Heart, Lung, and Blood Institute, 1988a), health-care providers have adopted and effectively used them. Bostick, Luepker, Kofron, and Pirie (1991) surveyed the same group of 241 physicians in 1987 and 1989. Their study showed marked shifts toward consensus with the recommendations of the National Cholesterol Education Program (NCEP) over the 2-year interval between surveys. This finding was felt to reflect that the NCEP guidelines were introduced between surveys and that physicians were responsive to them. Such studies suggest physician behavior is positively affected through educational programs and standardized clinical protocols. Data are needed on the impact of standardized health promotion and prevention protocols on the clinical practice of other health professionals.

Lack of Perceived Effectiveness as Counselors

Physicians frequently rated their behavioral counseling skills as low, especially in areas in which their personal knowledge was low (Mann & Putnam, 1985; Schwartz et al., 1991; Valente, Sobal, Muncie, Levine, & Antlitz, 1982). Even when physicians feel competent to counsel, they have low expectations of patient behavioral change (Mann & Putnam, 1985; Orleans et al., 1985).

Of certified nurse midwives surveyed, 72% reported that assisting patients in modifying health habits was an important part of their professional role. Despite a high level of confidence in their counseling abilities, they were somewhat skeptical about their counseling's effectiveness in getting patients to change personal health habits (Holcomb & Mullen, 1986).

Even the most effective smoking cessation counselors, for example, fail more than half the time. Thus, feedback can be disappointing, especially when the counselor expects a high success rate. This suggests that training programs should teach providers not only to be more effective counselors but also to have more realistic expectations.

Lack of Appropriate Training

Physicians report that they have not received adequate training about exercise science or behavioral counseling either in medical school or postdoctoral programs (Rosen et al., 1984; Wells, Lewis, Leake, Schleiter, & Brook, 1986). Several studies have evaluated the incorporation of health promotion and disease prevention curricula into residency programs (Kelly, 1988; Patterson, Fried, & Nagle, 1989; Rich, Schlossberg, Luxenberg, & Korn, 1989). The results indicate that improvements in physician health counseling behaviors followed the interventions.

Ackerman, Partridge, and Kalmen (1981) reported the results of a national survey of health education and counseling content in 266 baccalaureate nursing curricula in the United States. They concluded that these curricula should be restructured to develop nurses' health counseling competencies. The National League for Nursing (1983), a national accrediting body for nursing schools, now requires that nursing curricula include preparation of students in health promotion. Thus, many schools of nursing have revised curricula to integrate health education and counseling for health promotion and disease prevention into their programs (Benson & Williams, 1988; Richardson & Petrarca, 1990). There is a need to assess nurses prepared at the baccalaureate and graduate levels to determine the extent to which current curricula prepare them with the skills needed to deliver health promotion and prevention services, including physical-activity counseling.

In the next section we describe an experimental program to facilitate the integration of physical-activity counseling into primary-care practice. Although the program focuses on primary-care physicians, it advocates a team approach in which all primary-health-care providers could participate.

PACE: An Approach to Physical-Activity Counseling

Project PACE (Physician-Based Assessment and Counseling for Exercise) was developed in response to one of the U.S. Department of Health and Human Service's year 2000 health objectives (1991) and in collaboration with the Centers for Disease Control. Its aim is to develop programs and materials primary-care physicians can use when counseling apparently healthy adults about the adoption and maintenance of regular physical activity, with an emphasis on moderate-intensity activities.

The PACE materials include

- a tool designed to assess patients' level of physical activity or stage of readiness to engage in activity, as well as their potential risk for cardiac events associated with physical activity,
- three brief structured counseling protocols designed to address relevant issues at each stage of readiness,
- a physicians' manual describing how to use these materials, and
- a training manual.

The stages of change theory developed by Prochaska and DiClemente (1983) is the basis for the PACE program's assessment and intervention. The stages of change theory suggests that people make behavioral changes in stages and that different interventions are appropriate at each stage. It has proved to be an effective approach for physicians working with patients who smoke (Ockene, 1987).

Assessment Rationale

The first task of the PACE assessment is to determine the patient's level of physical activity. This finding determines the provider's choice of one of the three PACE counseling protocols. The second task is to assess the patient's general level of risk for a cardiovascular event associated with physical activity. This finding classifies the patient by risk status as follows:

- OK for moderate or vigorous activity,
- OK for moderate activity only, or
- must be tested before increases in physical activity of any type can be recommended.

The PACE Assessment

The PACE activity assessment tool is an 11-item self-report questionnaire (see Figure 8.1). It classifies patients as inactive or irregularly active, active in moderate activity, or active in vigorous activity. It further classifies the patient as

- a precontemplator,
- a contemplator, or
- an active

Precontemplators may realize that change is indicated, but they are not willing to consider making a change in their health behavior (e.g., ''I've never exercised, and I have no desire to start now''). *Contemplators* are considering making a change in their activity level, but they may not have the skills to do so (e.g., ''I've been wanting to start an exercise program, but I just can't get motivated''). *Actives* are doing some form of regular physical activity (e.g., ''Yes, I exercise

PAR - Q & YOU

(A Questionnaire for People Aged 15 to 69)

Regular physical activity is fun and healthy, and increasingly more people are starting to become more active every day. Being more active is very safe for most people. However, some people should check with their doctor before they start becoming much more physically active.

If you are planning to become much more physically active than you are now, start by answering the seven questions in the box below. If you are between the ages of 15 and 69, the PAR-Q will tell you if you should check with your doctor before you start. If you are over 69 years of age, and you are not used to being very active, check with your doctor.

Common sense is your best guide when you answer these questions. Please read the questions carefully and answer each one honestly: check YES or NO.

YES NO

☐ ☐ 1. Has your doctor ever said that you have a heart condition and that you should only do physical activity recommended by a doctor?

☐ ☐ 2. Do you feel pain in your chest when you do physical activity?

☐ ☐ 3. In the past month, have you had chest pain when you were not doing physical activity?

☐ ☐ 4. Do you lose your balance because of dizziness or do you ever lose consciousness?

☐ ☐ 5. Do you have a bone or joint problem that could be made worse by a change in your physical activity?

☐ ☐ 6. Is your doctor currently prescribing drugs (for example, water pills) for your blood pressure or heart condition?

☐ ☐ 7. Do you know of any other reason why you should not do physical activity?

(continued)

Figure 8.1 PAR-Q questionnaire.
Reprinted from the Canadian Society for Exercise Physiology (1994).

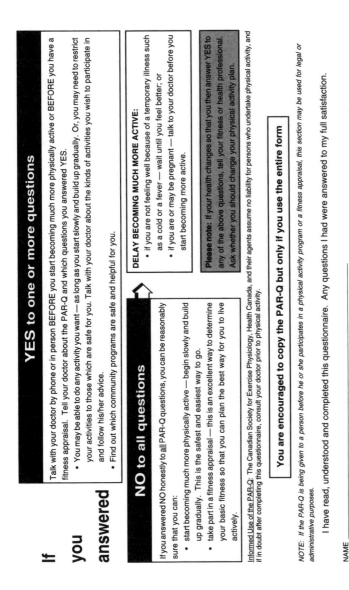

YES to one or more questions

Talk with your doctor by phone or in person BEFORE you start becoming much more physically active or BEFORE you have a fitness appraisal. Tell your doctor about the PAR-Q and which questions you answered YES.

- You may be able to do any activity you want — as long as you start slowly and build up gradually. Or, you may need to restrict your activities to those which are safe for you. Talk with your doctor about the kinds of activities you wish to participate in and follow his/her advice.
- Find out which community programs are safe and helpful for you.

If you answered

NO to all questions

If you answered NO honestly to all PAR-Q questions, you can be reasonably sure that you can:

- start becoming much more physically active — begin slowly and build up gradually. This is the safest and easiest way to go.
- take part in a fitness appraisal — this is an excellent way to determine your basic fitness so that you can plan the best way for you to live actively.

DELAY BECOMING MUCH MORE ACTIVE:

- if you are not feeling well because of a temporary illness such as a cold or a fever — wait until you feel better; or
- if you are or may be pregnant — talk to your doctor before you start becoming more active.

Please note: If your health changes so that you then answer YES to any of the above questions, tell your fitness or health professional. Ask whether you should change your physical activity plan.

Informed Use of the PAR-Q: The Canadian Society for Exercise Physiology, Health Canada, and their agents assume no liability for persons who undertake physical activity, and if in doubt after completing this questionnaire, consult your doctor prior to physical activity.

| You are encouraged to copy the PAR-Q but only if you use the entire form |

NOTE: If the PAR-Q is being given to a person before he or she participates in a physical activity program or a fitness appraisal, this section may be used for legal or administrative purposes.

I have read, understood and completed this questionnaire. Any questions I had were answered to my full satisfaction.

NAME _____

SIGNATURE _____   DATE _____

SIGNATURE OF PARENT _____   WITNESS _____
or GUARDIAN (for participants under the age of majority)

© Canadian Society for Exercise Physiology.   Supported by: Health   Santé
Société canadienne de physiologie de l'exercice   Canada   Canada

---

Figure 8.1   *(continued)*

a couple of times per week, and I really enjoy it''). Different counseling strategies are needed for each group, and they correspond to the three counseling protocols.

On the back of the assessment form is the Physical Activity Readiness–Questionnaire (PAR-Q) (Chisholm, Collis, Kulak, Davenport, & Gruber, 1975), a tool to assess the risk of a cardiac event during physical activity. The risk-assessment questionnaire asks about history of heart trouble, heart or chest pain, dizziness, blood pressure, musculoskeletal problems, other physical reasons why one should not follow an activity program, and whether the patient is over 35 years of age and unaccustomed to vigorous exercise.

The PACE assessment may be used in several ways. It is generally given to patients by a receptionist to complete while they wait for a medical appointment. It may also be mailed to patients with other questionnaires before the medical visit. The PACE assessment takes approximately 2 to 3 min to complete; the score ranges from 1 to 11. A score of 1 indicates the precontemplative stage, which fits approximately 10% of the general population. A score of 2 to 5 indicates the contemplative stage, which usually represents 50% of the general population. A score between 6 and 10 is desirable because moderate-intensity activity is considered desirable and is usual for 40% of the general population. A score of 11 indicates that the person exercises vigorously six or more times per week.

Following guidelines from the American College of Sports Medicine (1991), testers clear men under age 40 and women under age 50 with no more than two major risk factors (e.g., hypertension, hyperlipidemia, smoking, positive family history for cardiovascular disease, diabetes) for vigorous exercise. Those patients with more than two major risk factors or over the age criteria are restricted to moderate-intensity activity unless exercise stress testing is done. It is recommended that patients with disease or symptoms of cardiovascular disease receive further evaluation, including an exercise stress test.

The physician can look at the assessment form before entering the exam room and know which counseling protocol to use, based on the assessment score. Figure 8.2 shows how patients are moved through a PACE intervention.

Rationale for Counseling Protocols

It is assumed that merely telling people to become physically active is an insufficient intervention. The PACE counseling protocols are based on researchers' current knowledge about the determinants of physical activity (Dishman, 1988; Sallis & Hovell, 1990). Many of the determinants of physical activity can be modified, and the most powerful determinants were selected to be addressed in the counseling protocols. Recent evidence from a 2-year prospective study of physical-activity habits in a sample of community residents demonstrated that self-efficacy for exercise, social support for exercise, and perceived barriers were the strongest modifiable determinants of vigorous physical activity (Sallis, Hovell,

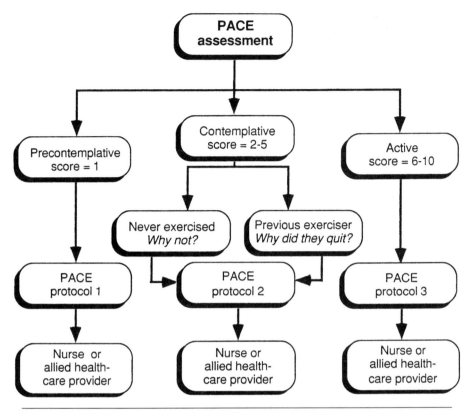

Figure 8.2   PACE assessment and counseling protocols.

Hofstetter, & Barrington, in press). These variables are systematically addressed in the PACE intervention.

Each protocol is designed to require 3 min or less during the health maintenance visit. Tailoring the content of the counseling to the stage of change ensures that counseling time is used wisely. Providers are encouraged to spend minimal time with precontemplators and actives and to concentrate on contemplators who are ready to change and may need more assistance.

How the PACE Protocols Are Used

Each protocol fits on a single piece of paper. The front includes questions relevant to activity for people at that stage of change. The back includes worksheets, information, and contracts of interest to patients at that stage of change. Protocols are printed with carbon copies so the provider has a copy for the chart. Counseling can be done by a physician, a nurse, or another member of the primary-care team.

Protocol 1

On the precontemplator's protocol, "Getting out of Your Chair," patients are asked to identify how they might benefit from activity and why they are not currently active. Providers are asked to give clear advice on ways physical activity would benefit the patient. Patients are asked to consider beginning a moderate physical-activity program and to state how they might benefit. The back of the protocol contains a summary of the benefits of physical activity and a worksheet that identifies potential barriers and suggests ways to get past them.

Protocol 2

On the contemplator protocol, "Planning the First Step," patients are asked to plan a realistic activity program. Such a plan includes the type of activity and specifies the times and days of the week they will do it, the duration and location of the activity, and who will support them. Patients also identify likely barriers to activity. Providers are asked to reinforce potential benefits to patients, advise them about what kind of activity is appropriate, emphasize the importance of obtaining social support, identify potential barriers, and schedule a follow-up appointment. After the plan is made, both patient and provider sign it as though it were a contract, indicating their commitment to carrying it out. On the back of the protocol are examples of moderate and vigorous activities. There are also a worksheet that asks patients to identify their two main benefits from regular physical activity, a roadblock worksheet, and an activity log.

Protocol 3

The final protocol is for actives and is called "Keeping the PACE." It is important to praise patients for their current activity and to review and make recommendations about their program. People in this stage, even long-term exercisers, are at risk for relapse to a sedentary lifestyle. The most important component of this protocol is relapse prevention. When inevitable interruptions in physical activity occur, patients are encouraged to not feel guilty but to restart activity right away. To avoid interruptions and relapses, patients are asked to anticipate barriers and develop solutions for surmounting them. The back of the protocol includes information about injury and tips for relapse prevention.

Who Can Implement the PACE Program?

The PACE program is designed to be used in a variety of settings by physicians, nurses, or allied health personnel. It is suggested that, no matter who provides most of the counseling, the physician verbalize support of physical activity because a direct recommendation made by a physician is an influential motivator (Gilmore, 1983; Mutual Life Insurance Company, 1978).

How Might the PACE Program Work in an Office Setting?

These materials can be used in several different ways. Because primary-care offices vary considerably in their organization, it is important that the program be flexible. In an office setting, a receptionist can give the assessment form to the patient to complete in the waiting room. The receptionist can scan the completed assessment form and put the appropriate protocol with the patient's chart for the physician to review. The physician then knows the patient's stage of change and can proceed with brief counseling. Another approach would be for the physician to recommend physical activity and to refer the patient to a nurse or exercise physiologist for counseling sessions.

The importance of follow-up cannot be overemphasized. We recommend a follow-up appointment after 1 month. Making a specific appointment for this purpose or asking about physical activity at subsequent appointments tells the patient that the issue is important. Follow-up appointments can be used to reevaluate the plan or solve problems.

The PACE program currently represents the state of the art in physical-activity counseling. In it, contemporary methods of behavior change are applied in a practical program designed to work within the constraints of primary-care practices. As with all intervention approaches, it is essential to document the effectiveness of both the protocols and the training program.

What Is Next? Possibilities for Physical-Activity Counseling

Although tremendous strides are already being made by primary-care providers in striving to achieve the physical-activity and fitness objectives of *Healthy People 2000: National Health Promotion and Disease Prevention Objectives* (1991), they must stretch further as a team to engage in visionary thinking about innovative uses of computer and telecommunications technology to enhance the effectiveness of their prevention and health promotion services. They should also consider the needs of special populations and how they might be creatively met. Some of these challenges are addressed in the following sections.

"High Tech" and Physical-Activity Assessment and Counseling

Emerging computer and telecommunications technologies offer unprecedented opportunities for innovation in counseling for, tracking, and assessing physical activity. The opportunity for patients to track their own physical activity is already present through a number of activity monitors the size of a calculator. Such monitors are relatively inexpensive ($40-$50) and comfortable to wear. Activity monitors that store computer-readable information about physical activity are also available. Monitors can be lent out and used periodically. This technology will empower patients by giving them more information about their level of physical activity during leisure and work. Patients will be able to bring their recording unit to the community clinic or physician's office for a computer readout, which will become part of their health record.

An increasing array of fitness assessment and exercise prescription software should be available in the near future to patients, enabling them to tailor an exercise program to their needs. Primary-care providers should develop this software in order to provide the public with high-quality products that optimize the benefits of physical activity and the chances of success in maintaining an exercise program while minimizing the hazards of injury.

In the future, primary care without walls will be a reality. Telecommunications technology will make it possible for primary-care providers to offer patients physical-activity counseling and exercise prescriptions in areas outside the office or clinic. Diagnostic parameters will be digitized for transmission over phone lines. Fiber-optic networks and satellite capabilities will enable live, interactive physical-activity counseling with patients in small rural clinics, community centers, or their homes. The exercise prescription—including illustrations of appropriate warm-up, cool-down, aerobic, and strength- and flexibility-building exercises—will be transmitted over telephone lines. National videoconferences on physical activity and fitness will be broadcast directly to patients, with opportunities for them to ask questions and receive immediate answers from health-care providers through interactive systems. Primary-care providers should be at the forefront of using "high tech" resources to improve health promotion and disease prevention services.

Populations With Special Needs for Exercise Counseling

Although the entire population of the United States is the target for interventions to increase physical activity, some groups merit special attention because of their developmental stage or the formidable barriers to exercise that they encounter. Adolescents and young adults, older adults, people with low incomes, and people with disabilities constitute such groups.

Adolescents and Young Adults

Adolescence and young adulthood are periods of marked decline in physical activity. Thus, they present a special challenge to health-care providers. In a survey of 362 college freshmen, Joffe, Radius, and Gall (1988) found that 58% reported having been admonished to exercise by health-care providers, but no data were available on how many followed the advice. In adolescence and young adulthood the educational demands of high school and college may decrease the time available for recreational activities. Parenting responsibilities in the young-adult years also minimize the time available for staying fit. Attention to maintenance of adequate physical activity during these developmental stages is critical to promoting good health and healthy aging.

Older Adults

Older adults also merit special attention for exercise counseling from primary-care providers because they seek health care at a high frequency. Remaining physically active can forestall the onset of disabilities and prevent the problems of disuse that are often confused with aging. The prevalence of a sedentary lifestyle increases with advancing age: 33% of people aged 45 to 64 report no leisure physical activity, and 43% of people over age 65 engage in no leisure physical activity (Caspersen, Christenson, & Pollard, 1986). There is increasing evidence for the positive physiological and psychological effects not only of vigorous but also of moderate activity, such as walking or gardening. Because of older adults' physical limitations, specially tailored exercise programs are essential. Such programs should provide exercises to increase strength and flexibility as well as aerobic capacity.

People With Low Incomes

People with low incomes also appear to exercise less than other segments of the population. Data from the 1985 National Health Interview Survey (National Center for Health Statistics, 1985) indicated that only 7% of low-income people age 18 and older engaged in vigorous exercise, and 32% reported that they did not engage in any leisure physical activity. Poor people's lack of resources, daily hassles, heavy work schedules, and family demands often restrict recreational sport and exercise options. In addition, their neighborhoods may not be safe for jogging or walking. Care must be taken to ensure that primary-care counseling for physical activity is not restricted to the affluent. Providers in public clinics, often nurses, need appropriate training and materials to support their physical-activity counseling.

People With Disabilities

Disabled people must often overcome considerable obstacles to maintain mobility and may expend considerable energy in carrying out the activities of daily living. This leaves little reserve for leisure physical activity. The stamina of people with disabilities is of special consideration, particularly early in the program, before energy reserves are improved. Assisting the patient in selecting feasible exercises that provide an early sense of accomplishment is important to ultimate success. Because disabilities vary widely and are often complex, primary-care providers may need to consult rehabilitation or exercise specialists to assist them in planning appropriate physical activity for the disabled. In 1985, 35% of people with disabilities reported no leisure physical activity (National Center for Health Statistics, 1985). The goal in *Healthy People 2000* is to decrease this figure to 20% (U.S. Department of Health and Human Services, Public Health Service, 1991).

Creating Facilitating Environments for Physical Activity

We are becoming increasingly aware of the importance of situational influences on the health behavior of people of all ages. Although primary-care providers are not environmental specialists, it is important for them to attend to the circumstances in which patients are asked to increase their physical activity. Patients' home environment or work setting may make it difficult for them to adhere to exercise programs despite their desire to do so (Ewart, 1991).

People are "social animals," and primary-care providers cannot ignore this fact in physical-activity counseling. A major consideration is the extent to which the patient's social network includes individuals who are physically active or encourage physical activity in others. This factor should be assessed by the primary-care provider. The patient may encounter resistance or ridicule in attempting to exercise if relatives and friends value a sedentary lifestyle and spending evenings with cronies at the local tavern or in front of the television. Possible sources of social support should be assessed. Would a spouse be supportive if included in the physical-activity counseling? Might an older child, a co-worker, or a friend join the patient in leisure physical activity? Could the patient join a community group of walkers or joggers? There are various ways of building supportive social environments for active lifestyles. The primary-care provider may be ineffective in counseling if these important aspects of the environment are not considered.

Primary-care providers should be aware of the range of physical-activity programs and facilities available in the community. This awareness includes having some knowledge about workplace exercise programs, school physical-education programs, YMCA and YWCA programs, and special community sports events. A periodically updated file that indexes such resources is valuable to the primary-care provider concerned with increasing the level of physical activity among patients of all ages. Primary-care providers should also be aware of the safety level of the environment in which patients live. High-crime environments may present formidable barriers to regular physical activity.

To be empowered to adopt a more active lifestyle, patients must have and be aware of options, have social support to exercise such options, and consider some of the options feasible. A health-strengthening environment, one in which healthy lifestyles can be enacted relatively unencumbered by social and physical barriers, is the goal of primary-care providers.

Directions for Future Research

Many research challenges are apparent from the gaps in knowledge that exist about

- patterns of physical-activity counseling by health-care providers,
- determinants of counseling behavior,
- strategies used in physical-activity counseling interactions, and
- the efficacy of counseling by primary-care providers.

The following questions need to be addressed through rigorous research:

- What is the content of physical-activity counseling by health-care providers?
- Do health-care providers have different physical-activity counseling styles?
- To what extent do health-care providers incorporate specific behavioral strategies into physical-activity counseling?
- Is physical-activity counseling by health-care providers developmentally appropriate?
- Is physical-activity counseling by health-care providers sensitive to the client's cultural background and socioeconomic status?
- What dimensions of health-care provider behavior in physical-activity counseling are most effective in helping patients initiate and maintain active lifestyles?

Physical-activity counseling is an important area of research and practice in primary care. The potential health impact of the wide adoption of active lifestyles by the American public is enormous (Hahn, Teutsch, Rothenberg, & Marks, 1990): Premature deaths from cardiovascular disease and other chronic diseases would significantly decline, disabilities caused by disuse would be reduced, and the population's energy level and vigor would be markedly enhanced. Primary-care providers can play a crucial role in developing and testing physical-activity counseling strategies, changing social norms about physical activity, creating environments that encourage active lifestyles, and helping patients gain the skills needed to remain optimally active throughout their lifespan.

References

Ackerman, A.M., Partridge, K.B., & Kalmen, H. (1981). Effective integration of health education into baccalaureate nursing curriculum. *Journal of Nursing Education*, **21**(1), 15-22.

American College of Sports Medicine. (1991). *Guidelines for exercise testing and prescription* (4th ed.). Philadelphia: Lea & Febiger.

Bandura, A. (1986). *Social foundations of thought and action: A social cognitive theory*. Englewood Cliffs, NJ: Prentice Hall.

Benson, A.M., & Williams, N.J. (1988). Wellness begins with the nursing student. *American Journal of Nursing*, **88**, 1711.

Bostick, R.M., Luepker, R.V., Kofron, P.M., & Pirie, P.L. (1991). Changes in physician practice for the prevention of cardiovascular disease. *Archives of Internal Medicine*, **151**, 478-484.

Brown, M.A., & Waybrant, K.M. (1988). Health promotion, education, counseling and coordination in primary health care nursing. *Public Health Nursing*, **5**, 16-23.

Canadian Society for Exercise Physiology. (1994). PAR-Q and YOU. Gloucester, ON: Author.

Caspersen, C.J., Christenson, G.M., & Pollard, R.A. (1986). Status of the 1990 physical fitness and exercise objectives—Evidence from NHIS-1985. *Public Health Reports*, **101**, 587-592.

Centers for Disease Control. (1990). Coronary heart disease attributable to sedentary lifestyle—Selected states. *Morbidity and Mortality Weekly Report*, **39**, 541-544.

Chisholm, D.M., Collis, M.L., Kulak, L.L., Davenport, W., & Gruber, N. (1975). Physical activity readiness. *British Columbia Medical Journal*, **17**, 375-378.

Dishman, R.K. (Ed.) (1988). *Exercise adherence: Its impact on public health*. Champaign, IL: Human Kinetics.

Division of Nursing, Bureau of Health Professions. (1990). [Survey data from state licensing and regulatory agencies]. Unpublished raw data.

Draye, M.A., & Peznecker, B. (1980). Teaching activities of family nurse practitioners. *Nurse Practitioner*, **5**, 28-33.

Ewart, C.K. (1991). Social action theory for a public health psychology. *American Psychologist*, **46**, 931-946.

Fasser, C.E., Mullen, P.D., & Holcomb, J.D. (1988). Health beliefs and behaviors of physicians' assistants in Texas: Implications for practice and education. *American Journal of Preventive Medicine*, **4**, 208-215.

Gemson, D.H., & Elinson, J. (1986). Prevention in primary care: Variability in physician practice patterns in New York City. *American Journal of Preventive Medicine*, **2**, 226-233.

Gilmore, A. (1983). Canada fitness survey finds fitness means health. *Canadian Medical Association Journal*, **129**, 181-183.

Hahn, R.A., Teutsch, S.M., Rothenberg, R.B., & Marks, J.S. (1990). Excess deaths from nine chronic diseases in the United States, 1986. *Journal of the American Medical Association*, **264**, 2654-2659.

Harris, S.S., Caspersen, C.J., DeFriese, G.H., & Estes, E.H. (1989). Physical activity counseling for healthy adults as a primary preventive intervention in the clinical setting. *Journal of the American Medical Association*, **261**, 3590-3598.

Holcomb, J.D., & Mullen, P.D. (1986). Certified nurse-midwives and health promotion and disease prevention: Results of a national survey. *Journal of Nurse-Midwifery*, **31**(3), 141-148.

Joffe, A., Radius, S., & Gall, M. (1988). Health counseling for adolescents: What they want, what they get, and who gives it. *Pediatrics*, **82**, 481-485.

Johns, M.B., Hovell, M.F., Ganiats, T., Peddecord, M., & Agras, W.S. (1987). Primary care and health promotion: A model for preventive medicine. *American Journal of Preventive Medicine*, **3**, 346-357.

Kelly, R.B. (1988). Controlled trial of a time-efficient method of health promotion. *American Journal of Preventive Medicine*, **4**, 200-207.

Lewis, C.E., Clancy, C., Leake, B., & Schwartz, J.S. (1991). The counseling practices of internists. *Annals of Internal Medicine*, **114**, 54-58.

Logsdon, D.C., Lazaro, C.M., & Meir, R.V. (1989). The feasibility of behavioral risk reduction in primary care. *American Journal of Preventive Medicine*, **5**, 249-256.

Mann, K.V., & Putnam, R.W. (1985). Physicians' perceptions of their role in cardiovascular risk reduction. *Preventive Medicine*, **18**, 45-58.

Mullen, P., & Tabak, G.R. (1989). Patterns of counseling techniques used by family practice physicians for smoking, weight, exercise and stress. *Medical Care*, **27**, 694-704.

Mutual Life Insurance Company. (1978). *Health maintenance: A nationwide survey of barriers toward better health and ways of overcoming them*. Newport Beach, CA: Pacific.

National Center for Health Statistics. (1985). *National health interview survey*. Hyattsville, MD: U.S. Department of Health and Human Services.

National Center for Health Statistics. (1990). *Health, United States, 1989* (DHHS Publication No. PHS 90-1232). Hyattsville, MD: U.S. Department of Health and Human Services.

National Heart, Lung, and Blood Institute. (1988a). *Report of the expert panel on detection, evaluation, and treatment of high blood cholesterol in adults* (DHHS Publication No. PHS 88-2925). Washington, DC: U.S. Department of Health and Human Services.

National Heart, Lung, and Blood Institute. (1988b). *The national report of the joint committee on detection, evaluation, and treatment of high blood pressure* (DHHS Publication No. PHS 88-1088). Washington, DC: U.S. Department of Health and Human Services.

National League for Nursing. (1983). *Criteria for the evaluation of baccalaureate and higher degree programs in nursing* (Publication No. 15-1251A). New York: Author.

Ockene, J.K. (1987). Physician-delivered interventions for smoking cessation: Strategies for increasing effectiveness. *Preventive Medicine*, **16**, 723-737.

Orleans, C.T., George, L.K., Houpt, J.L., & Brodie, K.H. (1985). Health promotion in primary care: A survey of U.S. family practitioners. *Preventive Medicine*, **14**, 636-647.

Patterson, J., Fried, R.A., & Nagle, J. (1989). Impact of a comprehensive health promotion curriculum on physician behavior and attitudes. *American Journal of Preventive Medicine*, **5**, 44-49.

Powell, K.E., Thompson, P.D., Caspersen, C.J., & Kendrick, J.S. (1987). Physical activity and the incidence of coronary heart disease. *Annual Review of Public Health*, **8**, 253-287.

Prochaska, J.O., & DiClemente, C.C. (1983). Stages and processes of self-change in smoking: Toward an integrative model of change. *Journal of Consulting and Clinical Psychology*, **51**, 390-395.

Repicky, P.A., Mendenhall, R.C., & Neville, R.E. (1980). Professional activities of nurse practitioners in adult ambulatory care settings. *Nurse Practitioner*, **5**(2), 27-34, 39-40.

Rich, E.C., Schlossberg, L., Luxenberg, M., & Korn, J. (1989). Influence of a preventive care educational intervention on physician knowledge, attitudes, beliefs, and practice. *Preventive Medicine*, **18**, 847-855.

Richardson, S.F., & Petrarca, D.V. (1990). Educating nurses in health promotion. *Journal of Nursing Education*, **29**, 351-354.

Roback, G., Randolph, L., & Seidman, B. (1990). *Physician characteristics and distribution in the U.S.* Chicago: American Medical Association.

Rosen, M.A., Logsdon, D.N., & Demak, M.M. (1984). Prevention and health promotion in primary care: Baseline results on physicians from the INSURE Project on lifecycle preventive health services. *Preventive Medicine*, **13**, 535-548.

Sallis, J.F., & Hovell, M.F. (1990). Determinants of exercise behavior. *Exercise and Sports Science Reviews*, **18**, 307-330.

Sallis, J.F., Hovell, M.F., Hofstetter, C.R., & Barrington, E. (in press). Explanation of vigorous physical activity during two years using social learning variables. *Social Science and Medicine*.

Schwartz, J.S., Lewis, C.E., Clancy, C., Kinosian, M.S., Radany, M.H., & Koplan, J.P. (1991). Internists' practices in health promotion and disease prevention: A survey. *Annals of Internal Medicine*, **114**, 46-53.

Sullivan, J.A. (1982). Research on nurse practitioners: Process behind outcome. *American Journal of Public Health*, **78**, 8.

U.S. Department of Health and Human Services. (1991). *Healthy people 2000: National health promotion and disease prevention objectives* (DHHS Publication No. [PHS] 91-50212). Washington, DC: U.S. Government Printing Office.

Valente, C.M., Sobal, J., Muncie, H.L., Levine, D.M., & Antlitz, A.M. (1982). Health promotion: Physicians' beliefs, attitudes, and practices. *American Journal of Preventive Medicine*, **2**, 82-88.

Wells, K.B., Lewis, C.E., Leake, B., Schleiter, M.K., & Brook, R.H. (1986). The practices of general and subspecialty internists in counseling about smoking and exercise. *American Journal of Public Health*, **76**, 1009-1013.

Wells, K.B., Lewis, C.E., Leake, B., & Ware, J.E. (1984). Do physicians preach what they practice? A study of physicians' health habits and counseling practices. *Journal of the American Medical Association*, **252**, 2846-2848.

Wells, K.B., Ware, J.E., & Lewis, C.E. (1984). Physicians' practices in counseling patients about health habits. *Medical Care*, **22**, 240-246.

Wirth, P., Kahn, L., & Storm, E. (1977). An analysis of 50 graduates of the Washington University PNP program. Part 3: Perceptions and expectations of their role in the health care system. *Nurse Practitioner*, **2**(8), 16-18.

Wyshak, G., Lamb, G.A., Lawrence, R.S., & Curran, W.J. (1980). A profile of the health-promoting behaviors of physicians and lawyers. *New England Journal of Medicine*, **303**, 104-107.

Kevin M. Patrick, MD, is the principal investigator of Project PACE and has contributed in many ways to this chapter. Greg Health, PhD, MPH, and Kimberly Yeager, MD, MPH, are colleagues at the Centers for Disease Control, and their assistance and guidance is appreciated.

CHAPTER *9*

Technological Supports for Sustaining Exercise

Guy Dirkin

Existing and emerging technologies can provide both new methods of supporting exercise and activity adherence at all fitness levels and more convenient methods of applying proven strategies. Technology may play a public-health role by helping increase the involvement of previously inactive individuals in moderate activity. It is my hope that the technologies outlined will provoke among readers speculation about both additional applications and the research validation of outcomes driven by technology.

The literature indicates that adherence to exercise can be facilitated through a variety of interventions (Dishman, 1991; King, 1991). One representative configuration of these interventions is the combined action of discrete, immediate, and frequent feedback with goal-setting, either in a context of social support or in the form of targeted communications designed to support sustained adherence.

The success of these strategies, even in elite performance environments, has been modest. In the public-health arena, the attempt to apply such techniques to health risk reduction has made still less impact. Two trends, coupled with increasingly sophisticated technologies, may be able to improve the effectiveness of these strategies.

The first trend is the acknowledgment of the existence of an activity continuum that ranges from almost complete inactivity to elite performance. Work by Blair and colleagues (see chapter 1) indicates that significant health benefits result from moderate levels of activity. Consequently, goals appropriate for elite performers on the continuum may not be applicable to the general population or even appropriate to meeting the public-health objective of overall risk reduction. Even with activity threshold guidelines reduced to a moderate level, the challenge remains of increasing lifestyle activity to achieve that level.

The second trend is an acknowledgment that positive internal feedback, although rewarding to many exercise participants, is not experienced equally (Dishman, 1993). The intrinsic rewards of exercise may not be sufficient to motivate people closer to the inactive end of the continuum. Many people prefer to combine exercise with other activities, such as reading while riding an exercise bicycle. At the moderate-activity area of the continuum, the need to increase the interest level and rewards associated with the overall exercise environment, outside of endogenous feedback, is evident.

Successfully employing technology to support exercise and activity adherence at all points along the activity continuum requires embracing new ways of fulfilling familiar functions. In goal-setting, technology, rather than a live counselor, can help participants develop appropriate personal goals through nonjudgmental probing and analysis. Technology can also provide discrete, frequent, and immediate feedback wherever and whenever participants require it. Critical information is no longer bound by site- and time-specificity. The system conforms to the needs of the participant. Technology can likewise support self-monitoring, a fundamental behavioral-change strategy, for those who find the process burdensome and a potential barrier to continued participation.

The technologies and applications I present in this chapter were evaluated using three criteria: cost, effectiveness, and access. At the high-activity end, technology must produce measurable results in people who are already highly fit; that is, it must be very effective. Cost (very likely high) may not be an issue and access will therefore be limited. At the low-activity end of the continuum, access will broaden as cost falls. Clearly, the greatest social utility will be served by developing technologies to support adherence that offer high access and effectiveness at a low cost per capita. The per capita qualification should be kept in mind when we examine the ability of expensive technologies to cost-effectively support large numbers of users.

How might existing and emerging technologies best serve the needs of individuals at all points along the activity continuum? The examples I give represent potential landmarks, not permanent boundaries. As such, they are sketched rather than exhaustively detailed. Although most of the core technologies—personal computers, Touch Tone telephones—are familiar, the key question is whether the applications described (or additional applications that occur to the reader) could successfully support the exercise adherence efforts of people who are not participating in the traditional paradigm.

All of the services outlined in this chapter could be targeted to reach participants at home, at work, or both places. The advantage of providing such services through the workplace is that doing so reduces the capital and labor overhead of a wellness or on-site fitness program. With data collection and analysis carried out remotely employers can, in effect, lease a wellness program without having to own all the necessary components or pay for the intensive labor.

Operational and configurative details aside, the behavioral function of the technology is to support goal-setting, offer precise and instantaneous feedback, and supply timely cues to assist in sustaining attention. Technology provides another means to achieve proficiency in the self-regulation and self-monitoring of cues critical to adherence and compliance: cues that the literature suggests steadily decline over time in the absence of external reinforcement.

Within the framework of this chapter, the function of technology is to address the issues raised in chapter 8. Can technology provide a means of overcoming the barriers that physicians cite as obstacles in counseling patients on physical activity? Such barriers include time and a lack of reimbursement, of standard protocols, of self-perceived effectiveness as counselors, and of appropriate training on the part of physicians in the area of activity counseling.

As I have suggested, the true cost of more complex technologies must be balanced with their ability to bypass such barriers. If, for example, the initial investment in a sophisticated computer-based health risk assessment system for a physician's office or work site appears high, its cost must be weighed against both what is currently offered (or not offered) and the long-term benefit of providing support. The value of gathering, analyzing, and disseminating data to individuals in previously unreached groups—opening as it does the possibility of creating large, albeit self-reported, databases—must also be considered.

As Prochaska and Marcus point out in chapter 6, the outcomes of computer-based counseling are very positive—better, in fact, than those involving human counselors. Although the topic is beyond the scope of this chapter, the unique character of the relationship between individuals and nonjudgmental support systems may provide the most fertile ground for developing successful adherence strategies.

This chapter examines technologies and applications in order of diminishing complexity of the end-user interface. Computers seem more complex to use than phones, phones seem slightly more complex than televisions, and printed materials seem quite simple. This structure also mirrors the level of investment required for the ownership of specific technologies. On average, computers cost the most, and printed materials cost the least. The combination of barriers to access represented by complexity and cost appear to suggest that computers would offer the fewest opportunities for providing support, whereas printed materials would provide the most. It becomes evident that all of the technologies incorporate strategies to overcome these barriers and provide cost-effective access and support to a broad range of participants: groups that, because of lifestyle, location, income, or health factors (too busy, too remote, too poor, too ill) are not being reached by more traditional means (King et al., 1992). Charting the effectiveness of the technologies is a task for future researchers (see chapter 10).

This chapter looks at the potential of personal computers, phones and phone-based systems (fax machines, beepers), television and television-based systems (video-on-demand, electronic games), and print communications and also offers a brief case study of a transferred technology—that is, a readily available and inexpensive technology—used in a community-based mall-walking program. Finally, I examine the implications, both practical and research-related, of evaluating the role of technology in enhancing exercise adherence.

Personal Computers

Although *personal computer* (PC) has come to mean any free-standing or networkable programmable data-processing device, it is defined here to include any device that collects personal data and produces output through computation. This definition thus includes such devices as heart-rate monitors, pedometers, and even timepieces built into medication vial caps that keep track of the last time the vial was opened. Although this last example might seem trivial, the increase in compliance such a simple device provides is significant (McKenney, Munroe, & Wright, 1992).

The combination of an unobtrusive data-collection device—such as a heart-rate monitor built into a wristwatch—and a basic data-processing system (a PC) could provide individuals with valuable information on their physical response to increased activity. Such a combination of elements could operate in a number of ways. Data could be collected through sensors on a wristband device and downloaded to a PC for comparison with the results of previous weeks. This PC could be owned by the participant, a community-based organization, the participant's employer, or a remote organization that the participant or workplace-based program reaches by modem. Existing systems, such as point of sale (POS) terminals in retail stores, could be used for data collection and processing. Data sent to a POS terminal would simply be downloaded with sales information in the course of daily operations. The use of existing wide area networks (WANs) opens the possibility for both national and cross-cultural data collection. The ability to easily and quickly transmit data renders nearly moot the question of where the processing will occur. Relieving individuals of the need to invest in a PC in order to participate considerably broadens the application of fitness-analysis software.

Linking exercise equipment directly to a PC, via cable or modem, can provide individuals with both immediate discrete feedback and cumulative analysis. In effect, the equipment becomes an input device. The PC then supports individuals by contributing to their self-competence in evaluating, prescribing, and planning an exercise program. The feedback contributes to motivation, thus increasing compliance.

On-line PC services already provide a continuous and ever-changing array of health and medical tips. The growing world network among computer users (directly analogous to the world community of ham radio operators), coupled with the rapid development of digital audio-processing capabilities, has already led to the creation of network-based, audio-only daily programming—in effect, a radio show aimed exclusively at computer network users. This method of information distribution, applied to the health-care and fitness community, opens the possibility of providing a growing database of answers to fitness and nutrition questions. Such a database could be accessed interactively by individuals using PCs or Touch Tone telephones. (The lines dividing areas of technology, already blurring, make describing discrete applications somewhat arbitrary. As an example, the PC industry's inability to successfully penetrate the home market is driving the development of "smart," or screen, phones, equipped with both monitors and keyboards. If bundled with a fax machine, the resulting device is almost indistinguishable from a combination PC, modem, and printer.)

The combination of a data-gathering device and touch tone telephone linked to a remote data processor can provide sophisticated analysis without requiring either substantial investment or impractical time demands of participants. Data gathered and analyzed in this fashion can be mailed or faxed directly to participants, to their workplace, or to community centers.

Data-gathering systems will likely grow smaller, cheaper, and more sophisticated, providing immediate feedback without requiring users to download or transmit data for analysis. Combining data gathering and entry with analysis, these devices could share data with health-care professionals to aid them in counseling individuals. For example, a heart-rate monitor could contain its own analysis and storage system. Users would be able to chart progress, receive immediate feedback, and download data to interested professionals.

More complex programs and systems, capable of conducting such tasks as health risk assessments, are and will be available through physicians' offices, community centers, and workplace wellness programs, as well as in commercial and retail settings, directing users toward everything from pharmaceuticals to fitness and wellness products. (As with all technology, there are issues of responsibility on the part of the supplier and trust on the part of the user. User suspicion that the system is "fixed" to produce results that favor the supplier of products would seriously compromise meaningful use.) Such systems could collect data and generate immediate feedback while establishing an ongoing record. The systems could use a variety of input systems to gather participant histories. A digitized or synthesized voice could walk a participant through the program, and visual cues on a touch screen could highlight choices for response. A low level of literacy need not be a barrier to access. Input could also be accepted through a traditional keyboard or a pen-based interface.

The flexibility of such systems should permit them to respond to participants at any stage of change—precontemplation, contemplation, preparation, action, maintenance, or termination (see chapter 6). The PACE assessment tool detailed in chapter 8 could be offered electronically, allowing participants to create a record while responding to the questions.

The multimedia and compact disc read-only memory (CD-ROM) capabilities of PCs provide users direct access to a broad range of health, fitness, nutrition, and medical information. Multimedia programming enables the user to explore information in a variety of forms: still and moving images as well as audio and text. CD-ROM provides a randomly accessible storage medium capable of holding the huge quantities of data required to drive multimedia applications. The combination of sound and motion offers the possibility of presenting, much in the manner of videotape, not only a follow-along in-home workout but also of adjusting it to meet the participant's growing competence and fitness. CD-ROM could provide a full range of progressively more intense workouts, precisely modulating each day's recommended program for increases in frequency, duration, and intensity. The ability to incorporate progress management may, by removing exercisers' perception of being stagnant, prove vital in sustaining long-term interest and adherence.

In the more distant future, there is the possibility of bringing current sophisticated performance analysis tools, such as motion evaluation, to the home, workplace, physician's office, or community center to assist individuals in clearly seeing and refining their physical activity. This technology could help temporarily or permanently disabled individuals develop workable physical coping strategies. Access to very precise information and expert system counseling could serve as a cost-effective middle ground for needs that exceed the competencies of a primary-care physician but may not require the services of a specialist.

Audio-only information could be programmed either randomly or deliberately into forms such as audiotapes or compact discs that could be used in tandem with physical activities such as walking, biking, and so on. The content of this information could range from counseling and coaching to modifying exercise intensity.

The "community" of the computer network also provides the opportunity for developing a new kind of a fitness club whose members might never meet face-to-face but could compare individual performance with the average performance of the group and offer one another support and encouragement.

One highly interactive and appealing area of computing is the video game. At present, the video game appears to enhance hand-eye coordination among the young as it contributes to their overall lack of fitness. Rather than ask avid game players to put down the control pad and go outside, technology can incorporate the game's high level of visual interactivity with exercise equipment, making activity an essential part of the game and, in effect, placing the player inside it. Virtual reality could bring the outdoors indoors by combining a video helmet and earphones with a piece of exercise equipment and thus transforming a treadmill, for example, into any environment one could walk or run through. By the same token, a stair-climbing, skiing, or rowing machine could take a user "virtually" anywhere, thus capitalizing on exercise-driven sensation seeking. Although these applications are tied to specific pieces of equipment, there is also the possibility of recreating "virtually" any sport that requires a partner, such as tennis, racquetball, or Ping-Pong. There are interesting ramifications in the potential for the video arcade to become an exercise environment.

The opportunity offered by the personal computer—which I have defined as a device as simple as an alarm clock built into a pill bottle (to gather data and provide feedback) to one as sophisticated as a fully interactive virtual-reality generator (to gather data and provide feedback on a considerably grander scale)— is its ability to adjust to the needs of the participant while providing structure for time management and readily analyzable data for use by both the participant and interested professionals. The ability of these systems to assemble a database for analysis from both a personal and a public-health perspective could simultaneously provide the opportunity to offer feedback in the form of incentives. Conceptually, there is no difference between tracking individual physical activity and tracking individual consumption of such services as airline travel or rental of hotel rooms or automobiles. The same mechanism that generates incentives for frequent users could be used to create incentives for frequent exercisers. As a later example will demonstrate, incentives that are not directly linked to physical activity may enhance adherence.

Phones and Phone-Based Systems

As I have mentioned, the Touch Tone telephone can be used as an input device for data that can be analyzed by a local or remote processor. From a public-health perspective, the value of the phone as a link to a variety of sophisticated analysis, support, and information resources lies in its near-universal penetration of all population groups. Even the homeless have access to public phones and, in pilot programs, have been able to access voice-mail systems for information on job openings. Just as the pill bottle alarm system can significantly increase compliance by reminding individuals of the last time they took their medication, a phone call can remind participants of previously agreed-upon activity goals. This approach can use automatic dialing and a digitized voice to reinforce messages and ideas discussed in a one-to-one counseling session with a physician, a nurse, a trainer, or another professional advisor. Though the same effect can be achieved with live operators, automation has proven more cost-effective.

A variation of this approach could use beepers. Key words from a counseling session can be transmitted at critical times throughout the day and thus reinforce an individual's goals. The meaning attached to the key word, as previously agreed upon by the client and counselor, can be a powerful behavioral trigger. Again, the cost is reasonable and the access is virtually universal.

Participants could also use Touch Tone telephones to transmit numeric data—possibly collected from a heart-rate monitor and entered manually on the phone—that, after analysis, could trigger the sending of specific messages to the participant. As the screen phone I have described becomes more common, it could be used to display information currently limited to PCs and televisions. A further step would cut the wires altogether by combining cellular phones with hand-held PCs, enabling individuals to input and receive information almost everywhere.

Exercise management's entry into the home through the use of phones will require the same type of paradigm shift on the part of potential users and suppliers that made remote banking through the automated teller machine (ATM) possible. Once consumers and banks were comfortable with the system, it rapidly became indispensable and ubiquitous. There is even the possibility of using a magnetically striped card-reader system like that used in ATMs to provide more immediate access to personal information or information about specific exercises. The system would recognize the user and begin the transaction—for example, providing a participant with a modified daily activity plan and an update on progress to date. A voice-mail option could enable participants to record questions that require more complex or qualitative responses. Counselors could leave answers in a participant's voice-mailbox for the following day. Such an application would allow counselors and clients to sustain a relationship that does not require them to be available to each other simultaneously.

The same approach could be applied to transmission of information over phone lines to fax machines, local area networks (LANs), and wide area networks (WANs). A daily or weekly activity plan could be generated, along with a daily or weekly meal plan or other health or disease management information. Analyses of changes in a participant's condition could also be charted and transmitted through the fax machine, LAN, or WAN to multiple recipients, including the client, the client's counselor, and the physician or trainer. Information supplied over the phone and fax could be provided in a variety of languages in order to make the service available to as many participants as possible.

These systems could be accessed by participants who are traveling and thus could help sustain adherence by providing a sense of continuity. In addition to meeting participants' needs, this approach has implications for health-care delivery and cost containment because it enables the system to hold participants more accountable. As I have mentioned, such close tracking could also provide data that could drive an incentive program to enhance compliance.

Telephone 900 numbers could offer low-cost access to high-level expertise. The 900-number system is gaining popularity as a means of providing information on a subscription basis—for example, to software users seeking technical assistance directly from a company. Such an approach could put exercising individuals in touch with live counselors who could answer their questions or help them overcome barriers to progress.

Special conference-call events—available through the same mechanism as pay-per-view television events and providing the same caliber of information as television-based postgraduate classes—could allow thousands of participants to listen in and possibly ask questions of sports figures, trainers, coaches, and exercise physiologists. Once the conference-call event has taken place, it could be made available at a reduced cost on a recorded basis over the phone, through the previously mentioned digitized computer "radio" network, as an audiocassette, or in transcript form.

Television and Television-Based Systems

The mechanisms for enabling participants to order specific programs through their cable system (pay per view) are already in place. As the system grows more sophisticated, it offers the opportunity to provide a wider range of material, making the television set capable of the type of access now available through the PC and soon to be available through the phone. This type of access (video-on-demand) transforms the television set into the equivalent of a computer monitor capable of displaying everything from sound-annotated text to full-color motion. The same possibilities discussed in the PC multimedia and CD-ROM section can be realized without the participant's having to purchase a PC. Rather than download data onto a hard drive, the user could capture data through a VCR.

The data-gathering systems I have described could output specific personal information through a television, allowing it to display an individual's progress as well as information appropriate to the individual based on that progress. Heart rates could be tied to levels of exercise and suggestions for different activities offered. Classes requested through the system would be tracked by the system. Attendance would, in effect, be taken each time a program was ordered. It would eventually be possible to draw correlations between the types of programs accessed and personal fitness data being input to determine levels of effectiveness and possibly compliance.

The technology that makes national call-in talk or shopping television programs possible could also be applied to more specific fitness messages. This is, in effect, the illustrated version of the conference call and 900-number possibilities I have raised.

Virtual-reality software could be used to link a television with a piece of exercise equipment to provide a more interactive experience, thus connecting activity to leisure. Until now, a dichotomy has existed between exercise performed for its own sake—as well as for the perceived benefits of increased attractiveness and decreased ill health—and exercise done because it fulfills the need to play. Virtual reality, by responding to the participant's actions, offers the potential to create an environment highly conducive to physical conditioning. The emerging technologies pose many interesting research opportunities, among them the chance to compare adherence sustained through feedback from the activity itself (the more traditional intrinsic reward approach) with that sustained by feedback from the virtual-reality environment (the technological approach).

Print Communications

Marketing companies can now individualize printed material with up to several hundred variables. Full use of such data has until recently been constrained by the inability of press technology to respond on a level much above that of a personalized letter (see chapter 7). The development of highly sophisticated, cost-effective programmable press technologies now makes possible the creation of truly special-interest publications—that is, those of interest to a single individual. Such publications could provide personalized cues, in the same vein as those sent by beeper, in a lasting glossy four-color form. Individualized information could be combined with general articles to yield a magazine responsive to the needs and progress of a single reader—literally, an interactive magazine.

The same data the participant finds in the magazine can be provided to interested professionals in a more concise form on paper, on diskette, or through a modem or fax. The opportunity to track the effects on adherence of such a publication opens a range of research possibilities, as does the linking of virtual reality and exercise. What is the difference between seeing something and hearing it? What are the effects of becoming a single-issue celebrity? What is the optimal reinforcement rate—weekly, monthly, bimonthly? What individual differences exist?

Transferred Technology

Technology can also be transferred from other areas and used in the service of exercise adherence. A mall-walking program in a large Midwestern city uses a time clock activated by magnetically striped cards—originally designed for use by security guards on their rounds—to track the activity levels of program members. Nonexercise-related incentives, such as discounts on merchandise purchased at the mall, are offered based on hours walked. The time clock eliminates the need for participants to write down their times or for program support staff to add up the hours. The resulting program offers both convenience and the beginnings of quantitative rigor. Concerns about the validation of the activity engaged in (i.e., time spent in the mall versus time engaged in exercise), could be answered with the incorporation of a device as simple as a heart-rate monitor.

Issues

Outcome validations of the technologies outlined in this chapter will require a well constructed multivariate approach, particularly where interactive effects are of interest. A key methodological issue, tied to validation, is whether the accuracy of self-reported data, gathered through the systems described, is sufficient to justify confidence in the data and outcomes. In addition to validating the efficacy and accuracy of the systems described, long-term studies should be conducted to determine whether initial results simply reflect the lure of the new and would decay over time or whether the flexibility of the systems is sufficient to sustain participants' interest.

Finally, the use of technology to support exercise adherence will require a shift in the way both participants and professionals engage in activity and counseling (King, 1991). This shift, as I have suggested, will be away from a time- and site-specific model (counseling occurs only face-to-face and in a counselor's office; exercise takes place only at certain times and in an exercise center)—to one that is not time- and site-specific (counseling can be provided through a variety of media; activity can be performed most anywhere).

These are admittedly oversimplified extremes, and I offer them only to highlight their fundamental differences. Nonetheless, the transition from building-based to community-based activity is already under way. Fully accomplishing this transition will require educators to play a key role as they prepare students to make use of whatever new technologies and combinations of technologies are eventually implemented.

Preliminary observations of the potential to improve adherence through technology are promising, although it is impossible to tell which of the possibilities outlined in this chapter will prove most useful. Only by openly exploring all of them and more will we learn whether the initial enthusiasm is justified or merely reflects an infatuation with gadgetry. It is clear, however, that the traditional model has failed for most segments of the population.

References

Dishman, R.K. (1991). Increasing and maintaining exercise and physical activity. *Behavior Therapy*, **22**, 345-378.

Dishman, R.K. (in press). Prescribing exercise intensity for healthy adults using perceived exertion and exertional symptoms. *Medicine and Science in Sports and Exercise*.

King, A.C. (1991). Community intervention for promotion of physical activity and fitness. *Exercise and Sport Science Review*, **19**, 211-259.

King, A.C., Bild, D., Dishman, R.K., Dubbert, P.M., Marcus, B.H., Oldridge, N.B., Paffenbarger, R.S., Powell, K.E., Yeaber, K., & Blair, S.N. (1992). Determinants of physical activity and interventions in adults. *Medicine and Science in Sports and Exercise*, **24**, S221-S236.

McKenney, J.M., Munroe, W.P., & Wright, J.T., Jr. (1992). Impact of an electronic medication compliance aid on long-term blood pressure control. *Journal of Clinical Pharmacology*, **32**, 277-283.

CHAPTER *10*

Social Marketing and Population Interventions

Robert J. Donovan
Neville Owen

As long as there have been social systems, there have been attempts to inform, persuade, influence, motivate; to gain acceptance for or adherents to certain sorts of ideas; to promote causes and to win over particular groups; to reinforce behavior or to change it—whether by favor, argument or force.–Young, 1989

The promotion of socially desirable causes is not new. In this century, particularly during and following the two world wars, there have been many systematic attempts to achieve both widespread public support for certain issues and widespread behavioral changes. These campaigns were largely developed and implemented by social-communication theorists with backgrounds in psychology and sociology. Aptly enough, these interventions were titled ''public communication campaigns'' (Rice & Atkin, 1989).

Social Marketing

In the late 1960s and early 1970s, using marketing techniques to plan and implement campaigns for social change increased substantially. Many factors inspired the broader use of marketing techniques in social-change campaigns. First, psychologists, sociologists, and health professionals realized that although they were expert in assessing what people should do, they were not necessarily expert in communicating their messages or in motivating and facilitating behavioral change (Manoff, 1985). Hence, they contracted the assistance of advertising and marketing professionals. Another factor was the move in public health toward the prevention of chronic illnesses such as heart disease and cancer—an approach based on epidemiological research about the relationships between habitual behaviors and long-term health outcomes (Wallack, 1983).

This awareness led to an emphasis (some would say an undue emphasis) on individual responsibility and individual behavioral change and hence a receptiveness to the discipline of marketing with its apparent philosophy of individualism and rational free choice. At the same time, social marketing had been criticized by people who felt that such a "philosophy" largely ignored the social, economic, and environmental factors that influence individual behaviors. Although some marketing campaigns were criticized because they tended to ignore the wider social, cultural, and economic environment, this criticism shows a lack of understanding of social marketing. That is, one of the fundamental aspects of marketing—and hence of social marketing—is an awareness of the total environment in which the organization operates and how this environment influences or can itself be influenced to enhance the marketing activities of the company or health agency (Kotler, 1988; Pride & Ferrell, 1980). Given marketing's roots in the behavioral science disciplines of psychology, sociology, anthropology, and communications (as well as in economics and statistics), it is not surprising that marketing principles have been applied to social-change campaigns. Perhaps what is surprising is that the field took so long to be accepted, no doubt because of many health educators' negative associations of marketing with commercialism (Manoff, 1985).

The term *social marketing* appears to have been first used by Kotler and Zaltman in the early 1970s to describe the application of the principles and methods of marketing to the achievement of socially desirable goals. Since Kotler and Zaltman's (1971) article, there has been rapid growth in the use of marketing techniques in the health field in the United States and other industrialized nations and also in third world countries. Large-scale health interventions were pioneered by the Stanford Heart Disease Prevention studies in the United States, similar programs in Finland, and a number of regional antismoking, immunization, nutrition, seat-belt use, and other campaigns in the United States (Fox & Kotler, 1980).

The last decade has seen a massive growth in mass-reach health promotion campaigns across a broad range of activities, including injury prevention, drinking and driving, seat-belt use, drugs, smoking, exercise, immunization, nutrition, and heart disease prevention (Fine, 1990; Kotler & Roberto, 1989; Manoff, 1985; Rice & Atkin, 1989). This has occurred particularly in countries such as Australia, Great Britain, and Canada, where governments finance extensive paid advertising for mass intervention campaigns. In the United States it has been government policy not to use paid advertising to promote health but rather to rely on voluntary media placement of public-service announcements (PSAs). The advent of AIDs, however, by highlighting the urgent need to reach and influence the behavior of large segments of the population quickly and cost-effectively, has led to questioning of this restrictive policy (Donovan, Jason, Gibbs, & Kroger, 1991).

The increasing use of marketing practices by nonprofit organizations for social-change objectives has led the American Marketing Association to redefine marketing from "the performance of business activities that direct the flow of goods and services from producer to consumer or user" (American Marketing Association, 1960, p. 15) to include the marketing of ideas: "the process of planning and executing the conception, pricing, promotion, and distribution of ideas, goods, and services to create exchanges that satisfy individual and organizational objectives" ("AMA board approves," 1985, p. 1). Social marketing is now a clearly established subsection of marketing and is defined as "the design, implementation, and control of programs aimed at increasing the acceptability of a social idea or practice in one or more groups of target adopters" (Kotler & Roberto, 1989, p. 24). Such an approach has clear implications for public campaigns to promote higher levels of participation in physical activity, as we will demonstrate.

Social marketing makes use of key concepts from mainstream product and service marketing:

- Market segmentation
- Market research
- Competitive assessment
- The use of product, price, promotion and distribution tactics
- Pretesting and ongoing evaluation of campaign strategies
- Models of consumer behavior adapted from the psychological and communications literature

Social marketing should not be confused with nonprofit organization marketing—that is, marketing practiced by arts and cultural groups, public universities and colleges, public-transport organizations, libraries, and various charitable groups. Although the principles of marketing apply as well to a self-employed tradesman as a large multinational consumer goods company, they in fact grew from the need to design, implement, and control the promotion and delivery of mass-produced goods to large sectors of the population. The discipline of marketing provides a systematic, research-based approach for the planning and implementation of mass intervention programs.

Old-style health-education programs tended to focus on direct interventions with high-risk individuals, who constitute a relatively small percentage of the population. Epidemiological evidence suggests, however, that substantial health benefits may be achieved through relatively small changes among large segments of the population (Rose, 1985). Furthermore, traditional health-education methods have had limited outcomes because of the limited ability of individual and group counseling resources to affect substantial proportions of the population and the limited ability of such programs to attract the interest of and spur attendance of people in hard to reach groups. There is now a well-developed public-health perspective on mass-reach campaigns that makes extensive use of marketing concepts and practice to overcome such limitations (Lefebvre & Flora, 1988; Winett, King, & Altman, 1990).

Social Marketing and the Limitation of Mass Media

For many health educators, social marketing is seen as synonymous with the use of mass media to promote socially desirable causes. This emphasis on mass media is not unexpected, given that many social marketers see their basic product as information (Wallack, 1983) or view social marketing as a means of working through channels of communication, with information as the primary resource (Young, 1989). In commercial marketing, however, the use of mass-media advertising and promotion is but one component of the total marketing process: the product must be designed to meet buyers' needs; it must be packaged and priced appropriately; it must be easily accessible; buyers should be able to try it (if a large commitment is required); intermediaries such as wholesalers and retailers must be established; and where relevant, sales staff must be informed and trained. Only after all these factors are in place are mass media used to make potential buyers

- aware of the product,
- aware of the product's benefits,
- aware of where it may be purchased, and
- interested (that is, motivated) enough to seek further information or to purchase or try the product.

In the same way, a campaign that aims to promote regular physical activity must be based on more than mass-media advertising. Programs and strategies must be offered at community level, in such a way that the activities promoted are within the target group's capacities; can be sampled before participants make a long-term commitment of funds, effort, or time; can be readily learned (that is, skills must be defined and training must be available); and must be accessible and affordable. Social marketing is by definition a far more comprehensive and effective approach than a mass-media campaign.

The relative importance of mass media in a social-marketing campaign can be illustrated by the hierarchical model shown in Figure 10.1 (after McGuire, 1988).

Mass media are most effective in the early stages of this hierarchy (exposure, attention, knowledge, and tentative attitude formation), whereas other elements of the marketing mix and environmental factors are far more influential at the later behavioral stages. Donovan and Robinson (1992) argue that one reason why many mass-media campaigns are deemed failures (Donohew, 1990) or appear to have limited impact (McGuire, 1986) is that they have been evaluated at the behavioral level rather than at higher levels in the hierarchy of effects. Figure 10.2 shows that a campaign's judged effectiveness depends on the level in the hierarchy where the campaign impact is measured and that even successful efforts at initial levels of the hierarchy must be sustained to achieve any significant impact at attitudinal and behavioral levels.

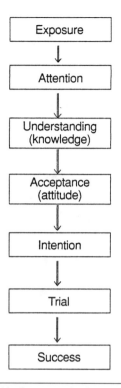

Figure 10.1   Steps in a hierarchical communication model.

Failure may also result because

- the messages failed to reach their target audience at a sufficient weight to have any impact (i.e., insufficient frequency of exposure and a limited reach),
- the messages were ineffective, or
- the expectation that media alone could influence the targeted behaviors was overly optimistic.

Research assessing the impact of mass media alone versus mass media plus community interventions (e.g., Egger et al., 1983) supports the view that although message and media weight effects may have been important determinants of the impact of some public-health campaigns, the primary limitation of such campaigns was probably their reliance on mass media alone.

Furthermore, in the debate on the effectiveness of media in achieving health behavior change, little attention has been devoted to the type of behavior targeted. When one-time behaviors have been targeted (e.g., HIV and STD testing, France, Donovan, Watson, & Leivers, 1991; Nicholas, Glover, Parr, Leonard, & D. Miller, 1987; cholesterol testing, Lefebvre & Flora, 1988; participation in smoke-free days, Donovan, Fisher, & Armstrong, 1984), success rates have been moderately to relatively high, especially when structural facilitators have been in place

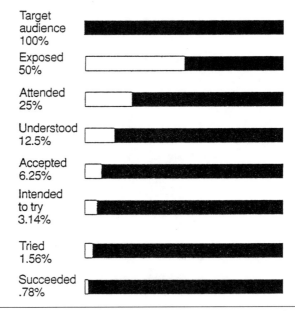

Figure 10.2   Campaign impact, given a 50% achievement rate, at each step in the hierarchy.

(e.g., easy access to testing services, intensive publicity to encourage social support for quitting smoking for a day).

When the targeted behavior is more complex, because of habituation or social or psychological addiction or because it is part of an associated cultural lifestyle, intervention has been less successful (e.g., drug-use behavior, abstinence from smoking, changes in diet, adoption of regular physical activity, seat-belt use). Even in these complex behavioral areas, it is clear that the more fully the social-marketing concept has been adopted in planning the campaign, the more successful the behavioral outcome is likely to be (McGuire, 1986; Wallack, 1990).

The adoption of regular physical activity may require not only substantial lifestyle changes but also development of skills, the economic ability to indulge in preferred exercise activities, and the availability of facilities that facilitate exercise adoption (e.g., running, walking, or cycling tracks; exercise equipment; day-care service). A comprehensive marketing perspective makes it clear that a mass-media campaign is but one component of any program to promote regular physical activity.

Mass Intervention Campaigns and the Promotion of Physical Activity

Although there have been a number of physical-activity campaigns at the work site, school, and community level, few mass intervention campaigns have been directed solely at the promotion of regular physical activity. Furthermore, these have generally been conducted at a national level and hence are difficult to evaluate (Powell, Stephens, Marti, Heinemann, & Kreuter, 1990). Although social-marketing strategies for exercise have been key components of mass-media oriented community-wide interventions to reduce cardiovascular risk (King, 1991), only limited evidence is available concerning what changes in exercise habits might be expected to result from large-scale campaigns concerned with exercise promotion. Much of the available information on effective exercise interventions comes from clinic-based investigations using high-risk individuals, from studies of participants in exercise rehabilitation programs, or from work-site programs (Iverson, Fielding, Crow, & Christenson, 1985; King, 1991; Lee & Owen, 1986a; Owen & Dwyer, 1988).

Mass-media communications about exercise and exercise-related community activities have been integral parts of the Stanford Heart Disease Prevention Program in California (Farquhar et al., 1990; Farquhar et al., 1984; Taylor & Owen, 1989), the North Karelia project in Finland (Puska et al., 1985), and other programs in the United States, Europe, and Australia (Iverson et al., 1985; King, 1991; Owen & Dwyer, 1988) that have focused on the assessment of changes in cardiovascular risk factors, dietary change, and reductions in the prevalence of cigarette smoking. Controlled research on changes in community exercise habits have been much less of a concern for these studies even though exercise activities have often been central elements of their programming.

The Minnesota Heart Health Program—a community-based research and demonstration project designed to modify cardiovascular risk, morbidity, and mortality in adults—has had an emphasis on exercise promotion and on the assessment of changes in physical activity and community awareness about exercise and health (Blake, Jeffery, Finnegan, 1987; Crow et al., 1986). Its education programs aimed to encourage all participants to initiate low- to moderate-intensity physical activity by reducing the use of labor-saving devices and by doing more incidental exercise. The Minnesota program conducted periodic fitness campaigns, the first of which had the following objectives:

- To increase awareness of the benefits of regular physical activity
- To neutralize perceived barriers to regular physical activity
- To increase opportunities for exercise participation
- To portray physical activity as sociable, enjoyable, and part of a balanced lifestyle

Data that documents changes in exercise prevalence or physical-fitness levels associated with these interventions are not yet available, but data do show changes in the intervention communities' exposure to exercise-related health messages, increased media coverage of community events related to exercise, and increased knowledge about exercise and health (Blake et al., 1987).

Other community-wide programs have used mass media and community events with the aim of increasing exercise participation. For example, the Participaction programs in Canada (Bell et al., 1979) and the Heart Week campaigns in Australia (Oldenburg, Bauman, Booth, & Owen, 1991) have demonstrated increased awareness of the campaign message and an increase in intentions to exercise. In Canada there is widespread awareness of the Participaction campaign, and increased levels of interest in exercising have been attributed to it. Population data on actual activity participation in Canada relative to other Western countries, however, show little direct evidence that the campaign has had a significant effect on exercise adoption (Powell et al., 1990). Two independent representative population surveys conducted before and after the Australian Heart Week campaign found no overall changes in reported exercise levels but did find significant changes among older people and the less educated (Booth, Bauman, Oldenburg, Owen, & Magnus, 1992).

A prerequisite for developing effective social-marketing strategies to increase participation in exercise is an understanding of the population prevalence of exercise habits and of the factors that may be related to different types and levels of participation—particularly the characteristics associated with physical inactivity. Psychological theory has been extensively used in investigations of community-based exercise programs (King, 1991; Lee & Owen, 1986a, 1986b; Owen, Lee, Naccarella, & Haag, 1987) but less extensively used in population exercise studies or in evaluations of mass-media interventions (King, 1991; Lee & Owen, 1986a).

Psychological theories of behavioral change and maintenance (particularly the Prochaska and DiClemente stages of change model; see chapter 6) have an important role to play in increasing our understanding of social-marketing strategies for exercise, as we will demonstrate.

Principles and Practices of Social Marketing

A number of aspects of marketing have been discussed in the context of social marketing (e.g., Hastings & Haywood, 1991; Kotler & Roberto, 1989; W. Lancaster, McIlwain, & J. Lancaster, 1983; Lefebvre & Flora, 1988; Manoff, 1985; Novelli, 1990; Solomon, 1989). The eight features of greatest value for the social marketing of exercise are summarized here and described in detail in the following sections.

1. The principle of differential advantage: an analysis of the marketer's resources versus those of the competition.
2. A consumer orientation: The essence of the marketing concept. Piercy (1991, p. 7) argues that "for all organizations the only thing that really matters . . . is . . . the long-term satisfaction of customers."
3. The concept of exchange: Marketing has been defined as the process of "facilitating and expediting exchanges" between consumers and the providers of goods and services (Pride & Ferrell, 1980, p. 7). Both sides trade something of value in return for something of value.

4. The principle of customer value: The notion that all elements of what is called the marketing mix (i.e., the product itself and its price, promotion, and distribution) contribute to the perceived value of a product or service a customer buys.
5. The principle of selectivity and concentration: The notion that the organization or health agency should identify, select, and concentrate on one or more segments of the market in which it has a differential advantage in delivering customer value.
6. The environment: Marketing activities occur in a dynamic environment that influences and is influenced by these activities.
7. The use of market research. Research is essential to establish consumer needs and desired benefits, to identify and profile various marketing segments, to test product offerings and marketing strategies, and to evaluate campaigns.
8. Strategic planning and integration: Marketing provides a systematic, integrated approach to planning and implementation: assessing needs, setting objectives, defining strategies and tactics, monitoring, and evaluating.

The Principle of Differential Advantage

In commercial marketing, organizations compare themselves with their competitors across a number of resource dimensions (e.g., financial, human, products, research and development, technology, expertise) in an attempt to find a differential advantage—an area in which the organization is better positioned than its competitors to profitably meet one or more groups of customers' needs. For example, an advantage may arise through lower production costs, more efficient technology, greater experience or expertise in an area, or superior marketing strength. An analysis of the organization's resources versus those of competitors helps ensure that resources are expended where they can have the greatest impact.

An obvious first step is to define the competition. In the commercial world, that would require defining what business the organization is in. In commercial terms, an organization's products and services compete with all products and services that can substitute for its own offerings. Kentucky Fried Chicken competes not only with other chicken fast-food outlets but also with any outlet offering the convenience of prepared food of acceptable quality at a moderate price, served quickly and at an accessible location. That is, the focus is not on the tangible product but on the overall benefits the consumer seeks (the core product). Focusing too much on the product has been termed "marketing myopia" (Levitt, 1960), which inhibits an organization's ability to succeed at the business of satisfying customers more than the competition can. Defining the competition provides a broader appreciation of goals and objectives and also helps identify what obstacles need to be overcome to achieve the organization's overall goals.

The differential advantage principle applies directly to the marketing of physical activity as a health promotion strategy. The weight of epidemiological evidence suggests that exercise promoters are primarily in the business of reducing the incidence of coronary heart disease (Blair et al., 1989; Powell et al., 1990) by increasing the proportion of the population who participate in regular physical activity at a level sufficient to gain cardioprotective benefits. The overall aim is to enhance health through the reduction of risk. The activity of exercise competes directly with all other people, activities, and organizations that aim to consume part of the individual's free time. Thus, competitors include not only the leisure, entertainment, and personal-development industries but also the individual's hobbies, interests, family demands, and community or social commitments.

The lessons for exercise promotion are twofold: First, people must be able to participate in an exercise program or follow a pattern of regular activity, formal or informal, that conflicts minimally with the demands of family or relevant others. Second, because exercise competes with other leisure activities, it must be seen to offer and deliver (for trial and maintenance, respectively) some of the benefits sought in other leisure activities: for example, relaxation, enjoyment, stimulation, excitement, social contact, or a break from routine. The specific benefits sought will vary between individuals: some desire competitive activities, some enjoy the social aspects, and some seek feelings of achievement (Donovan & Francas, 1990). In short, health benefits alone are insufficient reason for many to adopt and maintain a regular exercise program.

In analyzing the competition, promoters of physical activity need to determine their own strengths and weaknesses, so as to make maximal use of their resources. Strengths include the following:

- Physical activity is highly valued in most Western cultures, so most people already hold positive attitudes about exercise.
- Hospitals and medical practitioners are a major authoritative distribution channel.
- Physical activity has many benefits other than health.
- Many commercial organizations would be willing to cooperate in exercise promotion campaigns.
- There is a great variety of forms of exercise.

On the other hand, organizations should also be aware of weaknesses, some of which include

- a lack of skill in communicating with consumers,
- an inability to effectively use the existing health network, and
- a lack of sufficient funds for promotion, program development, and training.

The Marketing Concept: A Consumer Orientation

Marketing is not only a discipline but also an overall approach to business and human services. It is contrasted with production, product, and sales orientations (Kotler, 1989). Production-oriented companies tend to emphasize production efficiencies (availability and affordability), whereas product-oriented companies emphasize product quality (the "better mousetrap" philosophy that product improvement and quality are most important). Many health services operate on one or another of these philosophies (Lefebvre & Flora, 1988). A sales orientation tends to emphasize hard-sell techniques, sales promotions, and incentives to achieve a high level of sales. This orientation is most applicable to unsought goods and services and is characteristic of social advertising campaigns that emphasize incentives to achieve behavior change (see Winett et al., 1990).

The production, product, and sales orientations focus on the needs of the seller. In contrast, the marketing concept focuses on the needs of the buyer. It seeks profits or increased levels of participation in an activity or service through the identification of customer needs; the development of products and services to meet those needs; and the pricing, packaging, promotion, and distribution of products in accordance with consumer habits, aspirations, and expectations. That is, consumer needs are taken into account not only in the development of basic products and services but also in the way products are priced and packaged, where and how they are distributed, what sort of advertising messages will motivate the target audiences, and where and how often such messages should be exposed so as to reach and persuade a significant portion of the target audience to try the product.

One of the basic distinctions between social marketing and commercial marketing is that the former is usually based not on needs experienced by consumers but on those identified by health experts (Sirgy, M. Morris, & Samli, 1985). A marketing approach, however, emphasizes that the development, delivery, and promotion of the health messages must be carried out in accordance with consumers' needs. For example, messages about exercising must be in a language consumers understand, the promised benefits must be relevant, and the messages must be placed in media that consumers attend to.

The Concept of Exchange

Exchange has long been described as the core concept of marketing: "Marketing is the exchange which takes place between consuming groups and supplying groups" (Alderson, 1957, p. 15) and "Marketing is a social and managerial process by which individuals and groups obtain what they need and want through creating and exchanging products and values with others" (Kotler, 1989, p. 5). A market is defined as the aggregation of individuals willing and able to engage in exchanges. The essential factor that differentiates exchanges from other forms of need satisfaction is that both parties to the exchange gain and receive value (Houston & Gassenheimer, 1987). At the same time, each party perceives the offerings to involve costs. Hence, it is the ratio of perceived benefits to costs that determines choice between alternatives (Kotler & Andreasen, 1987). Kotler (1988) lists the following as conditions necessary for potential exchange:

- There are at least two parties.
- Each party offers something that might be of value to the other.
- Each party is capable of communication and delivery.
- Each party is free to accept or reject the offer.
- Each party believes it appropriate or desirable to deal with the other.

The lessons for social marketers are that we must offer something of perceived value to our target audiences and recognize that consumers must expend time, money, physical comfort, or psychological effort or make lifestyle changes in exchange for the promised benefits (Lefebvre & Flora, 1988). Furthermore, it must be remembered that all intermediaries enlisted in promoting higher levels of participation in physical activity (e.g., physicians, commercial health club operators, community health instructors, health promotion professionals' associations, volunteer workers, sponsors) also require something of value in return for their efforts (DeMusis & Miaoulis, 1988). Too often health promoters have assumed that the intermediaries' shared goal of public-health enhancement is sufficient to ensure their support. Each intermediary must be considered a target market, however, with needs and values that must be included in an exchange process. Hence, promotions to physicians that ask them to recommend exercise to their patients must be designed with physicians' needs in mind. For example, promotional materials should be easy to use and easy to distribute and should improve physicians' understanding of the area—that is, they should be of value to physicians.

Customer Value: The Concept of the Marketing Mix

There are two basic concepts to customer value. First, customers do not buy just products or services but rather benefits or bundles of benefits (K.J. Lancaster, 1966). Kotler (1988, p. 243) reports that Charles Revson of Revlon said, ''In the factory we make cosmetics; in the store we sell hope,'' and that Levitt made the point that although people buy a quarter-inch drill (the product), what they really want is a quarter-inch hole.

Second, the ''four *P*s'' of the marketing mix all contribute to customer value. The four *P*s are

- product (including brand name and reputation, packaging, range and types, and warranties),
- price (including the cost, credit terms, and ease of payment—for example, credit cards, electronic funds transfer at point of sale [EFTPOS],
- promotion (including advertising, sales promotions, publicity and public relations, personal selling), and
- place, or distribution (physical distribution, number and type of outlets, hours open, atmosphere in outlets, availability of public transport, and availability and ease of parking).

The marketing manager's task is to blend these four elements so as to provide maximal value to particular market segments. For example, products with a high price are accompanied by extensive advertising and promotion that attempt to justify the higher price, either objectively (e.g., by emphasizing "reinforced steel" or "powerful concentrated solvent") or subjectively through appeals to sensory attributes, social status, or lifestyle (e.g., Toyota's "oh, what a feeling" campaign or Mercedes' social status positioning). Time and effort costs are reduced by making the product easily obtained (e.g., with wide distribution or vending machines in appropriate locations), trialable before commitment (e.g., through sample packs, in-office or in-home demonstrations, or "7 days free trial"), easy to pay for (e.g., with credit card acceptance, layaway, or credit financing), and easy to use (e.g., with user-friendly packaging, instructions on use, or free training courses).

These two concepts (customer benefits; product, price, promotion, and place) are somewhat tied together by Kotler's (1988) concept of the core product, the augmented product, and the tangible product. For example, the tangible product might be a computer. The augmented product involves the buyer's total consumption system. For computers this involves after-sales service, training, warranties, software, a widespread consumer-user network, and so on. The core product might be better management decision-making. Many companies compete primarily not on tangible product features but on augmented product features (Levitt, 1969).

In exercise promotion the core product might be a longer, healthier life through cardiovascular disease risk reduction, the actual product might be an aerobics class, and the augmented product might include day-care facilities, off-peak discount rates, hygienic changing rooms, and a complimentary towel.

Market Segmentation: The Principle of Selectivity and Concentration

Lunn (1986) has described segmentation as one of the most influential aspects of the marketing concept. Market segmentation involves dividing the total market into groups of individuals who are more like one another than like individuals in other groups. The issue is to identify groups that will respond to different products or marketing strategies. The segmentation process involves three phases (Kotler, 1989):

1. Dividing the total market into segments and developing profiles of those segments
2. Evaluating each segment and selecting one or more segments as target markets
3. Developing a detailed marketing mix (i.e., the four Ps) for each segment

Most commercial organizations spend a great deal of money, time, and effort identifying segments and determining which ones will be most profitable. Selection is based primarily on the match between the company's resources and the target segment's needs and must take into account competitors' activities in the segments and the segments' characteristics, such as size, geographic location, and purchasing power and the extent to which its members can be reached and persuaded.

Segments can be described in many ways, with the major bases being

- psychographic (e.g., lifestyle, values),
- socioeconomic (e.g., lower, middle, or upper class; white collar or blue collar),
- geographic (e.g., Northeast, Midwest, Southwest),
- demographic (e.g., age, sex, income, family life cycle, ethnicity),
- purchasing behavior (e.g., light, medium, heavy), and
- benefits sought (i.e., motives for purchase).

For public-health campaigns, target groups are often described according to risk factors (e.g., smokers, the obese, the inactive, heavy drinkers, diabetics) or demographic groups that epidemiologically appear at higher risk (e.g., blue-collar groups for nutrition, exercise, and smoking campaigns; sedentary people for exercise and weight control; low-income single Hispanic mothers for family-planning campaigns; urban African-American youth for antidrug campaigns).

The psychographic, or lifestyle, approach has been favored by many marketers, who have used segment names such as "the affluent elderly," "the independent woman," and "new-age sensitive man," that have far more intuitive appeal than the traditional demographic descriptions. In lifestyle segmentation, respondents generally answer a large number (50 to 100) of questions about attitudes, beliefs, and behaviors. Cluster analysis is used to develop the segments. The segmentation can be based on general items or items specific to the topic at hand. Hence, some health researchers have segmented on the basis of attitudes about health issues (e.g., Slater & Flora, 1989). The resulting segments can then be described according to their risk factors, and certain segments may be targeted because they have a higher than average proportion of smokers or sedentary or obese people. This approach, however, has been criticized by Rossiter (1989) as "backward" segmentation, in which strategies are directed toward segments because they have a high proportion of, say, nonexercisers. Strategies are then developed based on the beliefs and attitudes of the overall segments rather than on the beliefs and attitudes of the nonexercisers within them. A more direct and efficient approach is to segment nonexercisers on the basis of their attitudes and beliefs about exercise and then to target strategies toward these subgroups.

Rossiter (1989) argues that because our objective is to change attitudes and purchasing behavior, we must first segment the market according to those two dimensions. The first step is to obtain the brand attitude–behavior segments shown in Figure 10.3. Motives for purchase and beliefs underlying (brand) attitudes are then established to assist the marketer in message strategy development. Selected target segments can be profiled demographically (to assist in media selection) and psychographically (to assist in message language and style). That is, demographics and psychographics should be used descriptively not prescriptively.

| | | Brand attitude | | | |
		Positive	Neutral	Negative	Unaware of brand
Behavior	Regular buyer (brand loyal)				
	Occasional buyer				
	Tried but discontinued				
	Never tried				

Figure 10.3   Brand attitude–behavior segmentation.

Sheth and Frazier (1982) have presented a similar attitude–behavior segmentation for social-marketing campaigns, along with suggested strategies for each of the segments (see Figure 10.4). For example, Sheth and Frazier state that segment 1 requires a reinforcement strategy, segment 4 an incentive strategy, and segment 6 a confrontational strategy.

For the mass marketing of regular physical activity, we strongly recommend that such a segmentation procedure first be applied to the general population. A large-scale survey should be carried out to determine

- the percentages of the population falling into each of the segments;
- the demographics, lifestyle, and media habits of each segment;
- the risk-factor profile of each segment;
- the predominant beliefs and attitudes toward exercise in general and toward specific forms of exercise among each segment; and
- perceived and actual sociostructural facilitators and inhibitors for exercise participation among each segment.

Qualitative research should be carried out with members of each segment to help researchers fully understand the nature of beliefs, attitudes, behaviors, and

| | | Attitude toward the behavior | | |
		Positive	Neutral	Negative
Behavior	Performs	1	2	3
	Does not perform	4	5	6

Figure 10.4   Sheth-Frazier segmentation.

motivations within each segment so that appropriate marketing and communication strategies can be developed for each.

Another useful segmentation model for social marketing derives from the work of Prochaska (1991; also see chapter 6 in this volume). Prochaska divides the total market into stages depending on individuals' progression toward adoption of the desired behavior, a concept similar to marketing's "buyer readiness" segmentation base (Kotler, 1989, p. 225). Prochaska's stages are

- *precontemplation*, in which individuals are not considering modifying their behavior;
- *contemplation*, in which people are considering adopting the recommended behavior, but not in the immediate future;
- *preparation*, in which people plan to try to adopt the recommended behavior in the immediate future (in the next 2 weeks);
- *action*, the 6-month period following trial and adoption of the recommended behavior;
- *maintenance*, a further period of 6 months until the recommended behavior is fully established; and
- *termination*, in which the problem behavior is eliminated, that is, people experience "zero temptation across all problem situations" (Prochaska, 1991, p. 806).

These stages are descriptive. In order to develop appropriate social-marketing strategies, researchers must understand the nature of beliefs, attitudes, facilitators, and inhibitors within each stage. The main points to note from the Prochaska model are that

- the evaluation of a social-marketing campaign should not be based on behavioral outcomes alone, and
- the relative proportion of the population in each segment should serve as a starting point for the campaign's overall objectives.

Recent population studies have focused on the prevalence and characteristics of Prochaska's stages of change in relation to cigarette smoking, on their implications for cessation campaigns (Beiner & Abrams, 1991; Owen, Wakefield, Roberts, & Esterman, 1992), and on psychological constructs that may identify the precursors of behavioral change (Pierce, Dwyer, Chamberlain, Aldrich, & Shelley, 1987). Research on the correlates of the stages of readiness to exercise is less advanced, but recent studies in Australia and elsewhere have begun to address these issues (see chapter 6 this volume; Marcus & Owen, 1992). Population prevalence studies of stages of change in exercise behavior have potential implications for exercise marketing strategies.

Understanding the distribution of exercise habits in the total population and the determinants of these levels is a key aspect of the market segmentation strategy for exercise. These exercise distribution issues show the necessary links between social marketing and behavioral epidemiology. Population prevalence data on the levels of exercise participation are available from a number of developed countries. Stephens (1987) deals with data showing that 15% to 20% of the adult populations of the United States and Canada are active at a level sufficient to strongly enhance cardiorespiratory fitness. Stephens found no consistent evidence that levels of participation in vigorous physical activity had increased recently, but he described findings that suggest a small but significant decline in the proportion of the U.S. population that take virtually no vigorous or moderate leisure physical activity.

Recent Australian surveys show similar levels of exercise participation (Bauman, 1987) and trends (Bauman, Owen, & Rushworth, 1990). An examination of pooled population data from five independent random surveys conducted from 1984 to 1987 found only slight increases in vigorous physical activity. The proportion of Australians who reported taking virtually no leisure-time exercise declined significantly, however (Bauman et al., 1990). The reported prevalence of being completely sedentary declined from 33% in July 1984 to just over 25% in January 1987. This rate is substantially similar to that found in North American surveys (Stephens, 1987; Stephens, Jacobs, & White, 1985).

If the inactive subgroup of the populations of industrialized countries is already beginning to change, it may be a cost-effective public-health strategy to attempt to accelerate this tendency. To use social-marketing strategies for this purpose, it will be necessary to determine who the inactive members of society are and to identify factors that may prevent them from exercising. Social-marketing strategies for exercise ought to focus primarily on the 30% of the adult population that is totally inactive. It has been argued that the greatest public-health benefits would accrue if, rather than attempt to persuade those who are already active to be more active, policies and campaigns to promote exercise participation were concerned with helping those who are completely sedentary participate in modest exercise (Owen & Dwyer, 1988; Owen & Lee, 1989). This focus is supported by more general public-health models (Jeffery, 1989; Winett, King, & Altman, 1990) and by recent evidence for the health benefits, particularly cardiovascular, of moderate activity and walking for exercise (Blair et al., 1989; Hardman, Hudson, Jones, & Norgan, 1990). There may be methodological advantages in studying sedentariness as a category rather than attempting to use data on continuous measures of activity for population studies of exercise habits (National Center for Health Statistics, 1989).

Thus, the focus of attention should not be on activities such as jogging and aerobic classes that the more visible, active exercisers engage in, but on inexpensive and convenient activities such as walking (which has considerable potential to reduce cardiovascular risk) and swimming, where the climate or facilities are appropriate. In fact, such activities may have a greater chance of being adopted by those who are physically inactive, particularly the socially disadvantaged (Morris, 1990). Owen and Bauman (1992) focused on the characteristics of those who are sedentary rather than on the predictors of participation in physical activity. This latter focus has tended to dominate research on the behavioral and public-health aspects of exercising. Owen and Bauman found that the factors that predicted reasons for inactivity were different from those that predicted inactivity itself.

The strengthening and refinement of population-focused exercise campaigns requires a more theoretically based understanding of the effects of campaigns themselves (Redman, Spencer, & Sanson-Fisher, 1990), particularly the characteristics that may influence people's willingness to take action in order to be more physically active. The stages of change model developed by Prochaska, DiClemente, and associates has been applied recently to representative population studies of change in smoking behavior (Owen & Davies, 1990; Owen et al., 1992) and of exercising (see chapter 6 this volume; Marcus & Owen, 1992).

Knowledge of the prevalence, sociodemographic characteristics, and attitudinal profiles of the stages of readiness to exercise has significant implications for the market-segmentation elements of social-marketing strategies. For example, those at the precontemplation stage in relation to exercise may best be influenced by an emphasis on the health and quality of life benefits of exercising, those at the contemplation stage may be more influenced by an emphasis on specific forms of exercise and the enhancement of their confidence that it is possible to exercise in comfort and safety, and those at the action stage may benefit from a focus on social support for continuing to exercise.

The Environment

Commercial marketers are keenly aware that the marketing process takes place in a changing environment and that this environment must be monitored continually, both to identify potential opportunities and to avoid potential and actual threats to the company and its products or sources. Environmental factors that influence the marketing of goods, services, and ideas include the following:

- political or legal (for example, exhaust emission requirements, antimonopoly laws, FTC rulings on the use of words such as *natural* and *fresh*)
- economic (the introduction of low-price alternatives during recessionary periods, changes in spending patterns)
- technological (changes in packaging and production methods, whole product categories such as typewriters becoming obsolete)
- social and cultural (changing attitudes toward "healthy" foods, the demand for environmentally friendly packaging and products, a yearning for traditional values)
- demographic trends (increases in single-person and single-parent households, the rapidly growing Hispanic population, the aging of the population)
- the consumer movement (safety demands, credit protection, guarantees)

All of these factors can affect the promotion of physical activity. For example, politicians can be lobbied to provide funds for exercise facilities; unions can bargain for exercise facilities to be provided at the work site; informal, low-cost methods of activity should be promoted during times of recession; home video workouts can take advantage of the widespread penetration of videocassette recorders; technological changes in resistance equipment can facilitate weight training; exercise can be presented as consistent with current attitudes toward health; cycling and walking can be promoted as nonpolluting transport modes; special programs can be designed for the relatively independent and healthy aged; and programs can take account, for example, of Hispanic (and other groups') cultural values and attitudes.

In order to promote participation in physical activity effectively, researchers must also take into account the physical environment. Indoor facilities must be available in very cold climates, and people who prefer to participate in outdoor activities such as cycling, jogging, and walking must be converted to indoor activities for the cooler months. Conversely, in very hot regions, people must be warned against exercising vigorously in high temperatures and must schedule their outdoor exercise during cooler evening and morning hours.

The Use of Market Research

Given all of the these factors, it is clear that effective marketing is a research-based process. Research is necessary to ascertain, in a theoretically informed and methodologically rigorous fashion, the needs of consumer segments; to test product and service prototypes among identified segments; to pretest advertising and other communication materials; to evaluate campaign outcomes; to monitor environmental influences; to assess media scheduling variables; to test packaging and price variations and the attractiveness of potential sales incentives; to provide feedback on competitive activity and consumer reactions to such activity; and to undertake test marketing activities. In short, research is necessary to effectively integrate all elements of the marketing mix (product, place, price, and promotion) so as to apply the organization's resources most efficiently toward meeting the needs of a defined segment or segments of a target audience. This is not to say that research has all the answers, however, or that it can always be afforded by potential users.

Research in social marketing is not so much concerned with the assessment of health needs and wants—these are defined primarily by epidemiological data—but with factors such as what health "products" (e.g., exercise, dietary fat reduction, smoking cessation) the community is most amenable to; what tangible products can be developed to facilitate the adoption of health-promoting behaviors or to reduce risk (e.g., no-tar cigarettes, low-fat foods, quit-smoking kits, exercise videos); what programs or services can be offered (e.g., weight control, aerobics classes, educational videos on exercise benefits, training videos on how to institute work-site exercise programs); how these products and programs should be packaged, priced, positioned, promoted, and distributed; how the message strategy should be developed; what other social and structural facilitators and inhibitors should be taken into account; who the relevant influencers and intermediaries are; what media (television, radio, press) and media vehicles (specific programs), if any, can be used to cost-effectively reach the target audience; and what competitive activities other marketers have undertaken.

The kind of research appropriate to the development and evaluation of social-marketing campaigns is illustrated by the National Research Council's publication on the evaluation of AIDS-prevention programs (Coyle, Boruch, & Turner, 1989). This identifies four types of research needs in health marketing:

1. Formative research, which attempts to answer the question: "What should be done, how, to whom, and in what way to be most effective?" It involves activities such as identifying and profiling priority target groups and developing and testing programs, communications, and other promotional materials.
2. Efficacy testing, which attempts to answer the question: "Can the strategy achieve its objectives?" That is, efficacy testing aims to determine whether the proposed products, programs, messages, and other strategies could be effective if implemented appropriately (is somewhat akin to test marketing).
3. Campaign process evaluation, which attempts to answer the question: "What was done, to whom, and how?" This research assesses whether the program was implemented as proposed and involves measures of exposure and program delivery.
4. Campaign impact and outcome evaluation, which attempts to answer the question: "What did we achieve with respect to our overall goals and objectives?" *Impact* refers to short-term intermediate effects such as changes in beliefs, attitudes, and some behaviors (e.g., enrolling in an exercise program), whereas *outcome* refers to a behavioral result (e.g., maintaining an exercise program for 6 months) or the result of the cumulative behavioral response (e.g., a decrease in CHD incidence). For many programs, for example, skin-cancer prevention and exercise promotions, the eventual outcomes of reduced CHD and reduced skin cancer would not be evident for some years and only after sustained programs. Hence, outcome evaluation generally focuses on short-term, intermediate objectives.

The major use of research in social-marketing campaigns has been primarily in the development and pretesting of message strategies (advertising, posters, brochures, PSAs); measures of exposure to campaign materials; and periodic or pre- and postsurveys to assess changes in attitudes, beliefs, and behaviors over the duration of the campaign. Formative research, especially qualitative exploratory research (most often using focus groups), is more prevalent than process and outcome research, and apart from the large-scale community studies we have mentioned, there is a lack of experimental controls in many studies (e.g., France et al., 1991; Nicholas et al., 1987). There is a clear need to increase the use of methodologically sound research in the social-marketing area.

An Integrated Planning Process

Although we have separately discussed a number of key marketing concepts, it is clear that they are interrelated and interdependent. Marketing is an integrated process, such that elements of the marketing mix, the company's or agency's resources, the use of market research, and the selection and concentration on specific market segments all combine to maximize the value of the company's or agency's offerings to the consumer and hence the company's profit or the intended changes in knowledge, attitude, and behaviors achieved by the health agency.

This integration strongly implies the need for a systematic strategic planning process, that includes the setting of clearly defined overall goals and of measurable objectives to meet those goals; the delineation of strategies and tactics to achieve the objectives; and management and feedback systems to ensure that the plan is implemented as desired, to avert or deal with problems as they arise, and to ensure that planned activities deliver the set objectives. These principles are basic to an effective campaign, whether the organization concerned is a commercial company or a health agency.

Developing a Mass-Media Strategy to Increase Participation in Regular Physical Activity

Social marketing is clearly more than delivering messages through mass media. The basic principles of social marketing apply equally to any component of the marketing mix, whether product development, message strategy, or message delivery. Program development, local community interventions, and sociostructural factors are dealt with elsewhere in this book. Hence the example in this section focuses on the mass media.

A focus on mass media is appropriate to mass intervention campaigns because information forms a major component of the exercise product, and hence the communication process is of primary importance. It is also appropriate because of the need to rapidly inform and motivate large sectors of the community about an issue while the programs and services are being offered. There is little point in developing programs, training personnel, and preparing videos for large groups of people if there are no means of informing people about such programs. Similarly, it does no good to have a mass-media campaign to encourage people to participate in exercise programs if adequate resources are not in place to facilitate and accommodate demand. Too often mass-media campaigns have been ineffective because other elements of the marketing mix were not in place.

Overall Roles of Mass Media

There are three major ways of using mass media:

1. Paid advertising and the voluntary placement of public service announcements (PSAs)

2. Publicity, both paid and unpaid
3. Health messages incorporated in mass market entertainment programs (dubbed *edutainment* by some writers; Donovan & Robinson, 1992)

Edutainment has been and is mainly used in third-world countries such as India and Mexico (Singhal & Rogers, 1990) but is receiving attention in both Australia and the United States (Davern, 1991; De Jong & Winsten, 1990).

Donovan and Robinson (1992) list the following advantages and disadvantages of these mass-media modes from the campaign manager's perspective. The primary advantage of paid advertising is control over message content, exposure (timing and "location"), and frequency; the major disadvantage is cost. Publicity and edutainment share the ability to reach large numbers of people in a relatively short time but have the disadvantages of less control over message content, exposure (especially PSA exposure), and frequency (unless the theme continues for several episodes in a soap opera). On the other hand, publicity releases (feature articles, talk-show appearances) are more credible than paid advertising and far less costly. While edutainment certainly builds awareness of an issue, there are no hard data on its effectiveness compared with that of more direct educational efforts in changing attitudes and behaviors (Singhal & Rogers, 1990).

Mass Media in the Social Marketing of Exercise

Donovan and Robinson (1992) list a number of roles that mass media can perform. For the general population the major roles of mass media in the promotion of exercise are

- to increase the salience of exercise as a health issue (i.e., agenda setting),
- to provide information on its primary health benefits,
- to communicate its nonhealth benefits,
- to arouse interest in exercise adoption (by way of points 2 and 3) and thus sensitize individuals to specific program promotions and face-to-face interventions, and
- to motivate some behavioral act such as trying a program, sending for information, calling a hot line, visiting a health club, or talking to others about exercise.

Not all of these roles apply equally to all segments of the population, however. For example, with regard to Prochaska's segments (see chapter 6), the major role for mass media in relation to precontemplators is to place the exercise issue on the agenda; in relation to contemplators, the role is to heighten interest and to motivate some intermediate behavioral objective such as seeking further information; for those in the preparation category, the aim is to initiate trial; for those in the maintenance category, mass media plays a reinforcement role. Table 10.1 illustrates these points.

Table 10.1   Prochaska's Stages and the Influence of Mass Media on Behavioral and Attitude–Belief Objectives

Stage	Behavioral objective	Attitudinal–belief objective
Precontemplation	—	Raise salience and relevance of issue
(Mass-media influence)	—	(High)
Contemplation	Intention to try	Increase personal relevance, decrease perceived inhibitors
(Mass-media influence)	(High)	(Moderate)
Preparation	Trial	Reinforcement of reasons for trial, build self-efficacy
(Mass-media influence)	(Moderate)	(Moderate)
Action	Adoption of behavior	Reinforcement of reasons for adopting, motivational and efficacy support
(Mass-media influence)	(Low)	(Low)
Maintenance	Maintaining new behavior	Reinforcement of reasons for adoption, increase salience of rewards for maintenance, reinforcement of self-efficacy
(Mass-media influence)	(Low)	(Low)

The maximal behavioral response pertaining to exercise that mass media can influence is the trial of an exercise activity—and then only for those in Prochaska's preparation group (i.e., those with positive attitudes toward adoption of exercise). An important point is that the objective of our message strategy is to form in the target audience's mind an intention to try to adopt an exercise program, not an intention to adopt the program outright. This important distinction is often overlooked by those who develop strategies based on attitude- and behavior-change models (Bagozzi & Warshaw, 1990).

Developing a Communication Strategy

Rossiter and Percy (1987) and Rossiter, Percy, and Donovan (1984) have presented a six-step model relating advertising exposure to company objectives and profits. The model is applicable to any message exposure, not only advertising. The six steps are listed on the left side of Figure 10.5. On the right are examples of the sorts of activities or measures appropriate to each step.

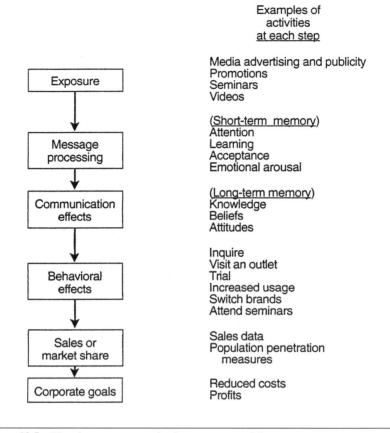

Figure 10.5   The six-step communication process model.

Figure 10.5 shows that the chain begins with exposure of the target audience to the message. Messages may be exposed in television advertisements, news items, magazine articles, promotions, videos, or face-to-face interventions. For advertising, the degree of exposure is determined by the media plan. Exposure leads to conscious processing of the message in short-term memory. This process involves attention to the message points, learning and comprehension, acceptance or rejection of the message, and emotional arousal.

Processing the message leads to long-term memory effects, which are called communication effects. The content of the message, the audience's initial attitudes and beliefs, the nature of the message exposure, and the degree of repetition of the message all affect what is stored in long-term memory and how easily it can be recalled later. The desired communication effect is encouraging various beliefs and attitudes about the subject of the message—in this case, health and fitness, physical activity in general, and specific types of exercise.

Such attitudes and beliefs, when recalled during decision-making, lead to behavioral effects such as inquiries, trial, increased frequency of purchase, or store visits. For exercise promotion, the desired effects would include sending for further information about exercise and health, deciding to visit a health club, or joining a corporate fitness program. The accumulation of such behavioral effects among the target audience leads to the achievement of the overall corporate objectives and goals, which for commercial concerns are usually profit objectives by way of sales and market-share objectives. In the health area, objectives usually relate to risk reductions, health cost reductions, or more positive life experiences.

In the planning chain, the commercial marketing manager and the social marketer begin by

1. defining overall corporate goals and specific measurable objectives,
2. selecting specific target audiences among whom to achieve these goals,
3. specifying behavioral objectives required of each of the target audiences,
4. delineating the beliefs and attitudes necessary to achieve the behavioral objectives,
5. generating the content and type of messages necessary to achieve those beliefs and attitudes, and
6. determining how, where, and how often the messages are to be exposed or delivered to specific target audiences.

Figure 10.6 shows the six-step planning process.

Communication Strategy as a Component of Social Marketing

Keep in mind that the communication strategy is only one of several factors that influence whether the behavioral objectives will be met. These other factors are shown in Figure 10.7 as product development and intervention strategies. By product factors, we mean developing programs and services, including training for the personnel necessary to deliver them. By intervention strategies we mean both structural and nonstructural facilitators that assist in the initiation and maintenance of exercise activity. Structural factors include access to facilities such as swimming pools, walking and jogging tracks, and change rooms. Nonstructural factors refer to group support, promotional activities, peer support, social interactions and so on.

Donovan Research (1987) has used this model to develop a communication strategy for the promotion of regular physical activity in Australia. Donovan's procedures are summarized as follows.

Step 1: Overall Goals.   In the Australian study the following goals were set:

- A substantial increase in feelings of well-being in the Australian population as a function of increased healthiness due to a more physically active lifestyle
- An increase in the health status of the general population and a decrease in the overall proportion defined as at risk because of a lack of physical activity
- Decreased national health costs

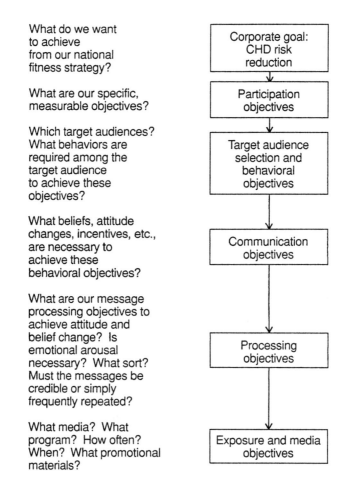

The left-side questions and right-side boxes read:

What do we want
to achieve
from our national
fitness strategy? → Corporate goal:
CHD risk
reduction

What are our specific,
measurable objectives? → Participation
objectives

Which target audiences?
What behaviors are
required among the
target audience
to achieve these
objectives? → Target audience
selection and
behavioral
objectives

What beliefs, attitude
changes, incentives, etc.,
are necessary to
achieve these
behavioral objectives? → Communication
objectives

What are our message
processing objectives to
achieve attitude and
belief change? Is
emotional arousal
necessary? What sort?
Must the messages be
credible or simply
frequently repeated? → Processing
objectives

What media? What
program? How often?
When? What promotional
materials? → Exposure and media
objectives

Figure 10.6   The six-step planning process.

Step 2: Participation Objectives.   The participation objectives for the first 12 months of an integrated exercise campaign were

- to increase by 25% the proportion of Australians currently participating at a sufficiently vigorous level to enhance or maintain cardiorespiratory fitness (i.e., from approximately 14% to 17.5% in the first year of the campaign), and
- to increase the proportion of Australians exercising at a moderate level by 25% (i.e., from 54% to approximately 67.5%).

Population data available at the time of the project were used to estimate the percentages of the population falling into the various cells of a modified Sheth-Frazier matrix shown in Figure 10.8. It should be noted that analyses of more recent Australian population data (Bauman et al., 1990; Owen & Bauman, 1992)

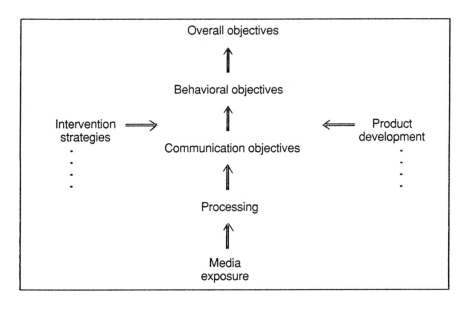

Figure 10.7   Communication strategy as a component of the marketing plan.

now support a much stronger focus on those who are totally inactive (see the bottom row of Figure 10.8), an idea advanced in earlier Australian behavioral work on exercise (Owen & Lee, 1984).

Figure 10.8 shows that 14% exercise at a vigorous level but that perhaps 3% of those who exercise vigorously hold neutral or mainly negative beliefs about exercising. That is, they probably do not enjoy the activity but continue to exercise for the benefit of risk-factor reduction. Another 19% are moderate exercisers but hold neutral to negative beliefs about exercise. Just under two thirds hold primarily positive beliefs about exercise, whereas just over one third hold primarily negative beliefs. The overall aim as described by Donovan Research (1987) was to move individuals toward segment A. (More recent population data would suggest a focus on moving those in segments E and F to segment C.) People in segments C and E require incentives to participate in (more) exercise. For those in cells D and F who are negative toward exercise, two strategies are feasible:

1. Change attitudes first, then induce a behavior change.
2. Encourage or ''enforce'' a behavior change and, through cognitive consonance (the tendency for consistency between attitude and behavior) or direct exposure to the benefits, induce a positive attitude.

Mass-media-based strategies must focus on the first strategy, whereas environmental change, intervention, and incentive strategies must focus on the second.

It may be noted that direct behavioral change is increasingly used in both the commercial and health-marketing areas (particularly in the latter, especially in

Exercise behavior . . .	Overall valence of attitudes and beliefs about exercise		Total
	Positive	Neutral or negative	Total
Exercise at or near level for maximal cardiovascular benefits	11% A	3% B	14%
Light to moderate exercise sufficient for some cardio-vascular benefits	35% C	19% D	54%
No exercise	16% E	16% F	32%
	62%	38%	100%

Figure 10.8   Target audience classification by attitude and behavior.

the area of cigarette smoking regulations (see Borland, Chapman, Owen, & Hill, 1990a, 1990b). In the exercise area, individuals are often cajoled by friends or co-workers to participate in a program or routine and, after they experience its benefits, maintain the behavior independently. This direct approach (Owen & Lee, 1989) can be successful, given that many exercise benefits are experienced only after time has elapsed. On the other hand, unless the activity is enjoyable, the direct approach will not work and may be counterproductive by lessening the likelihood that the individual will try again.

TARPAR: An Index for Target Audience Selection.   As we have noted, audiences selected for targeting by health campaigns have often been defined broadly, generally only behaviorally or demographically (e.g., all smokers for quit campaigns, all women for Pap smear campaigns, all food preparers for nutrition or low-fat campaigns). Very rarely are target audiences attitudinally defined. Consequently, scant attention is paid to whether target audiences are accessible through the usual media and whether media campaigns can be effective.

The Sheth-Frazier (1982) model provides a systematic procedure for describing various target segments in terms of attitudes and behavior (the ''diagnosis''), and it suggests strategies for achieving behavior change with each of the defined segments (the ''prognosis''). These suggested strategies include determining whether mass-media messages are an appropriate or cost-effective method of influencing the segments.

Given a population segmented into target audiences as illustrated in Figure 10.8 (see also Bauman et al., 1990; Owen & Bauman, 1992), the following factors could influence whether an audience is chosen for targeting by a health campaign:

- The number of people in the category: In general, the more people in the category, the higher its priority. Behavioral epidemiology studies with representative population samples allow accurate estimates.
- The proportion in that category classed as at risk (high or moderate): People at risk are those whose behavior, if modified, would provide the greatest reduction in health costs. In general, the greater this proportion, the potentially greater return, hence the higher the category's priority.
- The persuadability of the target audience: Persuadability is defined as the extent to which members of the target audience can be persuaded to alter their behavior (the less amenable, the greater the campaign cost). In general, the more amenable, the more likely it is that a media campaign can be effective.
- The accessibility of the target audience: The more accessible the target audience, the more likely an effective outcome and the higher the priority. This measure should take into account the relative cost of reaching the target audience via different media. For example, a target audience may be accessible, but the necessary media may be expensive.
- Additional resourses: Various target audiences might be amenable to a mass-media campaign and hence motivated to engage in regular physical activity, but new programs or facilities may be required to meet the demand. Similarly, inactives may be motivated only by programs not currently available. Hence, if resources are limited, this factor should be taken into acount.

These factors can be presented in the following formula, in which w_i indicates that different weightings may be applied to the factors:

$$\text{Priority} = f(w_1T, w_2AR, w_3P, w_4A, w_5R)$$
$$T = \text{total number in segment}$$
$$AR = \% \text{ at (high) risk}$$
$$P = \text{persuasibility}$$
$$A = \text{accessibility}$$
$$R = \text{additional resources required}$$

T and AR can be measured objectively, using representative population data and behavioral epidemiology research. P requires a subjective estimate based on qualitative attitudinal research and appropriate theoretical perspectives (as described in this chapter). A requires media exposure research, and R requires an analysis of existing resources and a survey of consumer preferences among the target audiences. AR can be calculated with respect to the population prevalence of the behavior under study (current physical activity; see the section on market segmentation) and with respect to other factors that enhance risk status such as smoking, excess alcohol intake, high cholesterol level, high blood pressure, or any combination of these.

The weights assigned to the different factors will vary by the area in question and the planner's specific needs, policies, and resources. For example, a population approach would assign a higher weight to T than to AR; a well-financed campaign would assign a higher weight to R than would a poorly-financed campaign.

Donovan Research (1987) selected several primary target audiences based on the need to attain the specific behavioral objectives we have noted earlier and on the following major measures: the number of people in the segment, the persuasibility of the segment (i.e., the nature of their current beliefs and behaviors), and the accessibility of the segment. The segments chosen as primary targets were

- people in segment C of Figure 10.8, who engage in moderate activity and have positive attitudes toward increased exercise (estimated 35% of population), and
- people in segment E of Figure 10.8, who are currently inactive but have positive attitudes toward engaging in exercise (estimated 16% of population).

The secondary target audiences were

- people in segment D of Figure 10.8, who engage in moderate activity and have negative attitudes toward their current exercise (and hence toward increased exercise levels). These people (estimated at 19% of the population) are at risk of dropping out, hence we need to maintain their level of exercise, and
- people in segments A and B of Figure 10.8, who currently engage in regular, vigorous exercise (14%). We wish to reinforce and maintain their behavior.

Inactive people who were negative toward participation in exercise (segment F of Figure 10.8) were not designated as a target group. Such people generally require a confrontational approach and a face-to-face intervention. The media communication strategy, however, could attempt to favorably predispose these inactive people toward such approaches.

To assist in marketers' message development, message execution, and media selection, each of the target audiences should be profiled, using the range of epidemiological, behavioral, attitudinal, and marketing studies we have described:

- Demographics and specific group identification (e.g., elderly, disabled, ethnic)—for target and media selection
- Media usage—for media selection
- Risk-factor status—for targeting specific behaviors and for medical promotions
- Other lifestyle factors—for message execution, that is, in order to communicate with language and symbols appropriate to the target audience

- Awareness of exercise benefits and beliefs about health, exercise, and fitness—for message strategy
- Awareness of health and other benefits of different types of exercise—for message strategy
- Knowledge of levels of exercise sufficient to provide cardiovascular fitness—for message strategy
- Reasons for participating in exercise or not, and perceived benefits and drawbacks of exercise—for message strategy
- Awareness of and access to specific exercise facilities and programs—for message strategy

Donovan Research (1987) carried out focus group research with members of target audiences in order to develop message strategies to overcome negative beliefs and attitudes and to clarify the relevant facilitators and inhibitors.

Step 3: Behavioral Objectives. Behavioral objectives are determined by the nature of the target audience. In Rossiter and Percy's (1987) terms, the following behavioral objectives apply:

- Trial (for inactives)
- Retrial (for lapsed exercisers and those in the early stages of exercise adoption)
- Increased intensity or frequency (for light exercisers)
- Maintenance (for those already engaging in exercise at a sufficient level)
- "Brand switching" (for those engaging in but not enjoying a particular activity)

Intermediate behavioral objectives for inactives include the following:

- Attending seminars or workshops on exercise (or health in general)
- Inquiring about health or exercise programs
- Sending for further information on exercise and exercise programs
- Asking friends about an exercise program
- Visiting an aerobics center or health club to look at the facilities and programs

Various behavioral stage models (Beiner & Abrams, 1991; DiClemente et al., 1991; Knapp, 1988; Owen & Lee, 1989; Prochaska, 1991) provide a framework for recommendations at the various stages of exercise adoption (e.g., incentives to try versus incentives to maintain the behavior, the need for skills training at the early stages of adoption). There has been more extensive development of many of these ideas in the smoking-cessation area (see Owen, 1989); many apply strongly to the social marketing of exercise.

Advertising and promotion strategies differ from intervention strategies and play different roles at each of the stages. Advertising has the greatest effect in initiating participation, whereas intervention strategies such as environmental supports and opportunities, feedback, goal-setting, and social support help to maintain behavior.

The behavioral objectives for the target audiences we have discussed are as follows:

• Moderately active postives: Depending on the type, frequency, duration, and intensity of current physical activity, these individuals (segment C of Figure 10.8) would be encouraged to increase their level of activity to that required for cardiovascular benefits. This includes the behavioral objective of gradually increasing the intensity level. For some individuals, the objective will be to switch to higher-intensity exercise (e.g., from leisurely to brisk walking). The specific behavioral changes required depend also on the various subgroups in these segments (e.g., the elderly, the disabled).

• Inactive positives: The primary behavioral objective for inactive positives (segment E of Figure 10.8) is to induce trial of some physical activity. Ongoing behavioral objectives then refer to retrial and skills learning of the chosen exercise activity. A further behavioral objective is for inactive positives to try a variety of exercise activities to ensure that the exercise activity chosen for regular adoption is enjoyable. Behavioral objectives include intermediate objectives such as visiting a fitness center or exercise program for further information, calling to inquire about program access, and inquiring about health and fitness. The final behavioral objective is the "purchase" (adoption) of a regular program of physical activity.

• Moderately active negatives: Those who exercise at a moderate level but hold negative beliefs and attitudes toward their exercise (segment D of Figure 10.8) do not enjoy the type of exercise they participate in or are subject to significant hassles from the home or from other activities that lead to time pressures (e.g., young mothers). The primary behavioral objective is to encourage people to try alternative activities that may be more enjoyable or to switch to alternative activities that may require less time and less pressure. Other behavioral objectives relate to learning time-management skills or involving relevant others in the exercise activity.

• Sufficiently active: The primary behavioral objective (see segments A and B of Figure 10.8) is maintenance of active behavior. Other behavioral objectives are favorable word-of-mouth and encouragement of others to exercise, particularly encouragement for those exercising at a light level to increase their intensity. A possible mechanism would be to encourage those exercising in a group to increase their group size by adding people from the pool of light exercisers.

• Inactive negatives: These people are not a prime target for the communication strategy to initiate any activity. Our primary objective is to ensure that inactive negatives (segment F of Figure 10.8) do not reject direct intervention strategies without giving some attention to the interventionist. In this sense our communication strategy aims to generate a favorable disposition on the part of inactive negatives toward listening to the interventionist's messages.

Step 4: Communication Objectives.   For all target groups the communication objectives are similar to the three major commercial objectives: brand awareness, brand attitude, and brand purchase intention. Such objectives would include

- increasing and maintaining awareness of the health and other benefits of exercise and the results of lack of exercise,
- creating or maintaining positive attitudes toward exercise and negative attitudes toward nonexercising (including perceptions of self-efficacy), and
- generating explicit intentions to try exercise among inactives, to increase the intensity of exercise among light exercisers, and to maintain exercise levels among those exercising vigorously.

A fourth major commercial advertising objective is purchase facilitation (Rossiter & Percy, 1987). This objective arises in the commercial world when various elements of the marketing mix inhibit purchase. For example, a product may not be widely distributed or may be available only in a few exclusive stores. In such a case, one of the advertising objectives may be to convince the target audience that it is worth the additional effort to obtain the product. The purchase facilitation objective is particularly relevant to exercise because, although many people claim to accept many of the benefits promised by exercise, various attitudinal and perceived structural inhibitors are believed to require too much effort relative to the expected return. This is further compounded by the delayed benefits of exercise—at least in the initial stages of adoption—whereas the benefits of not participating in exercise are situational and immediate. Hence, specific program promotions and exercise promotion in general must deal with this issue.

The specific message strategies for achieving these overall objectives among the target audiences are based on the motivations, beliefs, and attitudes of those audiences.

Category Versus Brand Communication Objectives.   In Rossiter and Percy's (1987) terms, the Australian strategy included two overall sets of communication objectives: those pertaining to the category (i.e., exercise and fitness per se) and those pertaining to brands within the category (i.e., different forms of exercise). Category communication objectives are targeted primarily toward nonexercisers, especially those in high-risk categories, and those with neutral or negative attitudes toward exercise. Brand communication objectives are directed primarily toward

- current exercisers (i.e., switching types of exercise maintains motivation and interest),
- lapsed exercisers who may be induced to try again by alternative exercises, and
- inactives with positive attitudes toward exercise in general.

Hence, our communication objectives can be restated as follows.

Awareness

Category: awareness of benefits of exercise and fitness per se
Brand: awareness of benefits of various types of exercise

Attitude

Category: increased positive attitudes toward exercise per se
Brand: increased positive attitudes toward different types of exercise

Intentions

Category: creating intentions to try exercise per se
Brand: creating intentions to try specific types of exercise

Facilitation

Category: exercise per se is worth the effort
Brand: a specific exercise is worth the effort

Donovan (1987) recommended that umbrella media campaigns emphasize category benefits (but not exclude brand benefits), that local promotions emphasize brand benefits, and that later stages of a campaign shift toward message executions that promote different brands but remain linked to the underlying health benefits.

Step 5: Processing Objectives.   Qualitative research on each of the target groups (Donovan, 1987) was used to determine the sorts of beliefs that needed to be addressed to achieve the desired behavioral objectives. For example, many moderate exercisers (e.g., hobby gardeners, once-a-week golfers or squash players) assumed that their low level of activity provided substantial cardiovascular benefits, when, in fact, it did not. Some inactives devalued the benefits of exercise and claimed that their healthy dietary habits precluded the need for an exercise routine. Others were inhibited from joining in aerobics programs because of the glamorous image associated with such exercise. A number of sources of information about attitudes and beliefs and facilitators and inhibitors exist (see Dishman et al., 1985; Donovan Research, 1987; Lee & Owen, 1986a, 1986b; Marcus & Owen, 1992).

The qualitative research for the Australian project probed current exercisers' motives for the adoption and maintenance of exercise and the benefits that exercisers seek and obtain from exercise participation. Nonexercisers were asked their reasons for not exercising, the circumstances surrounding previous attempts to exercise (if any), and reasons for lapsing. Exercisers' motives and benefits were tested against those of nonexercisers to assess what might influence them to try exercise.

The final message strategies adopted for the target audiences depend heavily on the motivations considered most relevant to achieving change within that group. This approach generally requires further segmentation of the primary target groups according to the benefits most appropriate to various subgroups. For example, middle-aged slightly overweight inactive positives might respond to messages stressing the likelihood of heart disease if no action is taken and of avoiding heart disease if an exercise program is adopted. Young inactive positives might respond to messages stressing weight control and muscle tone (i.e., appearance benefits).

At this stage in campaign development, advertising and public relations agencies would be briefed to generate materials such as advertisements (PSAs), posters, brochures, videos, press releases, and promotional events to be directed toward the target audiences. A common procedure for umbrella campaigns is to provide promotional materials without a source specified so that local groups (e.g., state health authorities, nonprofit health promotion organizations, associations of commercial fitness promotion operators) can customize the materials and use them to promote specific programs, events, or incentives. For example, an advertisement promoting the generic benefits of exercise could have an end tag promoting a swimming or cycling club, a fun run, or a commercial organization's aerobics classes.

The advertising and public relations agencies would be responsible for developing a media plan to cost-effectively reach the designated target audiences at an exposure frequency sufficient to have the desired communication and behavioral effects.

Integration.   Developing communication materials is only one element of a total campaign. If the campaign is to rely on voluntary media, it must be marketed to relevant media organizations. This marketing involves supplying materials in a format that facilitates their use and an accompanying message stating the expected community benefits as well as those that might accrue to the media organization's image by placing the materials.

All organizations involved in exercise need to be informed before the campaign launch so that local promotions can be planned and undertaken to support and to take advantage of the umbrella campaign. Similarly, additional skilled temporary personnel might be needed to handle increased inquiries and participation. In short, intermediary and structural elements must be in place before the launch of media components.

The Donovan Research (1987) model shows how specific aspects of exercise promotion, characteristics of target groups, and the stages and elements of a marketing strategy may be integrated. By treating exercise as a product in a marketing sense and using general marketing principles and social-marketing strategies, health professionals can gain unique insights into the many exercise promotion activities they might undertake and can learn how to approach the activities in an integrated fashion within a comprehensive framework.

Whereas the principles and practices of marketing are clearly applicable to the promotion of healthy lifestyles, it is a mistake to assume that social marketing is similar to commercial marketing in all respects. Even within the field of commercial marketing, different approaches are used for different products. Marketing low-cost, high-turnover supermarket goods is quite different from marketing more costly or complex products such as automobiles and financial services, just as the marketing of status-oriented personal products such as designer clothes and fashion jewelry is different from that used to sell functionally oriented products such as power tools, washing machines, and lawnmowers.

In short, although some of the principles of marketing are applicable, selling health or any other socially desirable product is not the same as selling soap (Wiebe, 1952) or other commercial products. The difference is greater for the selling of physical activity per se but smaller for commercial operators in the fitness industry. The point is that the marketing of any product must be based on an understanding of the consumer's decision making and consumption system with respect to that product. Bloom and Novelli (1981) and Rothschild (1979) list a number of important differences between marketing commercial products and socially desirable products such as exercise. The major differences are as follows:

- Commerical products tend to offer instant gratification, whereas the benefits of health behaviors are often delayed.
- Social marketing attempts to replace undesirable behaviors with those that often cost more time or effort and in the short term may be less pleasurable or unpleasant.
- Commercial marketing aims mostly at groups already positive toward the product and its benefits, whereas social marketing is often directed toward hard to reach or at risk people, who are frequently antagonistic to change.
- Health risk behaviors are often extremely complex personally and socially and far more complex than the behaviors involved in purchasing a commercial product.
- Intermediaries in commercial marketing are far fewer and generally easier to deal with (although perhaps more costly) than in social marketing.
- Defining and communicating the product is far more difficult in social marketing, especially when different experts have different views on the subject.
- The exchange process is far easier to define in commercial marketing than in social marketing.

The social marketing of exercise rests on a strong epidemiological rationale. Increasing evidence from the new, interdisciplinary field of behavioral epidemiology (see Jeffery, 1989; Owen, 1989) also deals with exercise prevalence, trends, and determinants (Bauman et al., 1990; Owen & Bauman, 1992; Stephens, 1987). This knowledge must be used in a more systematic fashion to inform exercise-marketing strategies. A strong set of social learning-based theoretical constructs also exists. Such knowledge is beginning to be applied to exercise participation as a public-health issue, but more research and applications are needed to develop these areas of exercise research and translate the relevant knowledge into effective interventions.

As this chapter and book make clear, promoting more widespread participation in appropriate forms of exercise is a key public-health priority. Social marketing relies on high-quality communication strategies and the availability of accessible and affordable exercise options. Key issues of social equity and access have been addressed in other papers (e.g., Owen & Bauman, 1992; Owen & Lee, 1989).

We hope it is clear that successful social marketing requires awareness of the social and environmental factors that may facilitate or limit participation in physical activity. We also hope that we have made clear that social marketing, if conducted honestly and vigorously, is a scientific and humane enterprise consistent with social justice and equity objectives as well as with effective approaches to producing population-wide reductions in disease risk.

References

Alderson, W. (1957). *Marketing behavior and executive action.* Homewood, IL: Irwin.

AMA board approves new marketing definition. (1985, March 1). *Marketing News*, p. 1.

American Marketing Association Committee on Definitions. (1960). *Marketing definitions: A glossary of marketing terms.* Chicago: American Marketing Association.

Bagozzi, R., & Warshaw, P.R. (1990). Trying to consume. *Journal of Consumer Research*, **17**, 127-140.

Bauman, A. (1987). Trends in exercise prevalence in Australia. *Community Health Studies*, **11**, 190-196.

Bauman, A., Owen, N., & Rushworth, R.L. (1990). Recent trends and sociodemographic determinants of exercise participation in Australia. *Community Health Studies*, **14**, 19-26.

Beiner, L., & Abrams, D.B. (1991). The contemplation ladder: Validation of a measure of readiness to consider smoking cessation. *Health Psychology*, **10**, 360-365.

Bell, R.D., Nixon, H.R., Struthers, J.K., Landa, S., Bailey, D.A., & Kisby, R. (1979). Participation Saskatoon: A media-oriented approach to fitness motivation. *Recreation Research Review*, **6**, 62-65.

Blair, S.N., Kohl, H.W., Paffenbarger, R.S., Clark, D.G., Cooper, K.H., & Gibbons, L.W. (1989). Physical fitness and all-cause mortality: A prospective study of healthy men and women. *Journal of the American Medical Association*, **262**, 2395-2401.

Blake, S.M., Jeffery, R.W., Finnegan, J.R., et al. (1987). Process evaluation of a community-based physical activity campaign: The Minnesota Heart Health Program experience. *Health Education Research*, **2**, 115-121.

Bloom, P.N., & Novelli, W.D. (1981). Problems and challenges in social marketing. *Journal of Marketing*, **45**, 79-88.

Booth, M., Bauman, A., Oldenburg, B., Owen, N., & Magnus, P. (1992). Effects of a national mass-media campaign on physical activity. *Health Promotion International*, **7**, 241-247.

Borland, R., Chapman, S., Owen, N., & Hill, D.J. (1990a). Changes in acceptance of workplace smoking following their implementation: A prospective study. *Preventive Medicine*, **19**, 314-322.

Borland, R., Chapman, S., Owen, N., & Hill, D.J. (1990b). Effects of workplace smoking bans on cigarette consumption. *American Journal of Public Health*, **80**, 178-180.

Coyle, S.L., Boruch, R.F., & Turner, C.F. (1989). *Evaluating AIDS prevention programs*. Washington, DC: National Academy Press.

Crow, R., Blackburn, H., Jacobs, D., Hannan, P., Pirie, P., Mittelmark, M., Murray, D., & Luepker, R. (1986). Population strategies to enhance physical activity: The Minnesota Heart Health Program. *Acta Medica Scandinavica*, **711**(Suppl.), 93-112.

Davern, J. (1991, May). *Promoting the compliance message in a popular drama series*. Paper presented at the Second National Immunization Conference of the Public Health Association of Australia, Canberra.

DeJong, W., & Winsten, J.A. (1990, summer). The use of mass media in substance abuse prevention. *Health Affairs*, pp. 30-46.

DeMusis, E.A., & Miaoulis, G. (1988). Channels of distribution and exchange concepts in health promotion. *Journal of Health Care Marketing*, **8**, 60-68.

DiClementa, C.C., Prochaska, J.A., Fairhurst, S.K., Velicer, W.F., Velasquez, M.M., & Rossi, J.F. (1991). The process of smoking cessation: An analysis of precontemplation, contemplation, and preparation stages of change. *Journal of Consulting and Clinical Psychology*, **59**, 295-304.

Dishman, R., Sallis, J.F., & Orenstein, E.R. (1985). The determinants of physical activity and exercise. *Public Health Reports*, **100**, 158-171.

Donohew, L. (1990). Public health campaigns: Individual message strategies and a model. In E.B. Ray & L. Donohew (Eds.), *Communication and health: Systems and applications* (pp. 136-152). Hillsdale, NJ: Erlbaum.

Donovan Research (1987). *A media based communication strategy to promote physical activity*. Canberra, Australia: Department of Arts, Sport, Environment, Tourism and Territories.

Donovan, R.J., Fisher, D.A., & Armstrong, B.K. (1984). "Give it away for a day": An evaluation of Western Australia's first smoke free day. *Community Health Studies*, **8**, 301-306.

Donovan, R.J., & Francas, M. (1990). Understanding communication and motivation strategies. *Australian Health Review*, **13**, 103-114.

Donovan, R.J., Jason, J., Gibbs, D., & Kroger, F. (1991). Paid advertising for AIDS prevention—Would the ends justify the means? *Public Health Reports*, **106**, 645-651.

Donovan, R.J., & Robinson, L. (1992). Using mass media in health promotion: The Western Australia immunization campaign. In R. Hall & J. Richters (Eds.), *Immunization: The old and the new*. Canberra, Australia: Public Health Association of Australia.

Egger, G., Fitzgerald, W., Frape, G., Monaem, A., Rubinstein, P., Tyler, C., & McKay, B. (1983). Results of a large scale media antismoking campaign in Australia: North Coast "Quit for Life" program. *British Medical Journal*, **287**, 1125-1128.

Farquhar, J.W., Fortmann, S.P., Flora, J.A., Taylor, C.B., Haskell, W.L., Williams, P.T., Maccoby, N., & Wood, P.D. (1990). The Stanford five city project:

Effects of community-wide education on cardiovascular risk factors. *Journal of the American Medical Association*, **264**, 359-365.

Farquhar, J.W., Fortmann, S.P., Maccoby, N., Wood, P.D., Haskell, W.L., Taylor, C.B., Flora, J.A., Solomon, D.S., Rogers, T., Adler, E., Breitrose, P., & Weiner, L. (1984). The Stanford five city project: An overview. In J.D. Matarazzo, S.M. Weiss, J.A. Herd, & N.E. Miller (Eds.), *Behavioral health: A handbook of health enhancement and disease prevention* (pp. 1154-1165). New York: Wiley.

Fine, S.H. (1990). *The marketing of ideas and social issues.* New York: Praeger.

Fox, K.F., & Kotler, P. (1980). The marketing of social causes: The first 10 years. *Journal of Marketing*, **44**, 24-33.

France, A., Donovan, R.J., Watson, C., & Leivers, S. (1991). A Chlamydia awareness campaign aimed at reducing HIV risks in young adults. *Australian Health Promotion Journal*, **1**, 19-28.

Hardman, A.E., Hudson, A., Jones, P.R.M., & Norgan, N.G. (1990). Brisk walking and plasma high density lipoprotein levels in previously sedentary women. *British Medical Journal*, **299**, 1204-1205.

Hastings, G., & Haywood, A. (1991). Social marketing and communication in health promotion. *Health Promotion International*, **6**, 135-145.

Houston, F.S., & Gassenheimer, J.B. (1987). Marketing and exchange. *Journal of Marketing*, **51**, 3-18.

Iverson, D.C., Fielding, J.E., Crow, R.S., & Christenson, G.M. (1985). The promotion of physical activity in the United States population: The status of programs in medical, worksite, school and community settings. *Public Health Reports*, **100**, 212-224.

Jeffery, R.W. (1989). Risk behaviors and health: Contrasting individual and population perspectives. *American Psychologist*, **44**, 1194-1202.

King, A.C. (1991). Community intervention to the promotion of physical activity and fitness. *Exercise and Sport Science Reviews*, **19**, 211-259.

Knapp, D.N. (1988). Behavioral management techniques and exercise promotion. In R.K. Dishman (Ed.), *Exercise adherence: Its impact on public health* (pp. 203-235). Champaign, IL: Human Kinetics.

Kotler, P. (1988). *Marketing management: Analysis, planning, implementation and control.* Englewood Cliffs, NJ: Prentice Hall.

Kotler, P. (1989). *Principles of marketing.* Englewood Cliffs, NJ: Prentice Hall.

Kotler, P., & Andreasen, A.R. (1987). *Strategic marketing for nonprofit organizations.* Englewood Cliffs, NJ: Prentice Hall.

Kotler, P., & Roberto, E.L. (1989). *Social marketing: Strategies for changing public behavior.* New York: Free Press.

Kotler, P., & Zaltman, G. (1971). Social marketing: An approach to planned social change. *Journal of Marketing*, **35**, 3-12.

Lancaster, K.J. (1966). A new approach to consumer theory. *Journal of Political Economy*, **14**, 132-157.

Lancaster, W., McIlwain, T., & Lancaster, J. (1983). Health marketing: Implications for health promotion. *Family and Community Health*, **5**, 41-51.

Lee, C., & Owen, N. (1986a). Exercise persistence: Contributions of psychological theory to the promotion of regular physical activity. *Australian Psychologist*, **21**, 427-466.

Lee, C., & Owen, N. (1986b). Uses of psychological theories on understanding the adoption and maintenance of exercising. *Australian Journal of Science and Medicine in Sport*, **18**, 22-25.

Lefebvre, R.C., & Flora, J.A. (1988). Social marketing and public health intervention. *Health Education Quarterly*, **15**, 299-315.

Levitt, T. (1960, July-August). Marketing myopia. *Harvard Business Review*, pp. 45-56.

Levitt, T. (1969). *The marketing mode*. New York: McGraw-Hill.

Lunn, T. (1986). Segmenting and constructing markets. In R.M. Worcester & J. Downham (Eds.), *Consumer market research handbook* (pp. 287-424). Amsterdam, Netherlands: North Holland.

Manoff, R.K. (1985). *Social marketing: New imperative for public health*. New York: Praeger.

Marcus, B., & Owen, N. (1992). Motivational readiness, self-efficacy, and decision-making for exercise. *Journal of Applied Social Psychology*, **22**, 3-16.

McGuire, W.J. (1986). The myth of massive media impact: Savagings and salvagings. In G. Comstock (Ed.), *Public communication and behavior* (Vol. 1, pp. 173-257). Orlando, FL: Academic Press.

McGuire, W.J. (1988). Theoretical foundations of campaigns. In R.E. Rice & C.K. Atkin (Eds.), *Public communication campaigns* (pp. 43-65). Newbury Park, CA: Sage.

Morris, N.N. (1990). Inequalities in health: Ten years and a little further on. *The Lancet*, **336**, 491-493.

National Center for Health Statistics. (1989). *Assessing physical fitness and physical activity in population-based surveys* (DHSS Publication No. 89-1253). Washington, DC: U.S. Government Printing Office.

Nicholas, H., Glover, L., Parr, D., Leonard, P., & Miller, D. (1987). *The effect of a government AIDS media campaign on a general population: Antibody test requests and reasons*. Paper presented at the Third International Conference on AIDS, Washington, DC.

Novelli, W.D. (1990). Applying social marketing to health promotion and disease prevention. In K. Glanz, F.M. Lewis, & B.K. Rimer (Eds.), *Health behavior and health education: Theory, research and practice* (pp. 342-369). San Francisco: Jossey-Bass.

Oldenburg, B., Bauman, A., Booth, M., & Owen, N. (1991). Increasing levels of physical activity in the Australian community. *Health Promotion Journal of Australia*, **1**, 15-18.

Owen, N. (1989). Behavioral epidemiology research and intervention studies to improve smoking-cessation services. *Health Education Research*, **4**, 145-153.

Owen, N., & Bauman, A. (1992). The descriptive epidemiology of physical inactivity in adult Australians. *International Journal of Epidemiology*, **21**, 305-310.

Owen, N., & Davies, M.J. (1990). Smokers' preferences for assistance with cessation. *Preventive Medicine*, **19**, 424-431.

Owen, N., & Dwyer, T. (1988). Approaches to promoting more widespread participation in physical activity. *Community Health Studies*, **12**, 339-347.

Owen, N., & Lee, C. (1984). *Why people do and do not exercise*. Adelaide, Australia: South Australian Department of Recreation and Sport.

Owen, N., & Lee, C. (1989). Development of behaviorally-based policy guidelines for the promotion of exercise. *Journal of Public Health Policy*, **10**, 43-61.

Owen, N., Lee, C., Naccarella, L., & Haag, K. (1987). Exercise by mail: A mediated behavior-change program for aerobic exercise. *Journal of Sport Psychology*, **9**, 346-357.

Owen, N., Wakefield, M., Roberts, L., & Esterman, A. (1992). Stages of readiness to quit smoking: Population prevalence and correlates. *Health Psychology*, **11**, 413-417.

Pierce, J.P., Dwyer, T., Chamberlain, A., Aldrich, R.N., & Shelley, J. (1987). Targeting the smoker in an antismoking campaign. *Preventive Medicine*, **16**, 816-824.

Piercy, N. (1991). *Market-led strategic change*. London: Thorsons.

Powell, K.E., Stephens, T., Marti, B., Heinemann, L., & Kreuter, M. (1990, June). *Progress and problems in the promotion of physical activity*. Paper presented at the World Congress on Sport for All, Tampere, Finland.

Pride, W.M., & Ferrell, O.C. (1980). *Marketing: Basic concepts and decisions*. Boston: Houghton Mifflin.

Prochaska, J.O. (1991). Assessing how people change. *Cancer*, **67**, 805-808.

Puska, P., Nissinen, A., Tuomilehto, J., Salonen, J.T., McAlister, A., Kottke, T.E., Maccoby, N., & Farquhar, J.W. (1985). The community-based strategy to prevent coronary heart disease: Conclusions from ten years of the North Karelia project. *Annual Review of Public Health*, **6**, 147-193.

Redman, S., Spencer, E.A., & Sanson-Fisher, R.W. (1990). The role of mass media in changing health related behavior: A critical appraisal of two models. *Health Promotion International*, **5**, 85-102.

Rice, R.E., & Atkin, C.K. (Eds.) (1989). *Public communication campaigns*. Newbury Park, CA: Sage.

Rose, G. (1985). Sick individuals and sick populations. *International Journal of Epidemiology*, **14**, 32-38.

Rossiter, J.R. (1989). Market segmentation: A review and proposed resolution. *Australian Marketing Researcher*, **11**, 36-58.

Rossiter, J.R., & Percy, L. (1987). *Advertising and promotion management*. New York: McGraw-Hill.

Rossiter, J.R., Percy, L., & Donovan, R.J. (1984). The advertising plan and advertising communication models. *Australian Marketing Researcher*, **11**, 36-58.

Rothschild, M.L. (1979). Marketing communications in non-business situations or why it's so hard to sell brotherhood like soap. *Journal of Marketing*, **43**, 11-20.

Sheth, J.N., & Frazier, G.L. (1982). A model of strategy mix choice for planned social change. *Journal of Marketing*, **46**, 15-26.

Singhal, A., & Rogers, E.M. (1990). Prosocial television for development in India. In R.E. Rice & C.K. Atkin (Eds.), *Public communication campaigns* (pp. 331-350). Newbury Park, CA: Sage.

Sirgy, M.J., Morris, M., & Samli, A.C. (1985). The question of value in social marketing: Use of a quality-of-life theory to achieve long-term satisfaction. *American Journal of Economics and Sociology*, **44**, 215-228.

Slater, M.D., & Flora, J.A. (1989). Health lifestyles: Audience segmentation analysis for public health interventions. *Health Education Quarterly*, **18**, 221-233.

Solomon, D.S. (1989). A social marketing perspective on communication campaigns. In R.E. Rice & C.K. Atkin (Eds.), *Public communication campaigns* (pp. 87-104). Newbury Park, CA: Sage.

Stephens, T. (1987). Secular trends in adult physical activity: Exercise boom or bust? *Research Quarterly for Exercise and Sport*, **58**, 94-105.

Stephens, T., Jacobs, D.R., & White, C.C. (1985). The descriptive epidemiology of leisure-time physical activity. *Public Health Reports*, **100**, 47-158.

Taylor, C.B., & Owen, N. (1989). Behavioral medicine: Research and development in disease prevention. *Behavior Change*, **6**, 3-11.

Wallack, L. (1983). Social marketing as prevention: Uncovering some critical assumptions. In T.C. Kinnear (Ed.), *Advances in consumer research* (Vol. 2, pp. 682-687). Chicago: Association for Consumer Research.

Wallack, L. (1990). Media advocacy: Promoting health through mass communication. In K. Glanz, F.M. Lewis, & B.K. Rimer (Eds.), *Health behavior and health education: Theory, research and practice* (pp. 370-386). San Francisco: Jossey-Bass.

Wiebe, G. (1952). Merchandising commodities and citizenship on television. *Public Opinion Quarterly*, **15**, 679-691.

Winett, R.A., King, A.C., & Altman, D.G. (1990). Extending applications of behavior therapy to large-scale intervention. In P.R. Martin (Ed.), *Handbook of behavior therapy and psychological science: An integrative approach* (pp. 473-490). Elmsford, NY: Pergamon Press.

Young, E. (1989). *Social marketing in the information era.* Paper presented at the American Marketing Association Conference, Ottawa, ON.

PART IV

Special Applications

CHAPTER *11*

The Natural History of Physical Activity and Aerobic Fitness in Teenagers

Han C.G. Kemper

It has long been recognized that physical activity is an important consideration during children's growing years to maintain normal growth and development (Bar-Or, 1983). Children are generally thought to be naturally physically active, but in recent years their activity levels have been a subject of great concern to health officials. Until a generation ago, physical activity was a natural part of life for most children. This is no longer so, and professionals are asking whether children and adolescents now get the physical activity required for healthy development.

The necessity for daily physical activity has been greatly reduced because of the mechanization and automation of work and leisure. Physical activity now depends on such factors as body build, physical fitness, and the availability of recreational and sport facilities. Physical inactivity is an important risk factor for coronary heart disease (CHD), and atherosclerosis starts soon after birth (Montoye, 1985). Many researchers have suggested that a sufficient amount and intensity of regular physical activity could decelerate this process (Powell, Thompson, Caspersen, & Kendrick, 1987). But an epidemiological prospective study, comparing many physically active children with a randomized group of less-active children over a long period, has never been conducted and apparently cannot be carried out (Mednick & Baert, 1981). There is also unfortunately no possibility of a double-blind study to measure the effects of physical activity. One way out of this difficulty is to measure the natural history of habitual physical activity in children longitudinally and to group individuals afterward according to registered activity patterns (Mirwald, Bailey, Cameron, & Rasmussen, 1981; Rutenfranz, Berndt, & Knauth, 1974; Rutenfranz et al., 1975; Sprynarova, 1974). Another possibility is to set up an experimental longitudinal study like the Canadian one in the Trois Rivières region (Jéquier et al., 1977), in which the effect of classes given additional physical education was compared with that of control classes over a couple of school years.

In the course of body growth and development come critical periods that determine whether individuals will later lead physically active lives (Masironi & Denolin, 1985):

- From ages 4 to 12, children first go to school and lose a considerable amount of play time.
- At age 12 children enter secondary school, with further restriction of free time by homework.
- At age 15 or 16 teenagers in European countries shift from bicycles to motorcycles, while teens in the U.S. shift from bicycles to automobiles.
- From age 18 young people further change to automobiles.

The consequences of such facts for the development of physical activity in children was illustrated by Rowland (1990), who showed the change in total daily energy expenditure (Figure 11.1). The total daily energy expenditure per kilogram of body weight (kcal/kg) diminishes rapidly between 6 and 14 years of age. The decrease is almost 50% in both boys and girls. In the same figure it can also be seen that boys are more active than girls at all ages; the difference is about 10%. During these growing years lifestyle seems to change considerably and thus perspectives on activity also change.

In this chapter I review the developmental changes in physical activity and aerobic fitness of boys and girls during the teenage period. I also present the

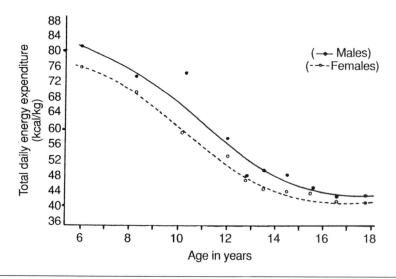

Figure 11.1   Total daily energy expenditure of boys and girls between ages 6 and 18. Reprinted from Rowland (1990).

results of a Dutch longitudinal study in which maximal aerobic power and habitual physical activity have been measured simultaneously (Kemper et al., 1985; Kemper, Snel, Verschuur, & Storm-vanEssen, 1990; Kemper & Verschuur, 1990).

Evaluating the natural history of physical activity and aerobic fitness in children requires valid and accurate measurement methods (Kemper, Verschuur, & deMey, 1989). The aerobic fitness of children can be measured by a maximal exercise test performed on a bicycle ergometer or treadmill. The maximal oxygen uptake ($\dot{V}O_2$max) is generally accepted as a valid and reliable method for measuring state of and change in aerobic fitness in both adults and children.

Daily physical activity however, is a difficult lifestyle parameter to measure because typically the measurement itself interferes with the normal physical-activity pattern of the child. Also, children's activities change from day to day and week to week, and they also depend strongly on seasonal influences.

From a physiological point of view, physical activities can be measured by energy expenditure. The methods adopted should meet at least four criteria. They should be

1. socially acceptable and interfere minimally with normal daily activity,
2. applicable over at least 24 hr in order to include school and leisure activities,
3. valid with respect to measurements of energy expenditure as the gold standard, and
4. acceptable in financial cost.

Available methods include measurements of oxygen uptake and heart rate (Åstrand & Rodahl, 1986), the use of doubly labeled water (Livingstone et al., 1990) and movement counters (Stunkard, 1960), and records of the intensity, duration, and frequency of exercise from diaries or questionnaires (Montoye & Taylor, 1984). The characteristics of the different methods with respect to these criteria are summarized in Table 11.1.

Data from the Amsterdam Growth and Health Study are used to illustrate different methods of measuring physical activity longitudinally in teenage boys and girls aged 12 to 21 years. This study started in 1976 with yearly measurements until 1980 and was continued with repeated measurements in 1985 and 1991 (Kemper, 1985). In this chapter I pay special attention to the problems of analyzing longitudinal data and to the effects that can interfere with the natural history. I conclude the chapter with an analysis of the relationship between the level of habitual physical activity (the independent variable) and maximal aerobic power (the dependent variable) (Kemper, 1985, 1986, 1991).

Table 11.1   Evaluation of Various Methods of Physical-Activity Measurement According to Four Criteria

Methods	Social acceptability	Applicability over 24 hr	Validity relative to energy expenditure	Financial cost
Measurements				
Oxygen uptake	X	X	XXX	X
Heart rate	XX	XX	XX	XX
Movement counters	XXX	XXX	X	XXX
Doubly labeled water	XXX	XXX	XXX	X
Self-reports				
Diary	XX	XX	XX	XXX
Questionnaire	XX	XXX	X	XX

Note. X = worst; XXX = best.

Analyzing Natural History From Longitudinal Data

In studies of growth and development, three classic designs have been widely used, namely, cross-sectional, time lag, and longitudinal (see Figure 11.2). In such studies each measurement taken on a subject at a particular moment is influenced by three factors:

1. Age of the subject, defined as the time between birth and time of measurement. Age effects produce the mean growth curve.
2. Birth cohort to which the subject belongs, which refers to the group of individuals born in the same year. Cohort effects can be used in studying secular trends.
3. Time of measurement is the moment at which the measurement is taken. Time of measurement effects have to do with changes in environmental conditions over a period of time (such as changes in methods of measurement).

These designs do not allow the three effects (age, time of measurement, and cohort) to be isolated (Schaie, 1965).

Multiple Longitudinal Design

The literature includes descriptions of several designs that attempt to address the problem of confounding effects (Kowalski & Prahl-Andersen, 1979; Rao & Rao,

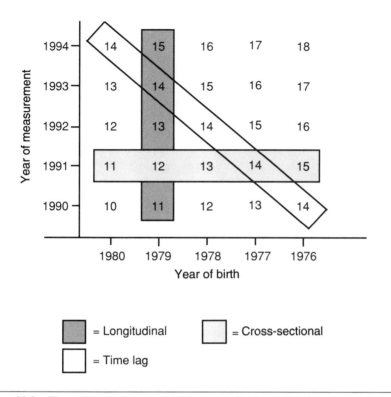

Figure 11.2   Three class designs graphed by year of subjects' birth and year of measurement. The resulting ages (in years) of the groups are plotted.

1966; Tanner, 1962). The design of the Amsterdam Growth and Health Study is multiple longitudinal, meaning that repeated measurements are taken on more than one cohort (Kemper & Hof, 1978), which has the advantage of isolating the main effect, for example, age effect, from interfering effects, such as time of measurement and cohort effects.

Cluster Effects

The first measurements were taken during 4 successive years, from 1976 to 1979. Original measurements were obtained for children from the first and second forms of a secondary school in Amsterdam. The two groups are referred to as clusters. The clusters were composed of children with an average age of 13 (C1) and 14 (C2) years in 1976 (see Figure 11.3). During the course of the study the composition of these clusters remained the same. Pupils who stayed in a class for a second year remained members of their original cluster. Because there were four times of measurement of two longitudinal studies conducted in parallel with a lag of one year in subjects' age, the study covered five age groups. Because

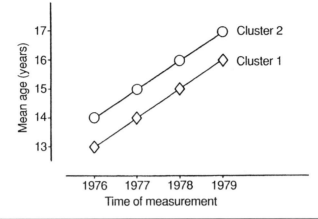

Figure 11.3   The multiple longitudinal study's design used two clusters.

of this overlap in ages, the two clusters can be compared with each other at three ages. A systematic difference between the two clusters at these three ages was called a cluster effect.

Time of Measurement Effects

It was possible to distinguish one of the interfering factors of a longitudinal study, namely, time of measurement (Veling & Hof, 1980). For example, 14-year-olds were measured in 1976 (C2) as well as in 1977 (C1). If no cluster effect was found, the time of measurement was blamed for a possible difference between the two groups. If no time of measurement or cluster effect appeared, the data were arranged in age groups, and a 5-year development pattern in a period of 4 years (Bell, 1954) could be estimated.

Testing or Learning Effects

Another problem that occurs with repeated measurements is that of a testing or learning effect. The measurement of many variables, physical as well as psychological, can bring about a change in motivation or habituation of the subject. This introduces differences between measurements that are solely due to changes in attitude toward the measurement procedure. Such testing effects may be positive (e.g., when habituation or learning is important) or negative (e.g., when motivation decreases). Repeated measurements may therefore have a disturbing influence on the quantity measured and diminish the external validity of the results.

Systematic testing effects can be estimated if the design also includes a control group in which repeated measurements are not made. In this study an identical cluster arrangement was made at a second school comparable with the first, but during the first 4 years of the study a different quarter of the pupils was measured every time (Figure 11.4). These measurements were comparable with those taken at the first school, except that they were not repeat measurements but came from independent samples. When one compares data from both schools, systematic divergence of mean values may be attributed to a testing effect.

Cluster effect, time of measurement effect, and testing effect—if established for a certain characteristic—will hinder the interpretation of individual and mean growth curves and thus the natural history of physical activity. When these effects were not found, the data were averaged and arranged according to age groups to facilitate the study of the development of children, irrespective of cluster and time of measurement.

Tails of the Mean Age Curve

The average age curve of, for example, the sum of four skinfolds (Figure 11.5) was more accurate in the middle part (ages 14 and 15) because observations of all three cohorts were available. The tails of the curve (ages 12 and 17), however, were estimates based on only a small group of children from one cohort. If, for example, the youngest members of the oldest groups deviated from the norm, it influenced the average age curve. To avoid misinterpretation, plots were made of the mean values of each cohort, and the cohorts were inspected for any typical deviations at the tails that could influence the developmental curves substantially.

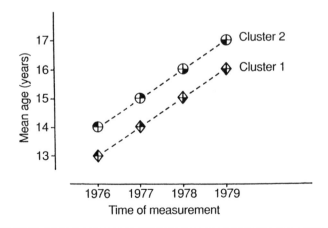

Figure 11.4   The study's control group consisted of two clusters and eight groups who were independently observed.

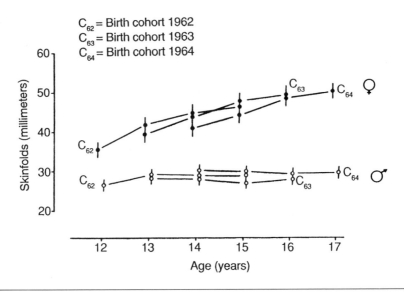

Figure 11.5   The tails of the average age curve are based on the data of only one cohort.
Reprinted from Storm-van Essen et al. (1985).

Individual Growth

The purpose of longitudinal studies is to investigate individual changes over time. This becomes difficult when the stochastic measurement error exceeds the change in time. The degree to which this affects a variable may be studied on the basis of interperiod correlation matrices (Veling & Hof, 1980). The interperiod correlation (IPC) is a coefficient of correlation between two periods of measurement for the variable. Hof and Kowalski (1979) have shown that under fairly realistic conditions, IPCs can be approximated by a linear function of the time interval (Figure 11.6). The intercept of the straight line is the correlation coefficient between two (independent) measurements (having an intermediate time interval equal to zero) and may be interpreted as the instantaneous measurement-remeasurement reproducibility. Therefore, it is a measure of the reliability of the measurement in question. The slope of the line or the decay in correlation per yearly time interval gives an impression of the interindividual change over time for the measurement in question. The ideal IPC matrix shows a line with an intercept of about 1.

Dropouts

The children studied were from two secondary schools in Amsterdam and Purmerend (a suburb of Amsterdam). The school in Purmerend (Ignatius College) served

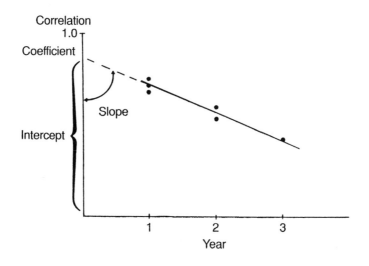

Figure 11.6   A plot of the interperiod correlation coefficients of a variable.

as a control school and was measured only between 1976 and 1977 and 1979 and 1980. The population of the longitudinal school (City College) in Amsterdam comprised 307 pupils in 1976 and 1977. During the first 4 years of the study a number of pupils withdrew from the sample. The main reason for withdrawal was leaving school. Because of the chance of selective dropout, this group was compared with the group of pupils who stayed in the sample for 4 years. We made this comparison on the basis of measurements from the 1st year (1976-1977) and used univariate or multivariate t-tests.

The fifth and sixth measurements of the longitudinal group were made in 1985 and 1991. The numbers of males and females who participated in the study and the percentage who dropped out are indicated in Table 11.2.

Methods

Here I describe the methods used to measure the subjects' aerobic fitness and physical activity. All measurements were performed in a mobile laboratory placed near the subjects' schools.

Maximal Aerobic Power

Maximal aerobic power was used as a valid measure of the subjects' aerobic fitness. Maximal aerobic power ($\dot{V}O_2max$) was measured directly, using a running test on a treadmill. Before the test, subjects were familiarized with the test procedure and warmed up during a 6-min submaximal treadmill run at a speed

Table 11.2 Number of Subjects (Male and Female) Who Stayed in the Longitudinal Study During Three Periods of Measurement and Number and Percentages of Dropouts

Measurement period	Females		Males		Total	
1977	159		148		307	
1980	131		102		233	
Dropouts 1977-80	28	(18%)	46	(31%)	74	(24%)
1985	107		93		200	
Dropouts 1980-85	24	(22%)	9	(10%)	33	(16%)
1991	100		82		182	
Dropouts 1985-91	3	(3%)	15	(18%)	18	(10%)
Total dropouts 1977-91	59	(37%)	56	(38%)	115	(37%)

of 8 km/hr. Every 2 min during the maximal test, the grade of the treadmill was increased by 2.5% or 5%, depending on the pupil's heart rate while running at 8 km/hr. The test was continued until pupils reached exhaustion (Kemper & Verschuur, 1980). To confirm their exhaustion, we used three criteria: a plateau in oxygen uptake, calculated as an increase of less than 150 ml per 2-min period; a heart rate that exceeded 90% of the maximal heart rate according to age; and a mean respiratory exchange ratio (RER) of more than 1.0 during the last minute (Kemper & Verschuur, 1987).

The subjects' oxygen uptake ($\dot{V}O_2$) was analyzed throughout the tests by the open-circuit technique, with the expired volume measured by a dry gas meter (Parkinson-Cowan, CD 4, Canada) and a two-way low-resistance breathing valve with a dead space of 35 ml. Samples of mixed expired air were analyzed for O_2 by a paramagnetic analyzer (Servomex, United Kingdom) and for CO_2 by an infrared analyzer (Mijnhardt, Netherlands). The accuracy of $\dot{V}O_2$max measurement with this system is comparable to that obtained from the classic method of collecting expired air in Douglas bags and analyzing it with the Scholander technique (Kemper, Binkhorst, Verschuur, & Vissers, 1976). Throughout the study, the exercise tests were supervised by the same research workers in the same mobile laboratory with the same equipment to minimize measurer influences on the results.

Physical Activity

Methods selected to measure physical activity should not interfere with a person's normal activity pattern and should obtain an estimate of the energy expenditure, which also reflects the intensity of the activity (Seliger, 1966). To give the researcher an impression of the daily activity pattern, the measurements should include school or work and leisure activities and should be applicable for at least 24 hr, all days of the week, and all seasons of the year (Edholm, 1966). In large group studies such as this one, the method must also be simple, cheap, and time efficient. These requirements and our need to limit the extent of the activity measurements because we used so many other variables led us to select three methods:

1. The eight-level heart-rate integrator (HRI), which has proved to be a reliable and simple method for recording heart rate (HR) (Saris, Snel, & Binkhorst, 1977; Verschuur & Kemper, 1985)
2. The pedometer, which was reduced in sensitivity (Verschuur & Kemper, 1980) in order to give a more reliable measurement of energy expenditure by only counting large movements (such as running) rather than small movements (such as walking)
3. A questionnaire-interview developed for this study, that aimed to trace activities with a minimal energy expenditure of four times the basal metabolic rate (4 METs) for 3 months before the interview

The three methods were applied once a year in winter (January through March). Physical activities during 2 randomly selected weekdays (approximately 48 hr) were measured simultaneously, using the HRI and the pedometer. The pedometer was also used to measure weekend activities, from Friday afternoon until Monday morning just before school started. The activity questionnaire was given during interviews that took place in the mobile laboratory, placed near the school.

Heart-Rate Integrator

The eight-level heart-rate integrator (Depex, De Bilt, the Netherlands) (Saris et al., 1977) is an electronic system about the size of a pack of cigarettes. Each R-R interval is measured by two chest electrodes and analyzed and stored in one of the eight registers of the integrator, which correspond to 40 to 69, 70 to 99, 100 to 124, 125 to 149, 150 to 176, 177 to 199, 200 to 224, and 225 to 300 beats/min. The eighth register range (225-300 beats/min) is used as a quality control of the ECG transmission and stores erroneous signals. The HRI was worn under subjects' clothes on a flannel belt around the waist (Figure 11.7). A readout unit (Depex, De Bilt, the Netherlands) gives the total number of beats counted in each register.

In order to transfer HR into aerobic energy expenditure, we determined the relationship between HR and oxygen uptake, which is linear between a HR of 110 to 120 and 170 to 180 beats/min (Åstrand & Rodahl, 1986), from the subjects' submaximal treadmill tests. The HR and oxygen uptake in steady state during running (8 km/hr) was measured at grades of 0, 2.5%, and 5%.

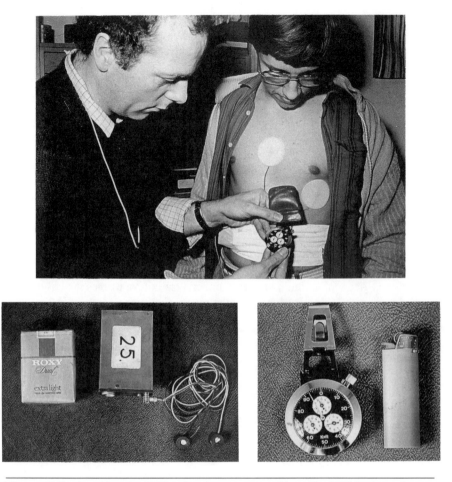

Figure 11.7   Attaching the HRI and pedometer to a subject. The HRI is about the size of a pack of cigarettes, the pedometer about the size of a lighter.

Pedometer

The pedometer (Kaspar & Richter, model 123, FRG, the Netherlands) measures vertical displacement. Attached to the body, it registers all movement of the center of gravity. Before application, we tested its accuracy (Kemper & Verschuur, 1977) and reduced its sensitivity so that it would start counting at a walking speed of 8 km/hr or more, a jogging pace, and would not register passive body movements such as riding in a car driving over a bumpy road (Verschuur & Kemper, 1980). The pedometer was worn in a leather cover and hung from the inside of the pupil's waistband (Figure 11.7). The activity score on the pedometer was the number of vertical displacements counted. The scores of 2 weekdays and 1 weekend were used.

The Activity Interview

The standardized activity interview covered the previous three months and was based on a questionnaire developed for this study. It was given by the same interviewer throughout the study. In order to classify the activities according to their energy cost, independent of body weight, we used the ratio between the work metabolic rate and the basal metabolic rate (1 MET; Andersen, 1971; Reiff et al., 1967). The interview was limited to activities with a minimal intensity level of approximately four times the basal metabolic rate (≥ 4 METs), which equals walking at a speed of approximately 5 km/hr. Below this level of intensity, physical activity will hardly contribute to a reasonable level of physical fitness. The scored activities were subdivided into three levels of intensity (light, medium to heavy, and heavy) in accordance with the three highest activity levels used by the World Health Organization (WHO; Andersen, 1971). They correspond to a relative energy expenditure of 4 to 7 METs for light activity, 7 to 10 METs for medium to heavy intensity activity, and 10 or more METs for heavy activity. The classification of activities into the three intensity levels was based on data from the literature (Andersen, 1971; Bink, Bonjer, & Sluys, 1966; Durnin & Passmore, 1967; Hollmann & Hettinger, 1976; Reiff et al., 1967; Seliger, 1966).

The interview gathered information on the average weekly time spent during the previous three months in each of the three activity categories, with a minimum of 5 min (Table 11.3). In addition, the active time for the total of these three categories was calculated. The energy expenditure per week above 4 METs, expressed as multiples of the basal metabolic rate (METs/week), was estimated by multiplying the time spent per level of intensity by a fixed value for the relative energy expenditure at that level—for example, 5.5 METs for light activity, 8.5 for medium to heavy, and 11.5 for heavy. The scores for the three levels were added, yielding a total METs/week score, a weighted activity score combining duration and intensity.

Interfering Effects

Inspections of the data on aerobic power and the three physical-activity measurements were conducted over the 4 measurement years between 1976 and 1980. Table 11.4 gives an overview of the interfering effects that appeared during this period. The measurement of $\dot{V}O_2max$ shows no interfering effect. The activity measurements (the pedometer week score) showed a significant time of measurement effect, illustrated in Figure 11.8. Although there is a general trend of lower mean week scores with increasing age of the three longitudinal cohorts and the control groups, this is not the case in all groups during the 2nd year of measurement (1978).

A possible explanation is provided by climatic conditions during the winter of 1978. In that year there was a longer period of frozen waters, so these Dutch youngsters were able to spend more time at their national sport, ice-skating.

Table 11.3 Classification of Sports and Leisure Activities Into Four Categories on the Basis of Average Intensity

Intensity	Activity	
Very light	Domestic:	Dish washing, dusting, floor sweeping
	Outdoor:	Sitting, standing, strolling
≤ 4 METs	Sport:	Billiards, bowling, bridge, checkers, chess, cricket, fishing, gliding, golf, sailing, shooting, skittle, t'ai chi ch'uan
Light	Domestic:	Beating carpets, carrying groceries, hammering, polishing floors, sawing, scrubbing floors
	Outdoor:	Bicycling, canoeing, rowing, walking
4-7 METs	Sport:	Ballet, baseball, bodybuilding, dancing (ballroom, modern, folk), gymnastics (rhythmic, remedial), hiking, horseback riding, softball, table tennis, tug of war, volleyball, waterskiing, weightlifting
Medium to heavy	Domestic:	Stair climbing
	Outdoor:	Basketball (dribbling, shooting), swimming
7-10 METs	Sport:	Badminton, fencing, gymnastics, mountaineering, scuba-diving, skating (figure, speed), skiing (alpine), tennis (outdoor or indoor) track and field (field event)
Heavy	Outdoor:	Basketball (game), running, soccer (game)
≥ 10 METs	Sport:	Basketball, canoeing, conditioning exercises, cycling (race), handball (European, indoor or outdoor), hockey (field, indoor or outdoor, ice, roller), jogging, kick boxing, netball (indoor or outdoor), martial arts (judo, jujitsu, karate, aikido, kendo, kung fu, tae kwon do), rowing, rugby, skiing (cross-country), soccer (indoor or outdoor), squash, swimming, track and field (track event), trampolining, water polo, wrestling

Note. Outdoor = unorganized recreational activity; Sport = activity in sports clubs.

The total time spent on physical activity, measured by the interview, revealed both a testing and a dropout effect. A testing effect was seen upon comparison of the longitudinal boys' total activity time per week spent above an intensity of 4 METs with that of control school boys (Figure 11.9). At age 12 to 13 the scores of the control group equal those of the longitudinal group. Thereafter they show a slight increase in the former and a decrease in the latter. In addition, it appeared that in girls the dropouts were significantly more active than the longitudinal group. Since the HRI and pedometer were applied only during a short period of time and were selected to be used only on a group level, the interperiod correlations are not applicable to these methods (see Table 11.4).

Table 11.4   Variables That Showed Interfering Effects in Boys and Girls During the First 4 Years of the Study

Interfering effects	$\dot{V}O_2$max		Pedometer		Heart-rate integrator		Activity interview	
	Boys	Girls	Boys	Girls	Boys	Girls	Boys	Girls
Time of measurement	−	−	+	+	−	−	−	−
Cohort	−	−	−	−	−	−	−	−
Testing	−	−	−	−	−	−	+	−
Dropout	−	−	−	−	−	−	−	+
Interperiod correlation	−	−	n.a.	n.a.	n.a.	n.a.	−	−

Note. − = no interfering effect; + = interfering effect; n.a. = not applicable.

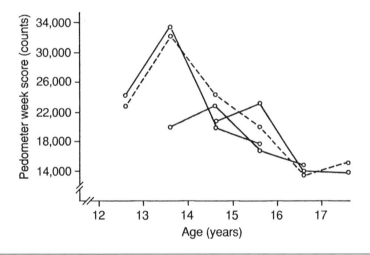

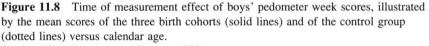

Figure 11.8   Time of measurement effect of boys' pedometer week scores, illustrated by the mean scores of the three birth cohorts (solid lines) and of the control group (dotted lines) versus calendar age.
Reprinted from Verschuur and Kemper (1985).

That interfering effects are revealed must be taken into account in interpreting the results of the age changes of physical activity in teenagers.

Results

Physical Activity Measured From HRI and Pedometers

In both girls and boys daily physical activity decreases from 12 to 17 years of age. This is the case in daily energy expenditure calculated as kJ per kg body

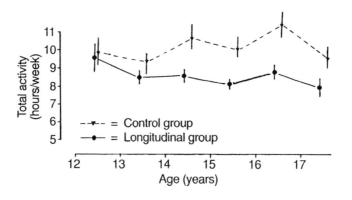

Figure 11.9   Mean and standard error of the total activity time per week spent above an intensity of 4 METs in longitudinal group boys (solid line) and control group girls (dotted line) versus calendar age.

mass from HRI (Figure 11.10) and calculated as week scores from pedometers (Figure 11.11). In girls the decrease is 23% in HRI scores and 52% in pedometer scores; in boys, 17% and 44%, respectively. Boys are significantly more active than girls before puberty (ages 13 and 14), but after puberty the differences become smaller.

When one takes the peak energy expenditure from the HRI by calculating the energy expenditure above 50% of $\dot{V}O_2$max, the rate of decrease with age is much faster (Figure 11.12) and the differences between boys and girls postpuberty is no longer significant.

Physical Activity Measured From Interview

The activity interview covered three areas of physical activity:

1. Activities in relation to school (including transportation, physical education)
2. Organized activities (memberships in sport clubs)
3. Unorganized activities (playing outdoors and leisure-time jobs)

1. School activities determine 50% of activity time in girls and 45% in boys, and these percentages do not change with age although total activity time is declining. Youngsters are physically active in going to and from school: At age 12 to 13, 70% to 80% go to school by bicycle and 10% by foot. A minority of boys and girls change to mopeds after age 16—3% of girls and 15% to 20% of the boys.

2. Only 15% to 20% of girls and boys' activities take place in sport clubs. A cross-sectional classification of sport participation in girls showed a decrease

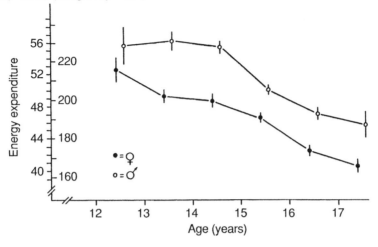

Figure 11.10   Mean and standard error of the energy expenditure calculated as kJ per kg body mass from heart rate in boys and girls versus calendar age.
Reprinted from Verschuur and Kemper (1985).

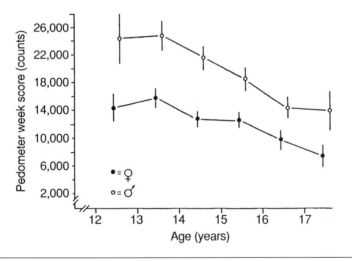

Figure 11.11   Mean and standard error of week scores measured from pedometers in boys and girls versus calendar age.
Reprinted from Verschuur and Kemper (1985).

from 61% to 44% between ages 13 and 17. In boys sport participation varied little over the same age period (55%-60%; Verschuur, 1987). These results are comparable with those of Backx, Erich, Kemper, and Verbeek (1989), who measured a rate of club membership in Dutch 8- to 16-year-olds of between 59%

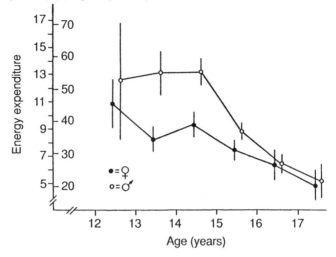

(kcal/kg body mass) (kJ/kg body mass)

Figure 11.12   Mean and standard error of energy expenditure above 50% $\dot{V}O_2$max from heart rate in boys and girls versus calendar age.
Reprinted from Verschuur and Kemper (1985).

and 75%. The highest participation rate was at age 10 (75%) and the lowest at age 15 (59%). A longitudinal analysis during the school years was used to indicate the stability of participation in sports. Approximately 25% of the teenagers were never members of a sport club. Only 30% of the girls and 40% of the boys played sports in a club during all 4 years of the study. Soccer was the most popular sport (30%-40%) in boys. Girls preferred dance and ballet (10%-15%).

3. Unorganized activities represent approximately 35% of girls' activity and 40% of boys'. In both girls and boys the total time spent on unorganized outdoor activities decreased by 50%. This decline, caused by a shift with age from playing games in the streets to shopping and dancing, is the most important change in these youngsters during their teens.

Subjects were given the activity interview four times between ages 13 and 17 and once again at age 21. In both girls and boys the same trend continues: From early teens to early twenties, subjects reduce their medium to heavy (7-10 METs) and heavy ($\geq$ 10 METs) activities. Only light activities (4-7 METs) increase with age.

The total activity score (Figure 11.13), measured as a weighted score of the duration and intensity of the activities, shows a rapid decrease between ages 13 and 17 in both boys and girls and thereafter a gradual decline till age 21. At all ages females are less active than males, but in young adulthood the differences are smaller and not significant.

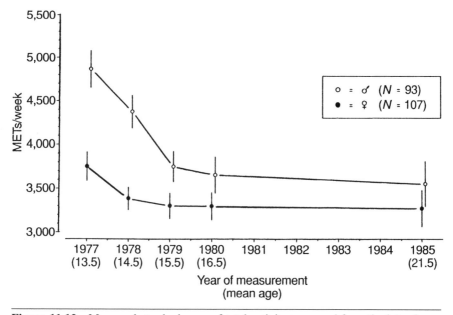

Figure 11.13   Mean and standard error of total activity measured from the interview as a weighted score of duration (min) and intensity (METs) of males' and females' activities versus calendar age.

Interrelation Between the Three Activity Methods

The three activity instruments indicate without exception a gradual decrease in habitual physical activity between ages 13 and 17 in both boys and girls. The extent of the decrease, however, depends on the method used. The pedometer week score shows the steepest decline (45%-50%), followed by the total time spent on activity per week as indicated by the interview (15%-20%). The daily energy expenditure (per kg body mass) from HRI decreases only slightly over the same age range (10%-15%).

These differences can be better understood if one realizes that all three instruments measured physical activity at different levels of intensity: HRI measures all daily activities, including sleep. The interview disregards very light activities and starts at 4 METs (walking). The pedometer, on the other hand, records only running (≥ 8 km/hr). Thus, the more the method records the heavier forms of physical activity, the more pronounced the decrease in daily activity. Moreover, the information gathered from the three activity methods overlaps only in part: The HRI and pedometer methods measure the activities of each individual during a relative short period of time. This time (2-4 days) is supposed to be representative of the whole year's activity. The activity interview is a method that looks back over the previous three months but is also more general, and the results are more dependent on the memory of the subject.

Table 11.5 presents Pearson correlation coefficients between the activity scores obtained from the same subjects by the three instruments. The correlations in

Table 11.5 Pearson Correlations Between the Three Activity Instruments

	HRI	Pedometer	Interview
Total energy week score from HRI	♀	.17	.16
Total week score from pedometer	.16		.20
Total weighted activity from interview	.18	.20	♂

Note. Mean values are for 4 years of measurement. Values of boys are in the lower right triangle, values of girls are in the upper left triangle.
Adapted from Kemper (1992).

boys and girls, averaged over the 4 school years, range between .16 and .20. These values are significant ($p < 0.05$) but explain only a small part of the total variation. These findings illustrate that it is not possible to use only one of the three methods and that a combination of measurement and observational methods are needed to obtain a valid picture of children's daily activity patterns.

The longitudinal approach revealed not only a gradual decline in physical activity but also that sport participation appears to be important at an early age to preserve an active lifestyle. The stability of the sports choices among long-term participants also seems to indicate that many (30%) children make their choices early in their teens. It stresses the importance of introducing children during school physical education to a variety of sports and other forms of movement in order to create opportunities for them to choose lifelong physical activity. Experimental studies of changes in physical activity reveal that effective strategies have in common a dimension of social reinforcement (Dishman, Sallis, & Orenstein, 1985). Schools could provide such reinforcement.

Aerobic Fitness

In Figure 11.14 the development of aerobic fitness between ages 12 and 21 is depicted as $\dot{V}O_2$max relative to body mass ($\dot{V}O_2$max/BM). Because no interfering effects could be demonstrated (see Table 11.4), the age trend shown is realistic. In boys, the $\dot{V}O_2$max/BM maintains a mean value of 59 ml/kg/min between ages 12 and 17 and thereafter declines to 52 ml/kg/min by age 21. In girls, there is a gradual decrease, from 50 ml/kg/min to 40 ml/kg/min by age 21.

The American College of Sports Medicine (1990) recommends that, in order to develop and maintain a reasonable level of aerobic fitness, people participate at least three times a week in physical activity with an intensity of 50% to 80% $\dot{V}O_2$max for 10 to 60 min. From our physical-activity data on medium to heavy activities as assessed by the activity interview (more than 180 min per week at ≥4 METs) and pedometer week scores (more than 18,000 per week), it appears

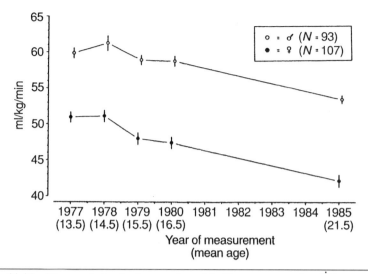

Figure 11.14   Mean and standard error of aerobic fitness measured as $\dot{V}O_2$max per kg body mass in males and females versus calendar age.
Reprinted from Kemper et al. (1989).

that boys maintain aerobic fitness throughout their teens until age 16 or 17 and that girls are at best fairly constant until age 14 or 15.

Relationship of Daily Physical Activity With Aerobic Fitness

To investigate the relationship between habitual physical activity (the independent variable) and $\dot{V}O_2$max (the dependent variable), we divided all girls and boys measured during the first 4 years of the Amsterdam Growth and Health Study into active and inactive groups (Verschuur, 1987). The selection was made on the basis of three activity variables:

1. Energy expenditure measured with HRI over 48 hr
2. Pedometer week scores
3. Total time spent in activity per week according to an activity interview

Active individuals were those who scored above the median in at least 3 of 4 years. Inactive ones were those who scored below the median in 2 of 4 years. Comparing active and inactive pupils over time, we found no differences in height, weight, or fat-free mass.

In contrast, parameters directly related to cardiorespiratory fitness are significantly related to the level of physical activity: Active girls and boys have significantly higher $\dot{V}O_2$max/BM than inactive ones. Again, the differences are small, and inactive children have a reasonably high aerobic fitness: for inactive boys, 55 ml/kg; for inactive girls, from 40 to 47 ml/kg. Because the differences in

$\dot{V}O_2$max/BM between active and inactive youngsters already exist at age 13, self-selection rather than training could be the cause.

Because physical activity was measured in 1985 with the same activity interview as in previous years, we divided the longitudinal group into sport participants and nonparticipants for the 8-year period between ages 13 and 21. The classification was made as follows: Sport participants were members of a sport club at least 3 of the initial 4 years (1977-1980) and also in 1985. The nonparticipants were not sport club members at least 3 of the initial 4 years or in 1985.

Figure 11.15 shows the maximal oxygen uptake per kg body mass for males and females who were sport participants or nonparticipants. Sport participants of both sexes have significantly higher aerobic fitness than nonparticipants. The differences are 3 to 5 ml O_2 per kg body mass, and because they do not change systematically with age, these results support the hypothesis that youngsters are more active because they have high aerobic fitness rather than the reverse—that they have high aerobic fitness because they are active.

Longitudinal measurement of the natural history of daily physical activity in Dutch youngsters shows that boys are more active than girls, especially in heavier activities ($\geq$ 10 METs). In both sexes the amount of activity declines dramatically from age 13 to 17. This was found to be the case by each of the three activity instruments: interview, heart-rate integrator, and pedometer. The instruments show relatively low intercorrelations, however, indicating that they overlap only in part.

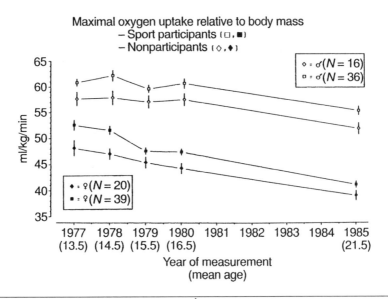

Figure 11.15   Changes in aerobic fitness ($\dot{V}O_2$max/BM) in males and females, sport participants and nonparticipants, between ages 13 and 21.

The activity methods also showed interfering effects, which seriously hinder measurement of the natural history of physical activity over time. During the teenage period, the development of aerobic fitness, measured as $\dot{V}O_2max/BM$, remains constant in boys and decreases in girls. By the time subjects reach their early twenties, aerobic fitness has declined in both sexes—in girls to a level lower than that recorded when they entered their teens.

Relatively active teenagers show higher aerobic fitness ($\dot{V}O_2max/BM$) than their relatively inactive counterparts between ages 13 and 17. This is also the case for sport participants and nonparticipants between ages 13 and 21.

Because the differences between active and inactive youngsters already exist from age 13, self-selection rather than training is thought to be the cause.

References

American College of Sports Medicine. (1990). Position statement on the recommended quantity and quality of exercise for developing and maintaining cardiorespiratory and muscular fitness in healthy adults. *Medicine and Science in Sports and Exercise*, **22**, 265-274.

Andersen, K.L. (1971). *Fundamentals of exercise testing*. Geneva: World Health Organization.

Åstrand, P.O., & Rodahl, K. (1986). *Textbook of work physiology*. New York: McGraw-Hill.

Backx, F.J.G., Erich, W.B.M., Kemper, A.B.A., & Verbeek, A.L.M. (1989). Sports injuries in school-aged children: An epidemiologic study. *American Journal of Sports Medicine*, **17**(2), 234-240.

Bar-Or, O. (1983). *Pediatric sports medicine for the practitioner*. New York: Springer-Verlag.

Bell, R.Q. (1954). An experimental test of the accelerated longitudinal approach. *Child Development*, **25**, 281-286.

Bink, B., Bonjer, F.H., & Sluys, H.vander. (1966). Assessment of the energy expenditure by indirect time and motion study. In K. Evang & K.L. Andersen (Eds.), *Physical activity in health and disease* (pp. 207-215). Oslo, Norway: Scandinavian University Books.

Dishman, R.K., Sallis, J.F., & Orenstein, D.R. (1985). Determinants of physical activity and exercise. *Public Health Reports*, **100**(2), 158-171.

Durnin, J.V.G.A., & Passmore, R. (1967). *Energy, work and leisure*. London: Heinemann.

Edholm, O.G. (1966). The assessment of habitual activity. In K. Evang and K.L. Andersen (Eds.), *Physical activity in health and disease* (pp. 187-197). Oslo, Norway: Scandinavian University Books.

Hof, M.A. van't, & Kowalski, C.J. (1979). Analysis of mixed longitudinal data sets. In B. Prahl-Andersen, C.J. Kowalski, & P. Heydendael (Eds.), *A mixed-longitudinal, interdisciplinary study of growth and development*. San Francisco: Academic Press.

Hollmann, W., & Hettinger, T. (1976). *Sportmedizin, Arbeits- und Trainung Grundlagen* [Sportsmedicine, occupational and training fundamentals]. Stuttgart: Schattauer Verlag.

Jéquier, J.C., Lavalée, H., Rajic, M., Beaucage, L., Shephard, R.J., & Labarre, R. (1977). The longitudinal examination of growth and development: History and protocol of the Trois Rivières regional study. In H. Lavallée & R.J. Shephard (Eds.), *Frontiers of activity and child health* (pp. 49-54). Ottawa, ON: Pelican.

Kemper, H.C.G. (Ed.) (1985). Growth, health and fitness of teenagers: Longitudinal research in international perspective. *Medicine and Sport Science* (Vol. 20), Basel: Karger.

Kemper, H.C.G. (1986). Longitudinal studies on the development of health and fitness and the interaction with physical activity of teenagers. *Pediatrician*, **13**, 52-59.

Kemper, H.C.G. (1991). Sources of variation in longitudinal assessment of maximal aerobic power in teenage boys and girls: The Amsterdam Growth and Health Study. *Journal of Human Biology*, **63**(4), 533-547.

Kemper, H.C.G. (1992). Physical development and childhood activity. In N.D. Norgan (Ed.), *Physical Activity and Health* (Symposium Vol. 34). New York: Cambridge University Press.

Kemper, H.C.G., Binkhorst, R.H., Verschuur, R., & Vissers, A.C.A. (1976). Reliability of the ergoanalyzer. *Journal of Cardiovascular Technology*, **4**, 27-30.

Kemper, H.C.G., Dekker, H., Ootjers, G., Post, B., Ritmeester, J.W., Snel, J., Splinter, P., Storm-vanEssen, L., & Verschuur, R. (1985). The problems of analyzing longitudinal data from the study "Growth and Health of Teenagers." In R.A. Binkhorst, H.C.G. Kemper, & W.H.M. Saris (Eds.), *Children and exercise XI: Vol. 15. International series on sport sciences* (pp. 233-251). Champaign, IL: Human Kinetics.

Kemper, H.C.G., & Hof, M.A. van't. (1978). Design of a multiple longitudinal study of growth and health in teenagers. *European Journal of Pediatrics*, **129**, 147-155.

Kemper, H.C.G., Snel, J., Verschuur, R., & Storm-vanEssen, L. (1990). Tracking of health and risk indicators of cardiovascular diseases from teenager to adult: Amsterdam Growth and Health Study, *Preventive Medicine*, **19**, 642-655.

Kemper, H.C.G., & Verschuur, R. (1977). Validity and reliability of pedometers in habitual activity research. *European Journal of Applied Physiology and Occupational Physiology*, **37**, 71-82.

Kemper, H.C.G., & Verschuur, R. (1980). Measurement of aerobic power in teenagers. In K. Berg & B. Eriksson (Eds.), *Children and exercise: Vol. 10. International series on sport sciences* (pp. 55-63). Baltimore: University Park Press.

Kemper, H.C.G., & Verschuur, R. (1987). Longitudinal study of maximal aerobic power in teenagers. *Annals of Human Biology*, **14**(5), 435-444.

Kemper, H.C.G., & Verschuur, R. (1990). Longitudinal study of coronary risk factors during adolescence and young adulthood—The Amsterdam Growth and Health Study. *Pediatric Exercise Science, 2*, 359-371.

Kemper, H.C.G., Verschuur, R., & deMey, L. (1989). Longitudinal changes of aerobic fitness in youth ages 12 to 23. *Pediatric Exercise Science, 1*, 257-270.

Kowalski, C.J., & Prahl-Andersen, B. (1979). General considerations in the design of studies of growth and development. In B. Prahl-Andersen, C.J. Kowalski, & P. Heydendael (Eds.), *A mixed-longitudinal, interdisciplinary study of growth and development* (pp. 3-13). San Francisco: Academic Press.

Livingstone, M.B.E., Prentice, A.M., Coward, W.A., Ceesay, S.M., Strain, J.J., Mekenma, P.G., Nevin, G.B., Baker, M.E., & Hickey, R.J. (1990). Simultaneous measurement of free-living energy expenditure by the doubly labeled water method and heart rate monitoring. *American Journal of Clinical Nutrition, 52*, 59-65.

Masironi, R., & Denolin, H. (1985). *Physical activity in disease, prevention and treatment.* Padua, Italy: Piccin.

Mednick, J.A., & Baert, A.E. (1981). *Prospective longitudinal research, an empirical basis for the primary prevention of psychosocial disorders.* London: Oxford University Press.

Mirwald, R.L., Bailey, D.A., Cameron, N., & Rasmussen, R.L. (1981). Longitudinal comparison of aerobic power in active and inactive boys aged 7 to 17 years. *Annals of Human Biology, 8*, 405-414.

Montoye, H.J. (1985). Risk indicators for cardiovascular disease in relation with physical activity in youth. In R.A. Binkhorst, H.C.G. Kemper, & W.H.M. Saris (Eds.), *Children and exercise XI: Vol. 15. International series on sport sciences* (pp. 3-25). Champaign, IL: Human Kinetics.

Montoye, H.J., & Taylor, H.L. (1984). Measurement of physical activity in population studies: A review. *Human Biology, 56*, 195-216.

Powell, K.E., Thompson, P.D., Caspersen, C.J., & Kendrick, J.S. (1987). Physical activity and the incidence of coronary heart disease. *Annual Review of Public Health, 8*, 253-287.

Rao, M.N., & Rao, C.R. (1966). Linked cross-sectional study for determining norms and growth rates—A pilot survey on Indian school-going boys. *Saykgya, 68*, 237-258.

Reiff, G.G., Montoye, H.J., Remington, R.D., Napier, J.A., Metzener, H.L., & Epstein, F.H. (1967). Assessment of physical activity by questionnaire and interview: In M.J. Karvonen & A.J. Barry (Eds.), *Physical activity and the heart.* Springfield, IL: Charles C Thomas.

Rowland, T.W. (1990). *Exercise and children's health.* Champaign, IL: Human Kinetics.

Rutenfranz, J., Berndt, I., & Knauth, P. (1974). Daily physical activity investigated by time budget studies and physical performance capacity of schoolboys. *Acta Paediatrica Belgica, 28*, 79-86.

Rutenfranz, J., Seliger, V., Andersen, K.L., Ilmarinen, J., Berndt, I., & Knauth, P. (1975). Differences in maximal aerobic power related to the daily physical activity in childhood. In G. Borg (Ed.), *Physical work and effort* (pp. 279-288). Oxford, UK: Pergamon Press.

Saris, W.H.M., Snel, P., & Birkhorst, R.A. (1977). A portable heart rate distribution recorder for studying daily physical activity. *European Journal of Applied Physiology and Occupational Physiology*, **37**, 19-25.

Schaie, K.W. (1965). A general model for the study of development problems. *Psychological Bulletin*, **64**, 92-107.

Seliger, V. (1966). Circulatory responses to sports activities. In K. Evang & K.L. Andersen (Eds.), *Physical activity in health and disease* (pp. 198-206). Oslo, Norway: Scandinavian University Books.

Sprynarova, S. (1974). Longitudinal study of the influence of different physical activity programs on functional capacity of boys from 11-18 years. *Acta Paediatrica Belgica*, **29**(Suppl.) 204-213.

Storm-vanEssen, L., Kemper, H.C.G., & Oojters, G. (1985). Purpose and design. In H.C.G. Kemper (Ed.), *Growth, Health and Fitness of Teenagers, Longitudinal Research International Perspective* (Vol. 20) (p. 21). Basel: Karger.

Stunkard, A.J. (Ed.) (1960). *Obesity*. Philadelphia: Saunders.

Tanner, J.M. (1962). *Growth at adolescence*. Oxford, UK: Blackwell Scientific.

Veling, S.H.S., & Hof, M.A. van't. (1980). Data quality control methods in longitudinal studies. In M. Ostyn, G. Beunen, & J. Simons (Eds.), *Kinanthropometry II: Vol. 9. International series on sport sciences* (pp. 436-442). Baltimore: University Park Press.

Verschuur, R. (1987). *Daily physical activity and health: Longitudinal changes during the teenage period*. SO, 12. Haarlem, Netherlands: de Vrieseborch.

Verschuur, R., & Kemper, H.C.G. (1980). Adjustment of pedometers to make them more valid in assessing running. *International Journal of Sports Medicine*, **1**, 87-89.

Verschuur, R., & Kemper, H.C.G. (1985). Habitual physical activity in Dutch teenagers measured by heart rate. In R.A. Binkhorst, H.C.G. Kemper, & W.H.M. Saris (Eds.), *Children and exercise XI: Vol. 15. International series on sport sciences* (pp. 194-202). Champaign, IL: Human Kinetics.

The Amsterdam Growth and Health Study was made possible by grants from the Dutch Prevention Fund (28-189A, 28-1106), the foundation for Educational Research (0255), the Dutch Heart Foundation (76.051-74.051), and the Ministry of Well Being, Health and Cultural Affairs. The author expresses his gratitude to the team of researchers and the 200 young men and women who participated in this study for almost 10 years.

CHAPTER *12*

Family Determinants of Childhood Physical Activity: A Social-Cognitive Model

Wendell C. Taylor
Tom Baranowski
James F. Sallis

Physical activity is an important component of the current and future health status of children (Sallis & McKenzie, 1991). With acceptance of this fact comes recognition of the need to understand the determinants of, or influences on, children's physical activity. The dynamics of children's and adults' physical activity may be quite different, and this chapter focuses on an issue of special importance regarding children's activity habits: the family. We review and critique family influences on children's physical activity. Recognizing the multiple influences on children's physical activity, we briefly review other domains of determinants. We also present recommendations for future research.

Definition of the Family

Many definitions exist for the term *family*. For our purposes, *family* is defined as two or more individuals who live in the same household, who have some common emotional bond, and who are interrelated by performing some social tasks in common (Baranowski & Nader, 1984a). This definition includes the nuclear family (father, mother, and children), single parents, adoptive parents, and multigenerational arrangements.

Physical-Activity Tracking

Because most of the health benefits of physical activity accrue to adults, an important issue in assessing influences on physical activity among children is to establish whether physically active children become physically active adults. The phenomenon of children's maintaining their relative ranking on a variable over time is called tracking. Studies are inconclusive on the stability of childhood activity into adulthood (Powell & Dysinger, 1987). These retrospective studies may not adequately test the hypothesis, however. Recently, R.R. Pate (personal communication, October 1991) reported correlations of .7 and higher in year to year levels of physical activity during childhood among children aged 3 to 7 years. Given error in measurement, which tends to attenuate such correlations, this is evidence for substantial year-to-year tracking in physical activity during childhood. More prospective studies are needed to determine whether activity tracks from youth to adulthood and to identify factors that may affect tracking.

Familial Aggregation of Physical-Activity Habits

It is important to establish whether families have common activity patterns. If no common activity patterns exist, it is unlikely that family members influence one another's activity behaviors. Familial aggregation of physical-activity habits has been reported in families of various ethnic backgrounds and with children of different ages. Since each method has associated biases, it is particularly important to demonstrate familial aggregation using alternative methods of assessing physical activity.

Using questionnaires of various descriptions, familiar aggregation of physical activity has been demonstrated among families with children aged 3 to 5 years (Willerman & Plomin, 1973), with seventh and eighth graders (Gottlieb & Chen, 1985), with children aged 12 to 14 years (Godin, Shephard, & Colantonio, 1986), and in Canadian families with children aged 10 years and older (Perusse, LeBlanc, & Bouchard, 1988; Perusse, Tremblay, LeBlanc, & Bouchard, 1989). Familial aggregation of physical activity has also been documented, using an interviewer-administered recall (Sallis, T.L. Patterson, Buono, Atkins, & Nader, 1988), a Caltrac accelerometer (Freedson & Evenson, 1991; Moore et al., 1991), and observation techniques (Sallis, T.L. Patterson, McKenzie, & Nader, 1988).

Studies with children of different ages, with families of different ethnic backgrounds, and with different methods of assessing physical activity consistently found significant familial resemblance in activity habits. The studies with the most reliable and valid methods (observation, mechanical instruments, and validated self-report measures) demonstrated significant familial associations, with most correlations in the range of .3 to .5. The mechanisms hypothesized to account for the aggregation of physical-activity levels within families include genetics (Bouchard, 1991; Kaprio & Koskenvuo, 1981; Perusse et al., 1989;

Scarr, 1966; Willerman & Plomin, 1973); environmental variables such as modeling, shared activities, social support, and encouragement (Perusse et al., 1989); and chance. Evidence for sibling aggregation of physical activity (Ruffer, 1965) and aggregation of change in family physical activity may be influenced by mechanisms other than parent to child aggregation. Nonetheless, the consistency of the findings suggests that family influences on children's activity are important across a wide range of ages.

Theoretical Perspective

No theory-based comprehensive review of the literature accounts for the documented family influences on children's physical-activity habits. Previous reviews have emphasized the development of children's sport-related social behaviors (Estrada, Gelfand, & Hartmann, 1988); family, peer, and school influences on sport socialization of children and adolescents (Lewko & Greendorfer, 1988); children and the sport socialization process (Coakley, 1987); and reviews of family aspects of physical activity in the context of health-related behaviors (Baranowski & Nader, 1984a, 1984b; Sallis & Nader, 1988). This review covers children's physical-activity habits and therefore includes discussion of both athletic competition and physical activity unrelated to sports socialization.

A theoretical approach to reviewing the literature provides a conceptual basis with which to understand the mechanisms of family influence. A theoretical perspective can suggest where the literature is deficient and thus guide future research. In this way, research findings can be interrelated and therefore build an integrated picture of influences on physical activity.

Many theoretical frameworks have been generated for use in analyzing and understanding family issues. Some are more academic (Burr, Hill, Nye, & Reiss, 1979); others, more clinical (L'Abate, 1985). Most could be applied to exercise behavior. For example, family systems theory (E.S. Epstein & Loos, 1989) postulates a complex theoretical framework of reciprocal relationships among family members, with subjective interpretations of family events at the core. Family systems theory suggests interventions to change the perceptions of the importance of physical activity by key family decision-makers. Family stress theory (Hansen & Johnson, 1979) has conceptualized how families respond to stressors. A possible application of family stress theory would be to examine under what circumstances a family initiates physical activity after a family member has a heart attack. Coercive family process theory (G.R. Patterson, 1982) focuses on the reward and punishment aspects of socialization behaviors within a family context. Studying or modifying parental practices that encourage or discourage physical activity would be an extension of coercive family process theory.

A more general conceptual framework, which combines cognitive, behavioral, and environmental factors, is social-cognitive theory (Bandura, 1986). This theory has been applied to numerous health behaviors (Parcel & Baranowski, 1981), and its reciprocal determinism aspect has been applied to families and health behaviors (Baranowski, 1990). Using social-cognitive theory permits the application of a rich conceptual framework shown to be useful in explaining and encouraging health behaviors (Perry, Baranowski, & Parcel, 1990).

Bandura's (1986) social cognitive theory suggests that behavior, cognitive and other personal factors (e.g., preferences, competencies, personality attributes), and environmental influences interact as determinants of each other. The determinants affect each other bidirectionally rather than unidirectionally. The mutual action between the three determinants is referred to as a triadic reciprocality model. Figure 12.1 illustrates the relationships among the three classes of determinants for one person in a triadic reciprocality model. The family perspective expands the focus of social-cognitive theory from the individual to two or more people. Figure 12.2 illustrates continuous reciprocal interactions among the home environment, parental cognitions and behaviors, and child cognitions and behaviors. The model in Figure 12.2 provides the theoretical foundation for this review.

Our primary interest in this review is the child's behavior. A child's cognitions are of interest only to the extent that they influence physical activity. Parents can affect a child's behavior directly (e.g., supplying a command) or indirectly, by changing the environment (e.g., purchasing and making available desired athletic equipment). Parents' cognitions can affect child behavior only when mediated by some form of parental behavior. An important aspect of this model is that children's behavior can affect parents' behavior, which may lead to a

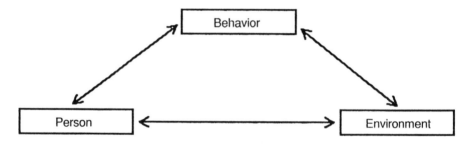

Figure 12.1   Bandura's model of triadic reciprocity.

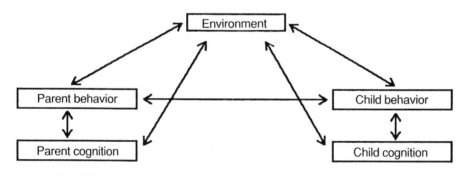

Figure 12.2   Social-cognitive theory—a socialization model of child behavior.

Family Determinants of Childhood Physical Activity 323

circular pattern of effects that either encourage or discourage physical activity. To understand family influences on children's physical-activity behavior, one must delineate the important aspects of the family environment, the child, and the parents and specify their reciprocal interactions.

Physical and Social Environment

Environmental factors can be categorized into physical, socioeconomic, and cultural components as well as social-cognitive components, including normative expectations, incentives, and rewards.

Effects on Physical Activity

The environment can be altered by parents and can facilitate or hinder physical activity. Access to facilities, equipment, and programs has been studied as an influence on sport socialization of youth.

Patriksson (1981) observed that the degree of involvement in sport, even for boys and girls with unusual physiological capabilities for sport, depends upon the environment: sports facilities, equipment, and transportation to sports grounds. The importance of the parental role is not in exerting an active influence but rather in supporting children and providing an environment that encourages physical activity (e.g., money for membership fees, transportation to playgrounds) (Patriksson, 1981). Coakley (1987) emphasized that access to equipment and facilities and opportunities to participate are important factors for sport socialization. Similarly, Butcher (1983) found that the child's total number of activities (interschool teams, intramural activities, and community activities) was most related ($r = .37$) to the amount of sports equipment available. Anderssen and Wold (1992) found that the most important determinant of physical activity among adolescents was direct parental help in exercising vigorously. Sallis et al. (1992) found that parent transportation was the parent behavior most consistently correlated with children's physical activity.

Facilities, the location of parks and schools, and opportunities to participate in games or sports were influential factors in the sport involvement of 9- to 12-year-old children (Greendorfer & Ewing, 1981). Time spent outdoors is a determinant of overall physical activity in young children (R.C. Klesges, Eck, Hanson, Haddock, & L.M. Klesges, 1990), and seasonal variations have been observed (U.S. Department of Health and Human Services, 1987). In some neighborhoods parents may restrict their children's time outdoors because appropriate and safe places are not available. Such restrictions may hinder children's physical activity. In adults proximity of physical-activity facilities was associated with activity levels (Sallis et al., 1990); however, this association has not been investigated in youth and families. Studies on environmental influences on physical activity have addressed participation in sports but rarely physical activity in general. Parental modifications of the familial environment have not been studied nor the ways they may influence children's interests and physical-activity patterns.

The social facilitation effect suggests that the presence of others can help or hinder an individual's performance (Zajonc, 1980). McKenzie, Sallis, Nader, Broyles, and Nelson (1992) revealed a negative adult social facilitation effect—that is, preschoolers' activity levels were lower when adults were present. Presumably, many of these adults were parents. The negative adult social facilitation effect was obtained both at home and during recess, which may indicate adults' desire to inhibit or control physical activity.

There may be critical periods in the development of an active lifestyle, and aspects of the environment may serve to inhibit or discourage lifelong physical activity. For example, many parents use playpens to limit the range of their children's physical activity (and thus protect their possessions from the child). This restriction of physical activity may dispose the child to learning nonactive methods of negotiating the environment.

Another interesting question concerns children's responses to different environmental conditions. Will children who are interested in physical activity find a way to be active even when their parents cannot afford equipment or membership fees? We suspect that children in families with limited resources have less opportunity for physical activity than those of families with abundant financial resources. Economic hardship may translate into a lack of transportation to facilities, limited financial resources for joining organized groups, and less leisure time available to participate. On the other hand, creative and makeshift environmental arrangements to accommodate children's physical-activity habits are legendary. For example, an Olympic long-jump champion began jumping at age 9 years into sand poured as a foundation for a building (Schoenfield, 1987).

Another issue is whether nonathletic children are disadvantaged by the lack of organized programs for nonelite athletes. Is a child's physical-activity behavior directly influenced by skill training and skill-acquisition opportunities? Research is lacking in all these areas. Conceptualization of environmental characteristics as they relate to the family and physical activity is a research priority. A central question is how proximity, access, and availability of facilities affect physical activity of children and their families.

Family and Socioeconomic Status

The family's socioeconomic status influences all aspects of the home's physical and social environment as well as environments the child is exposed to outside the home. Exposure to different kinds of sports, as well as the parent's interest in, time commitment to, financial resources for, and personal involvement in a child's physical-activity behavior, may be important. Access to equipment, programs, and safe places to be active is determined to a great extent by socioeconomic status. The literature on socioeconomic status and physical activity in children is characterized by different measures of physical activity and socioeconomic status. The results are similar, however; socioeconomic status is positively correlated with children's physical activity (Gottlieb & Chen, 1985; Shephard & Godin, 1986; Sunnegardh, Bratteby, & Sjolin, 1985; Tarbell et al., 1988). In the Sallis et al. (1992) study, however, parental education was generally not related to children's physical activity, but education was negatively associated with one measure of physical activity among girls. Overman and Rao (1981) reported that youth sport involvement and motivations were unrelated to socioeconomic status. In contrast with other studies, Overman and Rao's (1981) sample was high school seniors. By the time children reach this age, parental socioeconomic status may be a weak influence on sport involvement.

Social class may influence values about and perceptions of sports and physical activity. Watson (1977) found that middle-class parents evaluated Little League baseball as training in cooperation, whereas working-class parents saw it as training in learning to respond to authority.

None of these studies has sufficiently identified the mechanisms whereby socioeconomic status influences children's physical activity. For example, do affluent parents have different expectations or involvement with physical activity, compared with less-affluent parents? Do families of high socioeconomic status have more sports equipment or higher levels of membership in activity clubs or provide more encouragement to children than do low socioeconomic-status families? Are there differences in their active role models? Given the consistency of the association, this area appears to be a fruitful one for research.

Cultural and Ethnic Differences

Values related to culture and ethnic background influence the family environment. Research has not disentangled the possible confounding, additive, or interactive effects of socioeconomic status, race, and ethnic background as they relate to family influence on physical-activity patterns, and it may not yet be able to do so. The literature suggests that among preschoolers (McKenzie et al., 1992), Anglo-Americans were consistently more active than Mexican-Americans. Among children in seventh and eighth grades (Gottlieb & Chen, 1985), however, Anglo-Americans were more likely to participate in bicycling, running, swimming, tennis, roller-skating, and golf (individual, noncompetetive, aerobic activities) than African-Americans and Mexican-Americans. On the other hand, African-American children were more likely to participate in basketball and football (team sports), dancing, and skipping rope than Anglo- and Mexican-American children. Mexican-American children participated more in baseball than African- and Anglo-American children. Greendorfer and Ewing (1981) reported that sports involvement for African-American children was more influenced by facilities (the location of parks and schools), opportunities to participate in games or sports, and stronger values about sports (e.g., how important is it to the child, the child's father, etc., that the child be good in sports) than it was for

Anglo-American children, whose sports involvement was more influenced by teachers and fathers.

In a national survey (Wilson Sporting Goods Company, 1988) African- and Anglo-American girls were equally likely to be involved in sports, and their reasons for participating and quitting were the same. African-American girls participated more often through their school, however (65% versus 50%), whereas Anglo-American girls participated more often through private organizations (21% versus 7%). African-American girls were more likely than their Anglo-American counterparts to feel that "boys make fun of girls who play sports" (25% versus 1%) and more often had parents who felt sports were more important to boys than girls (30% versus 11%).

A topic related to socialization into sports is whether boys with above-average athletic skills from different racial or ethnic backgrounds are socialized into sports through different forms of encouragement, particularly from the family. The dynamics of socialization into sports may be quite different for various ethnic groups (Coakley, 1987). Some families may stress athletic competition as a viable channel to upward mobility, whereas other families may stress sports as an opportunity to develop as an individual and believe that seeking a professional career in sports is a "treadmill to nowhere" (Oliver, 1980).

Family values appear to be related to cultural and ethnic background. Such values may influence children's interests, attitudes, and physical-activity patterns. Research is needed to isolate the effects of socioeconomic background and cultural influences on children's physical-activity habits. Such information may be useful in targeting interventions to specific ethnic groups.

Normative Expectations

Social-cognitive theory refers to expectations as anticipatory aspects of behavior or determinants of behavior (Bandura, 1986). An individual anticipates many aspects of a situation and generates expectations before it occurs. Expectations are learned from previous experiences, observing others in similar situations, and hearing from others about such situations. The family, particularly parents, can convey explicit or subtle expectations to their children regarding participation in physical activity. These conveyed expectations are called normative expectations.

A national sample of parents found that mothers and fathers are eager for their children to be involved in physical activity whether or not they are active themselves (Perrier Corporation, 1984). The study showed that 93% of parents felt that their sons and daughters should "grow up with a deep concern about staying in top physical shape." In another study focusing on fathers, mothers, daughters, and sports, about one third of parents wanted their daughters to increase their involvement in sports (Wilson Sporting Goods Company, 1988).

Family expectations can be communicated by parents' enrolling their children in a class or activity. Similarly, expectations are communicated by parental constraints and "conditional permission" (Coakley, 1987). For example, a young child may ask a parent for permission to play. The child may hear, "I think it's great that you're going to play." Alternatively, the child may hear, "You have my permission as long as you 'stay close to the house' or 'keep your clothes clean' or 'don't play rough or get hurt' or 'watch your little brother' . . ." (Coakley, 1987, p. 46). Such conditional permission may influence skill development and constrain the nature of games and informal activities. Researchers contend that boys experience fewer parental constraints and have more opportunities to participate in both informal and organized sports than do girls (Coakley, 1987).

Active and sedentary children may differ in their perceptions of parental and peer expectations regarding physical activity (Godin & Shephard, 1984). Active children were more likely than sedentary children to report that parents and friends expected them to be physically active (Godin & Shephard, 1984). Parents' past athletic experience may lead to specific expectations for sons and daughters. Overman and Rao (1981) reported that parents' past athletic accomplishments had more influence on a child's sport involvement than perceived parental values about sports.

Family expectations have been associated with children's physical activity in several studies. The level of impact of expectations on physical activity is unclear. Also, the ways in which families communicate expectations to children have not been identified. Another research issue is how expectations change as children get older or perform well or poorly in physical activity or sports. The influence of expectations on physical activity within the family merits further study.

Incentives and Rewards

Social-cognitive theory describes incentives as inducements or motivators of behavior. Bandura (1986) explains cognitively based incentives thus:

> Through symbolic representation of foreseeable consequences, future outcomes can be converted into current guides and motivators of behavior. Here, the instigator to action is forethought rather than the sight of the actual incentives. The outcome expectations may be material . . . sensory . . . token . . . or social (e.g., positive and negative interpersonal reactions). (p. 233)

Within the context of the family, social incentives (e.g., anticipated respect and approval from family members) can be a powerful motivator of physical activity.

Outcome expectancies and perceived barriers are aspects of incentives and rewards. Tappe, Duda, and Ehrnwald (1989) assessed barriers to physical activity in high school students. Of nine barriers, time constraints and lack of desire were significantly different between low- and high-activity students. In an adult population (Steinhardt & Dishman, 1989) the family was perceived as beneficial (positive outcome expectancy) and as a limitation (barrier) to physical activity.

The positive factor was social time spent with family members; the barrier was family obligations (Steinhardt & Dishman, 1989).

Overall, the data are limited with respect to real and perceived incentives for physical activity in families. The potential power of family-controlled incentives is likely substantial because of the intimacy and duration of the relationships. Future research can identify the role, strength, and effectiveness of incentives within the family as determinants of physical activity.

Rewards and punishments are consequences or outcomes that follow actions or behaviors (from the child's perspective, rewards and punishments are the perceived incentives). Family members can reward and punish physical activity by word or action. In some cases parents may use physical activity itself as punishment (e.g., ''do 10 push-ups''). Rewards and punishments are likely strong influences on children's physical activity.

Most research on the consequences of children's participation in physical activity has studied the differences between active and inactive children and the effects of sports experiences (Coakley, 1987). A recent study (Taylor et al., 1991), however, with a national sample of third and fourth graders found that the children reported outcomes following physical activity as significant factors related to such activity. Outcomes included both negative consequences (e.g., teasing from friends) and positive ones (e.g., my parents cheer for me). Overall, the relationship between rewards, punishments, and physical activity within the family is an underdeveloped research area.

Parents' Attitudes and Behavior

Within social-cognitive theory, parents' attitudes and behaviors can affect children's physical activity through

- modeling,
- social influence, or
- social support processes.

These influences are reviewed in the following sections.

Modeling

Social-cognitive theory distinguishes among several modeling phenomena, each with different operating mechanisms (Bandura, 1986). Observational learning occurs when observers acquire cognitive skills and new patterns of behaviors by observing the performance of others. In observational learning, modeling teaches component skills. A second modeling phenomenon includes inhibitory and disinhibitory effects. In this instance, modeling strengthens or weakens inhibitions about previously learned behaviors. A third main function of modeling is response facilitation effects. In this case, others' actions serve as social prompts, inducements, or response-cuing effects for previously learned behaviors.

Observational learning is affected by the salience and complexity of modeled activities as well as the credibility and relevance of the model. In the family, parents are typically highly relevant and credible models, at least for younger children. For older children, peers become increasingly important. Children are exposed to frequent and lengthy contact with parental and sibling models. Therefore, children can be profoundly influenced by the modeling of family members.

No literature specifically addresses modeling and physical activity. The potential for modeling effects within the family can be assessed by reviewing the literature on parental exercise patterns, parental exercise with children, and studies identifying modeling as a variable of interest. Such papers provide a conflicting pattern of results.

The National Children and Youth Fitness Study II (NCYFS II) (U.S. Department of Health and Human Services, 1987) reported that 42.1% of mothers and 48% of fathers of children in grades 1 through 4 did not participate in moderate to vigorous physical activity in a typical week; 28.6% of mothers and 29.9% of fathers exercised 3 or more days per week. Thus, most parents do not model regular physical activity.

In a small observational study, Baranowski, Hooks, Tsong, Cieslik, and Nader (1987) found that fathers were absent at the times children were physically active, thereby minimizing the possibility that fathers are models for children's physical activity. The NCYFS II (1987) reported that 58.1% of mothers and 61.7% of fathers did no exercise with their child in a typical week. Only 10.7% of mothers and 11.3% of fathers exercised 3 or more days per week with their child. The frequency of parents' exercising with their children was correlated with the frequency with which parents themselves exercised. The correlation between total days that either parent exercised with the child and mother's exercise days was .30; the correlation with father's exercise days was .29. NCYFS II concluded that parents do not spend much time exercising with their children and that those who do provide positive role models because of their own exercise behavior.

Another study found similar results: "Among parents who participate in sports and athletics, 58 percent spend more than half of that time participating together as a family. At least some time is spent participating with the family by 90 percent of all active parents" (Perrier Corporation, 1984, p. 7). Similarly, Godin and Shephard (1986) found that the strength of seventh to ninth graders' intention to exercise was associated with the father's current physical-activity habits ($p <$ .05). Gottlieb and Chen (1985) and Anderssen and Wold (1992) found that parental exercise is related to overall frequency of exercise in adolescents.

Sallis et al. (1992) did not find a significant association between parent and child activity levels. There was weak and inconsistent evidence linking the frequency of parents playing with the child to child self-reported physical activity. In a study of preschool children, vigorous parental activity was a significant contributor to moderate child activity during free-play periods at preschools.

Though the studies to date generally indicate that parental modeling is an important correlate of child physical activity, playing with the child is a related mechanism for influencing child activity that needs to be studied more.

The literature suggests that most parents are not physically active and that active parents are more likely to exercise with their children. Because so few parents are active, the potential effects of parental modeling of physical activity within the family are not being realized. More research is needed to clarify which mechanisms of family physical-activity modeling are most influential. The consistency of parent-child correlations of physical-activity levels suggests that parental modeling is a very important influence.

Social Influence (Encouragement, Persuasion, Nagging, Sanctions)

Parents may exert direct social influence over children's physical activity through encouragement, discouragement, pressure, and direct prompts to promote or inhibit activity. Few studies clearly conceptualize and operationalize parents' social influence on children's physical-activity patterns, with notable exceptions (Klesges et al., 1984; Klesges et al., 1990; Klesges, Malott, Boschee, & Weber, 1986; McKenzie et al., 1991). Empirical studies suggest that the success of parental attempts to influence directly a child's physical-activity level is inconsistent.

Some studies suggest that parental social influence is effective. Dennison, Straus, Mellits, and Charney (1988) found that the parental encouragement adults reported receiving as children contributed significantly to discriminant scores that identified physically active and inactive adults. Also, using discriminant function analysis, Lewko and Ewing (1980) reported that socialization influences differ for children in high and low sport involvement groups. For boys, the father's influence was a significant factor discriminating high and low sport involvement. For girls, the influence of each family member (mother, father, brother, sister) was a significant variable. Similarly, L.H. Epstein, Smith, Vara, and Rodefer (1991) showed that parental prompts for children to play outdoors, rather than watch television or play video games, increased children's level of physical activity. Anderssen and Wold (1992) found that parental encouragement was an important correlate of adolescents' physical activity.

In an early series of studies, Klesges et al. (1984, 1986) reported that young children's activity patterns were related to parental behaviors such as encouraging and discouraging physical activity. In the 1986 study, parental encouragement to be active correlated with the intensity of the activity, but additional analyses revealed that parental encouragement was related to extreme levels of children's activity ($r = .47$, $p < .01$) but not to minimal ($r = .03$) or moderate ($r = .09$) levels. Similarly, McKenzie et al. (1991) found a correlation ($r = .43$) between prompts to be active and preschoolers' overall physical activity at home.

Other studies suggest that parental social influence is limited or ineffective. Klesges et al. (1990) found parental commands or encouragement to be active unrelated to children's activity level. In contrast to their earlier studies, which suggested that parental interaction was related to children's activity level, the number of encouragements by parents was quite small. The markedly different levels of encouragement may account partly for the discrepant findings. Also, Sallis et al. (1992) found that the more concrete the parental support, the more likely that it was related to children's physical activity. Parental activity and encouragement were not related to children's behavior. Playing with the child was related in some cases, however, and transporting the child was most often related to children's physical activity.

Determining parental influences on children's activity levels is not simple. The inconsistent findings suggest that the mechanisms of influence are complex and that perhaps interactions occur among several variables.

One obvious factor is the child's age. As children make the transition to school, they become part of a wider social network. By ages 6 and 7 children engage in a broad range of relationships and thus experience greater exposure to other social influences (Lewko & Greendorfer, 1988). Therefore, direct social influence prompts from parents may be successful at certain ages and not at others. As the child matures, negotiation may be more important than direct social influences.

Nagging, sanctions, discouragement, and other negative behaviors merit study. Klesges and colleagues (1984, 1986) have studied the discouragement of physical activity. Limited research has been conducted in the area of how children perceive parental social influences. Parents may not be aware of any difference between pressure, which can be destructive, and encouragement, which can be positive. The child's perception of parental behavior is a factor in the success of social influence efforts by parents.

Social Support

Social support is any behavior that assists another person in achieving desired goals (Caplan, Robinson, French, Caldwell, & Shinn, 1976), and it has been subdivided into informational, material, and emotional support (Caplan et al., 1976). At times it is difficult to separate social influence from social support. In the context of the family and physical activity, social support can take a variety of forms: for example, parents' providing information on physical activity, viewing a child's play or practice, discussing physical activity with the child, offering to exercise with the child, and assisting the child (e.g., providing transportation to practice) in physical-activity interests.

Routh, Walton, and Padan-Belkin (1978) found that 5-year-olds were significantly more active when their mothers were present. The Wilson Sporting Goods Company (1988) (in a study of daughters only) found that 44% of daughters said parental participation in their sports activity was the encouragement they remembered the most.

Several studies have demonstrated that active children perceived more parental encouragement than inactive children. Melnick, Dunkelman, and Mashiach (1981) found that mothers of 12- and 13-year-old track and field athletes, gymnasts, and swimmers gave their children significantly more encouragement ($p < .001$) for participation in physical activity than parents of a control group. Treiber, Baranowski, Braden, Strong, and Levy (1991) reported that social support for exercise in an adult sample was positively correlated with physical activity. Ethnic background, sex, and specific types of support were important mediators of the relationship, however.

The Child

The child's personal atributes can be influenced by the family and may in turn be related to physical-activity habits. The psychological factors that have been studied include

- personality characteristics,
- knowledge,
- attitudes,
- beliefs,
- values,
- self-efficacy, and
- intentions.

Personality Characteristics

Several personality characteristics have been studied, including achievement motivation, stress tolerance, social adequacy, self-confidence, and independence. Most studies (Butcher, 1985; Dekker, Ritmeester, & Snel, 1985) in children have found nonsignificant or weak associations between personality attributes and physical activity.

Physical Activity, Knowledge, Beliefs, and Behavior

Studies on the relationships between physical activity, knowledge, and behavior in youth suggest that knowledge about the health effects of physical activity is not important (O'Connell, Price, Roberts, Jurs, & McKinley, 1985) but that knowledge of how to be physically active may be a significant influence (Gottlieb & Chen, 1985). A variety of measures of attitudes toward physical activity have consistently been weak or moderate correlates of physical activity in youth (Desmond, Price, Lock, D. Smith, & Stewart, 1990; Ferguson, Yesalis, Pomrehn, & Kirkpatrick, 1989; Godin & Shephard, 1986; Neale, Sonstroem, &

Metz, 1970). Shephard and Godin (1986) reported that during adolescence (Grades 7 to 9), prior experience with physical activity had a significant influence ($p < .001$) upon intentions to exercise. Also, students with a high intention to exercise had strong positive beliefs about the value of physical activity ($p < .001$). No research has been reported on the effects of family variables on these characteristics.

Self-Efficacy and Intentions to Exercise

Self-efficacy (i.e., confidence in one's abilities) regarding physical activity (Reynolds et al., 1990), intentions about exercise (Ferguson et al., 1989; Godin & Shephard, 1986; Greenockle, Lee, & Lomax, 1990), and satisfaction with one's sports skills (Butcher, 1983) are specific beliefs about one's physical activity that have been strongly associated with or predictive of the physical activity of adolescents. No studies have reported the influence of family variables on these characteristics.

In summary, enduring personality traits are probably not strong influences on children's physical activity. Knowledge, beliefs, and attitudes about physical activity are in general weak or inconsistent correlates. Only specific beliefs about personal physical activity have been strongly associated with physical activity in multiple studies. Reliable and valid measures of activity-specific psychological variables must be developed for children and adolescents. Social-cognitive theory variables—for example, behavioral capability (skill development), intrinsic motivation, and self-efficacy—should be studied in relation to children and physical activity as well as the ways such factors are influenced by family variables.

Family-Based Interventions to Promote Physical Activity and Treat Obesity in Youth

Because of the strong and consistent associations that exist between parent and child physical activity, there has been a great deal of optimism about the potential effectiveness of family-based physical-activity interventions. At least three family-based health promotion programs with healthy families have been reported. The programs were based on social-cognitive theory and included training in both physical-activity and self-management skills, but none showed any effect on child or parent physical activity (Baranowski et al., 1990; Nader et al., 1983, 1989). Although these studies led to diminished expectations for the efficacy of family-based interventions, they have identified barriers that must be overcome if family interventions are to become effective. Most families do not want to participate in intensive health promotion programs (Crockett, Perry, & Pirie, 1989), so recruitment is difficult. Even after families are recruited, however, the most obvious barrier is the difficulty of getting families together for face-to-face interventions. If families do not attend sessions, the efficacy of the interventions is necessarily reduced. The problems faced by studies of freestanding health promotion programs suggest that it may be more fruitful to organize family interventions in locations where families are already together, such as in churches. Alternatively, other school and community organizations could promote family involvement in children's physical activity through approaches that did not include face-to-face meetings.

In contrast to programs for healthy families, family-based interventions for high-risk children have succeeded. A.C. Taggart, J. Taggart, and Siedentop (1986) reported on a program for children who scored low on health-related fitness tests. The intervention was an intensive clinically oriented program in which counselors trained parents to set up contracts for their children's increased physical activity. Children earned rewards by increasing their activity levels. All children showed substantial increases in physical activity as well as in fitness scores.

Several studies have documented the effectiveness of family-based interventions for treating obese children. Behaviorally oriented family-based treatments are more effective than nonbehavioral interventions (L.H. Epstein et al., 1985) and control conditions (Israel, Stolmaker, Sharp, Silverman, & Simon, 1984; Kingsley & Shapiro, 1977). Training in both general parenting and weight-reduction skills produced superior weight loss in children at follow-up (Israel, Stolmaker, & Andrian, 1985). L.H. Epstein, Koeske, and Wing (1984) and colleagues reinforced both children and adults for behavior change, and this approach was more effective than reinforcing children only. This family-based diet and physical-activity program for obese children led to weight loss that was partially maintained for a 10 year period (L.H. Epstein, Valoski, Wing, & McCurley, 1990).

Two studies of family-based obesity treatment of adolescents have been reported. Brownell, Kelman, and Stunkard (1983) found that more weight loss occurred when parents and adolescents were seen separately than when they were seen together. Coates, Killen, and Slinkard (1982) found no difference at follow-up between adolescents who were treated with or without their parents. Thus, there is little support for joint parent and adolescent treatment of obesity.

Family-based clinical programs for high-risk children can be effective in treating activity-related conditions such as obesity, and the data on maintenance of results are encouraging. Family-based physical-activity interventions for healthy children have not been shown to be effective. Research is needed to develop methods of involving families in physical-activity promotion programs.

We have reviewed the literature on family determinants of childhood physical activity. Our theoretical approach was social-cognitive theory (Bandura, 1986), which explains human functioning as the reciprocal interaction of three determinants: behavior, cognition, and environment. We adapted social-cognitive theory to develop a socialization model of child behavior (Figure 12.2). In this framework, the environment influences parents' and children's behaviors and cognitions, that in turn cause reciprocal interactions among the components of the model. Most of the existing research has focused on the parent's influence on the child's behavior. Our model suggests that the child's behavior can influence the parent's behavior as well. Reverse socialization and reciprocal effects refer to the ways in which children influence their parents' involvement in physical activity (Berlage, 1982; Snyder & Purdy, 1982). For example, the family lifestyle (e.g., providing transportation, changing mealtimes, rearranging vacation plans and work routines) is altered to accommodate a child's practice sessions, lessons, and games. A child's participation in sports can result in greater parental interest in attending athletic events, reading about sports, and watching sports on television. As a result, parents learn about and become more involved in sports because of their children's participation (Snyder & Purdy, 1982).

We recognize that the family is only one of several influences on a child's physical-activity habits. As children mature, particularly during adolescence, parental influence weakens. Peers and other personal and environmental factors become influential in shaping children's behavior (Buhrmester & Furman, 1987; Godin et al., 1986; Higginson, 1985; Patriksson, 1981). This transfer of influence in regard to children's activity and sports has not been described.

The school environment can be key in influencing the activity patterns of youth (Gilliam & MacConnie, 1984; Parcel et al., 1987; Simons-Morton et al., 1990). Coaches (Coakley, 1987; Higginson, 1985), teachers (Godin & Shephard, 1984; Patriksson, 1981), physicians, and other adults (e.g., youth leaders) can play pivotal roles in influencing children's physical-activity habits.

Genetics, or the inheritability of activity (Scarr, 1966), is another determinant related to the family. Obviously, however, genetics is not an appropriate target for intervention programs. Therefore, our review emphasized social environmental variables, which are amenable to change.

The influence of the family is thought to be central to the development of several health behaviors in children (Baranowski & Nader, 1984a). Some researchers believe that the surest way to instill positive attitudes toward physical activity in children is to place them in homes in which the parents are physically active (Pate & Blair, 1978). Other scientists are concerned about the eroding influence of the family (Rowland, 1990). The competing social forces that work against the family and its vital role of influencing a child's behavior include financial insecurity, marital stress, job priorities, less time available for family activities, and less cohesive families. Cratty (1973) asserted that "children do not seem to be taught to play vigorously in formal ways by their brothers, sisters, and parents. They seem instead to catch the mood of the family toward play and sports" (p. 211). Steinhardt and Dishman (1989) reported that the family offers benefits (time spent with family members) and barriers (family obligations) to physical-activity participation. These observations and findings underscore the complexity of family influence.

Research based on our socialization model of child behavior can help investigators better understand the mechanisms of influence within the family, the complexity of its influence, and the changing trends within families. Family-based interventions have not been consistently successful. A better understanding of family influences on physical activity in children should help health professionals identify optimal ages and improve techniques for interventions.

The sport socialization literature has contributed to our understanding of the processes that lead children into sports involvement. The research investigating involvement in physical activity apart from sports is not extensive, and the family determinants of nonsport physical activity may be quite different from those of socialization into sports.

The literature reviewed indicates that families can influence children's physical activity in many ways. Parents and siblings are powerful role models. Families control important aspects of the physical environment that can affect physical activity. Family socioeconomic status and cultural background are associated with many determinants of children's physical activity. Parents can exert direct influence through encouragement, discouragement, persuasion, sanctions, and support. Thus, a wide variety of mechanisms of family influence has been identified. Other hypothesized mechanisms have not yet been studied. It is not possible to conclude which mechanisms are more powerful for specific subpopulations of children, however, partly because of the limited number of variables in each study.

We recommend a social-cognitive approach to the study of family determinants of children's physical activity. Within this framework, multifactorial studies with children who vary by age, sex, ethnic background, motor ability, and type of physical activity (Butcher, 1983; Melnick et al., 1981) are needed. Specific types of influence and reciprocal interactions can be studied in relation to a variety of child characteristics. The objective is to understand the complex mechanisms of influence within the family in order to design better programs and to promote physical activity that all family members can enjoy.

References

Anderssen, N., & Wold, B. (1992). Parental and peer influences on leisure-time physical activity in young adolescents. *Research Quarterly for Exercise and Sport*, **63**(4), 341-348.

Bandura, A. (1986). *Social foundations of thought and action*. Englewood Cliffs, NJ: Prentice Hall.

Baranowski, T. (1990). Reciprocal determinism at the stages of behavior change: An integration of community, personal and behavioral perspectives. *International Quarterly of Community Health Education*, **10**(4), 297-327.

Baranowski, T., Hooks, P., Tsong, Y., Cieslik, C., & Nader, P.R. (1987). Aerobic physical activity among third to sixth grade children. *Journal of Developmental and Behavioral Pediatrics*, **8**(4), 203-206.

Baranowski, T., & Nader, P.R. (1984a). Family health behavior. In D. Turk & R. Kerns (Eds.), *Health, illness and families* (pp. 51-80). New York: Wiley.

Baranowski, T., & Nader, P.R. (1984b). Family involvement in health behavior change programs. In D. Turk & R. Kerns (Eds.), *Health, illness and families* (pp. 81-107). New York: Wiley.

Baranowski, T., Simons-Morton, B., Hooks, P., Henske, J., Tiernan, K., Dunn, J.K., Burkhalter, H., Harper, J., & Palmer, J. (1990). A center-based program for exercise change among Black-American families. *Health Education Quarterly*, **17**, 179-196.

Berlage, G.I. (1982). Children's sports and the family. *Arena Review*, **6**(1), 43-47.

Bouchard, C. (1991). Heredity and the path to overweight and obesity. *Medicine and Science in Sports and Exercise*, **23**(3), 285-291.

Brownell, K.D., Kelman, J.H., & Stunkard, A.J. (1983). Treatment of obese children with and without their mothers. *Pediatrics*, **71**, 515-523.

Buhrmester, D., & Furman, W. (1987). The development of companionship and intimacy. *Child Development*, **58**, 1101-1113.

Burr, W.R., Hill, R., Nye, F.I., & Reiss, I.L. (Eds.) (1979). *Contemporary theories about the family* (Vols. 1 & 2). New York: Free Press.

Butcher, J. (1983). Socialization of adolescent girls into physical activity. *Adolescence*, **18**(72), 753-766.

Butcher, J. (1985). Longitudinal analysis of adolescent girls' participation in physical activity. *Sociology of Sport Journal*, **2**, 130-143.

Caplan, R.D., Robinson, E.A.R., French, J.A.P., Jr., Caldwell, J.R., & Shinn, M. (1976). *Adhering to medical regimens: Pilot experiment in patient education and social support*. Ann Arbor, MI: University of Michigan, Institute for Social Research.

Coakley, J.J. (1987). Children and the sport socialization process. In D. Gould & M.R. Weiss (Eds.), *Advances in pediatric sport sciences: Vol. 2. Behavioral issues* (pp. 43-59). Champaign, IL: Human Kinetics.

Coates, T.J., Killen, J.D., & Slinkard, L.A. (1982). Parent participation in a treatment program for overweight adolescents. *International Journal of Eating Disorders*, **1**, 37-47.

Cratty, B.J. (1973). *Psychology in contemporary sport: Guidelines for coaches and athletes*. Englewood Cliffs, NJ: Prentice Hall.

Crockett, S.J., Perry, C.L., & Pirie, P. (1989). Nutrition intervention strategies preferred by parents: Results of a marketing survey. *Journal of Nutrition Education*, **21**, 90-94.

Dekker, H., Ritmeester, J.W., & Snel, J. (1985). Personality traits and school attitude. In H.C.G. Kemper (Ed.), *Growth, health, and fitness of teenagers* (pp. 137-147). New York: Karger.

Dennison, B.A., Straus, J.H., Mellits, E.D., & Charney, E. (1988). Childhood physical fitness tests: Predictor of adult physical activity levels? *Pediatrics*, **82**(3), 324-330.

Desmond, S.M., Price, J.H., Lock, R.S., Smith, D., & Stewart, P.W. (1990). Urban black and white adolescents' physical fitness status and perceptions of exercise. *Journal of School Health*, **60**, 220-226.

Epstein, E.S., & Loos, V.E. (1989). Thoughts on the limits of family therapy. *Journal of Family Psychology*, **2**, 405-421.

Epstein, L.H., Koeske, R., & Wing, R.R. (1984). Adherence to exercise in obese children. *Journal of Cardiac Rehabilitation*, **4**, 185-194.

Epstein, L.H., Smith, J.A., Vara, L.S., & Rodefer, J.S. (1991). Behavioral economic analysis of activity choice in obese children. *Health Psychology*, **10**(5), 311-316.

Epstein, L.H., Valoski, A., Wing, R.R., & McCurley, J. (1990). Ten-year follow-up of behavioral, family-based treatment for obese children. *Journal of the American Medical Association*, **264**, 2519-2523.

Epstein, L.H., Wing, R.R., Woodall, K., Penner, B.C., Kress, M.J., & Koeske, R. (1985). Effects of family-based behavioral treatment on 5- to 8-year-old children. *Behavior Therapy*, **16**, 205-212.

Estrada, A.M., Gelfand, D.M., & Hartmann, D.P. (1988). Children's sport and the development of social behaviors. In F.L. Smoll, R.A. Magill, & M.J. Ash (Eds.), *Children in sport* (3rd ed.) (pp. 251-262). Champaign, IL: Human Kinetics.

Ferguson, K.J., Yesalis, C.E., Pomrehn, P.R., & Kirkpatrick, M.B. (1989). Attitudes, knowledges, and beliefs as predictors of exercise intent and behavior in school children. *Journal of School Health*, **59**, 112-115.

Freedson, P.S., & Evenson, S.K. (1991). Familial aggregation and physical activity. *Research Quarterly for Exercise and Sport*, **62**(4), 384-389.

Gilliam, T.B., & MacConnie, S.E. (1984). Coronary heart disease risk in children and their physical activity patterns. In R.A. Boileau (Ed.), *Advances in pediatric sport sciences: Vol. 1. Biological issues* (pp. 171-187). Champaign, IL: Human Kinetics.

Godin, G., & Shephard, R.J. (1984). Normative beliefs of school children concerning regular exercise. *Journal of School Health*, **54**, 443-445.

Godin, G., & Shephard, R.J. (1986). Psychological factors influencing intentions to exercise of young students from grades 7 to 9. *Research Quarterly for Exercise and Sport*, **57**, 41-52.

Godin, G., Shephard, R.J., & Colantonio, A. (1986). Children's perception of parental exercise: Influence of sex and age. *Perceptual and Motor Skills*, **62**, 511-516.

Gottlieb, N.H., & Chen, M.S. (1985). Sociocultural correlates of childhood sporting activities: Their implications for heart health. *Social Science in Medicine*, **21**(5), 533-539.

Greendorfer, S.L., & Ewing, M.E. (1981). Race and gender differences in children's socialization into sport. *Research Quarterly for Exercise and Sport*, **52**, 301-310.

Greenockle, K.M., Lee, A.A., & Lomax, R. (1990). The relationship between selected student characteristics and activity patterns in a required high school physical education class. *Research Quarterly for Exercise and Sport*, **61**, 59-69.

Hansen, D.A., & Johnson, V.A. (1979). Rethinking family stress theory: Definitional aspects. In W.R. Burr, R. Hill, F.I. Nye, & I.L. Reiss (Eds.), *Contemporary theories about the family* (Vol. 1) (pp. 582-603). New York: Free Press.

Higginson, D.C. (1985). The influence of socializing agents in the female sport-participation process. *Adolescence*, **20**(77), 73-82.

Israel, A.C., Stolmaker, L., & Andrian, C.A.G. (1985). The effects of training parents in general child management skills on a behavioral weight loss program for children. *Behavior Therapy*, **16**, 169-180.

Israel, A.C., Stolmaker, L., Sharp, J.P., Silverman, W.K., & Simon, L.G. (1984). An evaluation of two methods of parental involvement in treating obese children. *Behavior Therapy*, **15**, 266-272.

Kaprio, J., & Koskenvuo, M. (1981). Cigarette smoking, use of alcohol, and leisure-time physical activity among same-sexed adult male twins. In L. Gedda, P. Parisi, & W.E. Nance (Eds.), *Twins research 3: Part C. Epidemiological and clinical studies: Vol. 69. Progress in clinical and biological research* (pp. 37-42). New York: Liss.

Kingsley, R.G., & Shapiro, J. (1977). A comparison of three behavioral programs for the control of obesity in children. *Behavior Therapy*, **8**, 30-36.

Klesges, R.C., Costes, T.J., Moldenhauer-Klesges, L.M., Holzer, B., Gustavson, J., & Barnes, J. (1984). The FATS: An observational system for assessing physical activity in children and associated parent behavior. *Behavioral Assessment*, **6**, 333-345.

Klesges, R.C., Eck, L.H., Hanson, C.L., Haddock, C.K., & Klesges, L.M. (1990). Effects of obesity, social interactions, and physical environment on physical activity in preschoolers. *Health Psychology*, **9**, 435-449.

Klesges, R.C., Malott, J.M., Boschee, P.F., & Weber, J.M. (1986). The effects of parental influences on children's food intake, physical activity, and relative weight. *International Journal of Eating Disorders*, **5**(2), 335-346.

L'Abate, L. (Ed.) (1985). *The handbook of family psychology and therapy* (Vols. 1 & 2). Homewood, IL: Dorsey Press.

Lewko, J.H., & Ewing, M. (1980). Sex differences and parental influence in sport involvement of children. *Journal of Sport Psychology*, **2**, 62-68.

Lewko, J.H., & Greendorfer, S.L. (1988). Family influences in sport socialization of children and adolescents. In F. Smoll, R. Magill, & M. Ash (Eds.), *Children in sport* (pp. 287-300). Champaign, IL: Human Kinetics.

McKenzie, T.L., Sallis, J.F., Nader, P.R., Broyles, S.L., & Nelson, J.A. (1992). Anglo- and Mexican-American preschoolers at home and at recess: Activity patterns and environmental influences. *Journal of Developmental and Behavioral Pediatrics*, **13**, 173-180.

McKenzie, T.L., Sallis, J.F., Nader, P.R., Patterson, T.L., Elder, J.P., Berry, C.C., Rupp, J.W., Atkins, C.J., Buono, M.J., & Nelson, J.A. (1991). Beaches: An observational system for assessing children's eating and physical activity behaviors and associated events. *Journal of Applied Behavior Analysis*, **24**, 141-151.

Melnick, M.J., Dunkelman, N., & Mashiach, A. (1981). Familial factors of sports giftedness among young Israeli athletes. *Journal of Sport Behavior*, **4**, 82-94.

Moore, L.L., Lombardi, D.A., White, M.J., Campbell, J.L., Oliveria, S.A., & Ellison, R.C. (1991). Influence of parents' physical activity levels on activity levels of young children. *Journal of Pediatrics*, **118**, 215-219.

Nader, P.R., Baranowski, T., Vanderpool, N.A., Dunn, K., Dworkin, R., & Ray, L. (1983). The Family Health Project: Cardiovascular risk reduction education for children and parents. *Developmental and Behavioral Pediatrics*, **4**, 3-10.

Nader, P.R., Sallis, J.F., Patterson, T.L., Abramson, I.S., Rupp, J.W., Senn, K.L., Atkins, C.J., Roppe, B.E., Morris, J.A., Wallace, J.P., & Vega, W.A. (1989). A family approach to cardiovascular risk reduction: Results from the San Diego Family Health Project. *Health Education Quarterly*, **16**, 229-244.

Neale, D.C., Sonstroem, R.J., & Metz, I.F. (1970). Physical fitness, self-esteem, and attitudes toward physical activity. *Research Quarterly for Exercise and Sport*, **40**, 743-749.

O'Connell, J.K., Price, J.H., Roberts, S.M., Jurs, S.G., & McKinley, R. (1985). Utilizing the health belief model to predict dieting and exercising behavior of obese and nonobese adolescents. *Health Education Quarterly*, **12**, 343-351.

Oliver, M.L. (1980). Race, class and the family's orientation to mobility through sport. *Sociological Symposium*, **30**, 62-86.

Overman, S.J., & Rao, V.V. (1981). Motivation for and extent of participation in organized sports by high school seniors. *Research Quarterly for Exercise and Sport*, **52**, 228-237.

Parcel, G.S., & Baranowski, T. (1981, May/June). Social learning theory and health education. *Health Education*, pp. 14-18.

Parcel, G.S., Simons-Morton, B.G., O'Hara, N.M., Baranowski, T., Kolbe, L.J., & Bee, D.E. (1987). School promotion of healthful diet and exercise behavior: An integration of organizational change and social learning theory interventions. *Journal of School Health*, **57**, 150-156.

Pate, R.R., & Blair, S.N. (1978). Exercise and the prevention of atherosclerosis: Pediatric implications. In W.B. Strong (Ed.), *Atherosclerosis: Its pediatric aspects* (pp. 251-286). New York: Grune & Stratton.

Patriksson, G. (1981). Socialization to sports involvement. *Scandinavian Journal of the Sports Science*, **3**(1), 27-32.

Patterson, G.R. (1982). *A social learning approach: Vol. 3. Coercive family process*. Eugene, OR: Castalia.

Perrier Corporation. (1984). *Fitness in America: The Perrier Study*. New York: Garland.

Perry, C., Baranowski, T., & Parcel, G. (1990). How individuals, environments and health behaviors interact: Social learning theory. In K. Glanz, F.M. Lewis, & B.K. Rimer (Eds.), *Health behaviors and health education, theory, research and practice* (pp. 161-186). San Francisco: Jossey-Bass.

Perusse, L., LeBlanc, C., & Bouchard, C. (1988). Familial resemblance in lifestyle components: Results from the Canada Fitness Survey. *Canadian Journal of Public Health*, **79**, 201-205.

Perusse, L., Tremblay, A., LeBlanc, C., & Bouchard, C. (1989). Genetic and environmental influences on level of habitual physical activity and exercise participation. *American Journal of Epidemiology*, **129**(5), 1012-1022.

Powell, K.E., & Dysinger, W. (1987). Childhood participation in organized school sports and physical education as precursors of adult physical activity. *American Journal of Preventive Medicine*, **3**, 276-281.

Reynolds, K.D., Killen, J.D., Bryson, S.W., Maron, D.J., Taylor, C.B., Maccoby, N., & Farquhar, J.W. (1990). Psychosocial predictors of physical activity in adolescents. *Preventive Medicine*, **19**, 541-551.

Routh, D.K., Walton, M.D., Padan-Belkin, E. (1978). Development of activity level in children revisited: Effects of mother presence. *Developmental Psychology*, **14**, 571-581.

Rowland, T.W. (1990). *Exercise and children's health*. Champaign, IL: Human Kinetics.

Ruffer, W.A. (1965). A study of extreme physical activity groups of young men. *Research Quarterly*, **36**, 183-196.

Sallis, J.F., Alcaraz, J.E., McKenzie, T.L., Hovell, M.F., Kolody, B., & Nader, P.R. (1992). Parental behavior in relation to physical activity and fitness in 9-year-old children. *American Journal of Diseases of Children*, **146**, 1383-1388.

Sallis, J.F., Hovell, M.F., Hofstetter, C.R., Elder, J.P., Hackley, M., Caspersen, C.J., & Powell, K.E. (1990). Distance between homes and exercise facilities related to frequency of exercise among San Diego residents. *Public Health Reports*, **105**(2), 179-185.

Sallis, J.F., & McKenzie, T.L. (1991). Physical education's role in public health. *Research Quarterly for Exercise and Sport*, **62**, 124-137.

Sallis, J.F., & Nader, P.R. (1988). Family determinants of health behaviors. In D.S. Gochman (Ed.), *Health behavior* (pp. 107-124). New York: Plenum.

Sallis, J.F., Patterson, T.L., Buono, M.J., Atkins, C.J., & Nader, P.R. (1988). Aggregation of physical activity habits in Mexican-American and Anglo families. *Journal of Behavioral Medicine*, **11**(1), 31-41.

Sallis, J.F., Patterson, T.L., McKenzie, T.L., & Nader, P.R. (1988). Family variables and physical activity in preschool children. *Journal of Developmental and Behavioral Pediatrics*, **9**(2), 57-61.

Scarr, S. (1966). Genetic factors in activity motivation. *Child Development*, **37**, 663-671.

Schoenfield, A. (1987). Children in sports. *Olympic Message*, 9-16.

Shephard, R.J., & Godin, G. (1986). Behavioral intentions and activity of children. In J. Rutenfranz, R. Mocellin, & F. Klimt (Eds.), *Children and exercise XII: Vol. 17. International series on sport sciences* (pp. 103-109). Champaign, IL: Human Kinetics.

Simons-Morton, B.G., O'Hara, N.M., Parcel, G.S., Huang, I.W., Baranowski, T., & Wilson, B. (1990). Children's frequency of participation in moderate to vigorous physical activities. *Research Quarterly for Exercise and Sport*, **61**, 307-314.

Snyder, E.E., & Purdy, D.A. (1982). Socialization into sport: Parent and child reverse and reciprocal effects. *Research Quarterly for Exercise and Sport*, **53**, 263-266.

Steinhardt, M.A., & Dishman, R.K. (1989). Reliability and validity of expected outcomes and barriers for habitual physical activity. *Journal of Occupational Medicine*, **31**, 536-546.

Sunnegardh, J., Bratteby, L.E., & Sjolin, S. (1985). Physical activity and sports involvement in 8- and 13-year old children in Sweden. *Acta Paediatrica Scandinavica*, **74**(6), 904-912.

Taggart, A.C., Taggart, J., & Siedentop, D. (1986). Effects of a home-based activity program: A study with low-fitness elementary school children. *Behavior Modification*, **10**, 487-507.

Tappe, M.K., Duda, J.L., & Ehrnwald, P.M. (1989). Perceived barriers to exercise among adolescents. *Journal of School Health*, **59**, 153-155.

Tarbell, S.E., Freedson, P.S., Ellison, R.C., Vickers-Lahti, M., Garrahie, E.J., & Marmor, J.K. (1988). *Interrelationship between psychosocial factors and indices of physical activity and body fat in young children.* Paper presented at the Toronto Conference, Toronto, ON.

Taylor, W.C., Parcel, G.S., Elder, J.P., Stone, E.J., Perry, C.L., Oliveria, S.A., & Johnson, C.C. (1991). *Development and evaluation of an instrument for assessing physical activity reinforcement in children.* Manuscript submitted for publication.

Treiber, F.A., Baranowski, T., Braden, D.S., Strong, W.B., & Levy, M. (1991). *Social support for exercise: Relationship to physical activity in young adults.* Manuscript submitted for publication.

U.S. Department of Health and Human Services. (1987). National Children and Youth Fitness Study II. *Journal of Physical Education, Recreation, and Dance*, **58**, 85-96.

Watson, G. (1977). Games, socialization and parental values: Social class differences in parental evaluation of Little League baseball. *International Review of Sport Sociology*, **12**(11), 17-47.

Willerman, L., & Plomin, R. (1973). Activity level in children and their parents. *Child Development*, **44**, 854-858.

Wilson Sporting Goods Company. (1988). *The Wilson report: Moms, dads, daughters and sports.* River Grove, IL: Author.

Zajonc, R.B. (1980). Compresence. In P.B. Paulus (Ed.), *Psychology of group influence* (pp. 35-60). Hillsdale, NJ: Erlbaum.

We gratefully acknowledge the assistance of Ms. Sema Spigner and Ms. Kathye Brewer in typing the manuscript and of Ms. Sharon Snider in reviewing it for APA style requirements.

CHAPTER 13

Determinants of Exercise in People Aged 65 Years and Older

Roy J. Shephard

Surveys of both single communities (e.g., the Tecumseh Study, Montoye, 1975) and of representative national samples (e.g., the Canada Fitness Survey, 1983) have shown a progressive reduction of habitual physical activity with age. The final years of life are marked by a major deterioration of health and consequent demands for expensive medical services (Canada Health Survey, 1982), although there is growing evidence that regular exercise can delay the functional losses that lead to dependency and institutionalization (Shephard, 1991). It is thus important to analyze the causes of the trend toward a restriction of exercise behavior in senior citizens and to seek methods of preventing or reversing the age-related decline in habitual activity.

The behavioral model of Fishbein and Ajzen (1975) has been adapted to exercise (Godin & Shephard, 1985, 1990b). It provides a convenient framework for the present analysis (Figure 13.1). According to this model, a behavioral intention (e.g., an intention to exercise) is formed through a weighted appraisal of attitudes toward the specific behavior and perceived subjective norms for this behavior. The individual's attitude toward a specific act at any given age depends on the summed product of beliefs that the behavior in question will contribute to specific outcomes and an evaluation of the desirability of such outcomes. For example, a person might believe that participation in a biweekly exercise class at the local seniors' center would increase social contacts, and they might evaluate this as a desirable personal outcome. Subjective norms reflect the summed products of the individual's beliefs that specific referents, such as a spouse or friend, think he or she should perform the behavior in question and the individual's

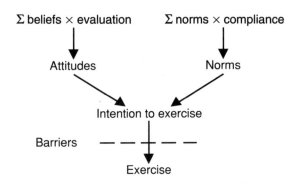

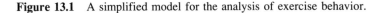

Figure 13.1   A simplified model for the analysis of exercise behavior.

motivation to comply with a referent's perceived wishes. For example, an 80-year-old woman might think that her doctor wants her to be very cautious about participating in a regular biweekly exercise class, and she might also have a strong motivation to comply with this perceived normative medical recommendation.

External Variables Influencing Exercise Intentions

Godin and Shephard (1990b) have shown that, in the case of exercise, the Fishbein and Ajzen model does not provide a complete description of the reasoned behavioral process. External variables, such as habits, personality characteristics, and socioeconomic status influence various steps in the formation of a behavioral intention. Physical and psychological barriers, real and perceived, also limit the translation of a behavioral intention to exercise into the overt behavior of participation.

We will now examine the way in which these several influences operate in the senior citizen.

Age

Senior citizens do not form a homogeneous group (Shephard, 1987). Gerontologists commonly distinguish between the young old, who have no obvious limitation on physical activity; the middle old, who suffer from physical limitations; and the very old, who are almost totally dependent. Representatives of the three subgroups are concentrated in successive age ranges (65-74 years, 75-84 years, and over 85 years, respectively), but much individual variation of physical activity exists among people of any given age, and it is better to base a classification on what individuals can accomplish (i.e., according to functional age) than on calendar age.

There are few formal studies comparing physical-activity patterns across the three subgroups of seniors. Sedentary individuals may show a brief phase of increased physical activity as they seek new interests around the time of retirement (Shephard, 1987), but casual observation strongly suggests that the age-related trend of a decline in habitual physical activity then continues and even accelerates. A volunteer bias may exaggerate activity patterns in the older representatives of some test samples. The nature of habitual physical activity commonly changes as people age. For example, in the city of Tecumseh (Michigan) Montoye (1975) found that participation in 8 of 10 active pursuits declined with aging; on the other hand, older individuals showed some increase in participation (although not necessarily in energy expenditure) in walking and gardening. In a national sample of Canadians, Stephens and Craig (1990) found a progressive decline in participation in swimming and cycling with age. Although 44% of men and 50% of women aged 25 to 44 years swam, less than 20% of men and 20% of women over 65 swam. Likewise, 50% of men and 46% of women aged 25 to 44 years reported cycling, but less than 20% of men and less than 15% of women over age 65 did. The figures for walking were 62% and 78% versus 77% and 81%, and for gardening, 66% and 62% versus 77% and 57%.

Gender

Until recently, men have claimed to view physical activity as a means to health, whereas women have reported valuing exercise more as a means of social interaction or improving their appearance (Shephard, Morgan, Finucane, & Schimmelfing, 1980). Older people often espouse traditional values, and one might thus anticipate a persistence of such gender-related differences among senior citizens. Stephens and Craig (1990), however, noted relatively small differences in motives for exercising between men and women over age 65. Feeling better physically (men, 58%; women, 55%) and improving fitness (men, 51%; women 53%) were valued about equally, whereas looking better/achieving weight control (men, 31%; women, 44%) and socializing (men, 25%; women, 31%) were only slightly more common motives for women.

When the Fishbein behavioral model was applied to subjects aged 45 to 74 years, Godin and Shephard (1986c) found that this model explained more of the variance in exercise intentions in men than in women, and in their sample men tended to report stronger exercise intentions than women (1.6 versus 1.1 on a 7-point scale of −3 to +3, nonsignificant). A difference in this direction would be expected if men were interested in exercise for health reasons, whereas women attended classes for social interaction that was not closely linked to the act of exercising.

Socioeconomic Status

Younger adults show quite marked socioeconomic gradients of physical-activity patterns (Stephens & Craig, 1990). Although a difference in disposable income may contribute, it does not seem to explain the entire gradient because low-income groups in Canadian society still find substantial sums to spend upon such passive recreational devices as motor homes, powerboats, and snowmobiles (Shephard, 1986). Possible influences favoring the development of physical-activity habits in the upper echelons of society include greater education, more awareness of the health benefits of exercise, stronger social norms of active leisure, greater access to transportation, and an exercise environment that often offers greater acceptance to those of high socioeconomic status. A comparison of people who failed to complete high school with university graduates indicated that the differences in participation were larger for cycling (30% versus 56%) and swimming (32% versus 56%) than for the more readily available pursuits of walking (68% versus 75%) and gardening (60% versus 58%).

There are no formal studies relating activity to education and income after retirement, but informal observations suggest that the socioeconomic gradients of active leisure established during working life persist into retirement.

Habit

Habit is an important determinant of most types of future behavior (Triandis, 1977). In the case of exercise, both early life experiences (Harris, 1970; Schreyer, Lime, & Williams, 1984; Sofranko & Nolan, 1972; Yoesting & Burkhead, 1973) and more recent involvement in physical activity (Oldridge, 1981; Valois, Sheph-ard, & Godin, 1986) influence compliance and adherence to current programs (Table 13.1). Statistical analysis reveals no significant age and habit interaction, however, suggesting that the impact of habit upon reasoned behavior is unaffected by the individual's age.

Personality

An individual's personality can influence the development and evaluation of beliefs, perception of and compliance with behavioral norms, and perhaps most importantly, reaction to barriers, real or perceived, that threaten the translation of an exercise intention into overt behavior.

Subjects with a favorable attitude toward exercise are more likely to become active if they have an internal rather than an external locus of control (Sonstroem & Walker, 1973) and thus see themselves as controlling the environment, rather than being controlled by it.

Although two recent studies found no relationship between perceived physical ability and either the attitude-behavior relationship (Godin & Shephard, 1986a) or physical-activity patterns (Valois et al., 1986), all of the subjects involved were of working age rather than retirees, and few had any overt physical disabilities. Moreover, the type of activity being considered was health-related exercise rather than competitive sport (as in the study of Ryckman, Robbins, Thornton, &

Table 13.1 Relationship of Physical Activity to Perceived Physical Ability and Activity Habits

Perceived physical ability	Current physical-activity score		
	Weak habit	Moderate habit	Strong habit
Low	4.2 ± 5.3	9.9 ± 6.0	14.6 ± 3.8
High	4.1 ± 4.5	12.2 ± 4.9	13.9 ± 4.1
All subjects	4.1 ± 5.1	10.9 ± 5.6	14.3 ± 3.9

Note. Physical activity (in arbitrary units) is average for a 2-month period. Perceived physical ability was observed over the preceeding 4 months. Subjects covered three age ranges (< 30 years, 30-45 years, and > 45 years), with no differences of effect related to age. Data from Valois et al. (1986).

Cantrell, 1982), in which the expected influence of perceived self-efficacy upon participation was demonstrated. Stephens and Craig (1990) noted that the percentage of individuals who perceived little control over the choice to be active increased from 19% of men and 28% of women aged 20 to 24 years to 45% of men and 42% of women over age 65.

An individual's locus of control usually becomes externalized as physical disabilities develop (Goldberg & Shephard, 1982). Such a shift probably has a negative influence upon the translation of exercise intentions into exercise behavior among the frail elderly, thus affecting participation not only in sports, such as masters' competitions, but also in more moderate health-related activity.

Another group of factors that influences the usefulness of the standard behavioral model includes the individual's attitudes toward targets, people, and institutions in various situations. The interaction of age with such external factors remains unclear.

Finally, there is the issue of meshing the demands of the proposed exercise program with individuals' personality characteristics, such as location on the extroversion-introversion continuum. Extroverted individuals respond positively to group programs, but introverts react more favorably to individual exercise programs (Massie & Shephard, 1971). To the extent that individual exercisers face fewer practical barriers than those who seek organized group programs, it may be easier for introverts than for extroverts to translate an exercise intention into exercise behavior.

Godin and Shephard (1990a) noted that in one sample of employees ranging in age from 20 to 65 years, variables external to the standard Fishbein model (particularly age and sex) had a much greater impact upon behavioral intentions than the model's intrinsic components (Table 13.2). Plainly, the fraction of the total variance described by existing models of reasoned behavior remains small, and there is room for imaginative research.

Table 13.2   Standardized Beta Weights for a Multiple Regression Model Predicting Intentions to Exercise

Variable	Standardized beta weight
Fishbein variables	
Normative belief (nb)	.050
Motivation to comply (mc)	.078
nb.mc	.054
Age	−.294[a]
Female sex	−.131
Education	.088

Note. Subjects were 190 employees aged 20 to 65 years; cumulative r^2 = .104.
[a]$p < .001$.
Data from Godin and Shephard (1990b).

Attitudes Toward Exercise

One basic tenet of Fishbein's model of reasoned behavior is that an individual carries out a personal cost-benefit analysis before initiating a given behavior. He or she forms a positive attitude toward a particular behavior, such as undertaking a given type of exercise, if it is perceived to have more beneficial than harmful consequences for the individual concerned.

A number of studies have examined seniors' beliefs about exercise by using open-ended questions. Sidney and Shephard (1977) designed an experimental exercise program for university retirees. They found that for men the rank ordering of stated reasons for participation were improved fitness or health, availability of an instructional program, "to assist science," improved appearance or control of body weight, and availability of exercise testing. For the women the perceived reasons were fitness or health or the availability of an instructional program, psychological well-being, availability of exercise testing, fun or curiosity, and socializing. The Canada Fitness Survey (1983) classified stated reasons for exercising according to age. Many items, such as "feeling better" or "improving flexibility," showed little age gradient. One item ("a doctor's advice") increased sharply in importance among older respondents, whereas three other items ("pleasure, fun, and excitement"; "learning new things"; and "challenging one's abilities") became less important among older subjects. More recently, Stephens and Craig (1990) found the strongest age gradient in "exercise as a means of getting outdoors," which was reported by 31% of men and 36% of women aged 20 to 24 years but by 59% of men and 54% of women over age 65. The Norwegian Confederation of Sports (1984) observed an increasing appreciation of the contribution of exercise to health and a diminished valuation of the fun and enjoyment of exercise among the older members of the population they sampled.

The Kenyon Inventory of Attitudes Toward Physical Activity (Kenyon, 1986) has been criticized because it fails to focus on an individual's attitudes toward participation in a particular type of physical activity under specific circumstances (Godin & Shephard, 1986a). Nevertheless, scores from this device support the view that senior citizens, relative to teenagers and middle-aged adults, place increasing value on exercise as an aesthetic experience and as a means to health and fitness, whereas they show decreased interest in exercise as the pursuit of vertigo (Sidney, Niinimaa, & Shephard, 1983; Sidney & Shephard, 1977).

When a sample of adults aged 45 to 74 years responded to an objective 7-point Likert-type scaling of exercise beliefs (Godin & Shephard, 1986c), the dominant items were to control body mass, look younger, fill recreational time, be healthy, be energetic, and improve physical fitness (Table 13.3). A multivariate analysis in which all 14 beliefs were considered jointly confirmed the statistical significance of the differences seen in univariate comparisons between those with high and low exercise intentions [$F(13,69) = 3.24$]. Although exercise as a means to good health remained a significant factor in this analysis, it was less important than had been suggested by open-ended questioning. Other trends regarding differences of belief between the groups with high and low exercise intentions, although not statistically significant, were generally in the expected directions.

Table 13.3   Scores on an Intention to Exercise Scale in Relation to Specific Beliefs About Exercise

	Intention to exercise	
Belief about exercise	Low	High
Control body mass	0.06	1.29[a]
Look younger	0.06	1.29[a]
Fill recreation time	−.25	0.99[a]
Be healthy	1.94	2.50[b]
Be more energetic	1.38	2.07[b]
Improve appearance	0.63	1.56[b]
Live longer	1.25	1.10
Relieve tension	1.63	1.66
Be tired	1.69	0.90
Feel good	1.81	2.14
Meet people	0.44	0.91
Consume time	1.25	1.17
Improve thinking	0.69	1.11
Be physically fit	1.44	1.90

Note. Beliefs were measured with an arbitrary 7-point scale (−3 to + 3).
[a]$p < .01$.
[b]$p < .05$.
Data From Godin and Shephard (1986c).

The belief that exercise would increase longevity was not held particularly strongly by those with a marked intention to exercise. Likewise, the belief that exercise would make participants feel good seemed less well developed in the 45- to 74-year-old subjects than in younger exercisers, perhaps because the former were finding it physically more difficult to undertake the prescribed exercise or exercise was becoming less comfortable. The perception of the time demands of the program did not differ with the strength of exercise intentions, perhaps because a work-site program was readily available to these subjects.

Fishbein's model considers attitude toward activity as the summed product of individual beliefs and their personal evaluation (Godin & Shephard, 1986c). There is quite a substantial zero-order correlation between the summed product and an independent assessment of attitude toward physical activity in people aged 45 to 74 years ($r = .522$, Godin & Shephard, 1986c), showing that the model accounts for a substantial fraction of the variance in attitudes of older people.

Subjective Norms for Exercise

Fishbein and Ajzen (1975) postulated that behavioral intentions would be significantly strengthened if the people under study both perceived that their significant others wished them to adopt a given behavior and were strongly motivated to comply with the perceived desire. In the case of exercise for senior citizens, the behavioral norm of an active lifestyle is unfortunately weak in many societies. Until recently the overall subjective norm has been that retirement provides an opportunity for people to "slow down" and "take a well-earned rest." It is thus not surprising that the perceived attitudes of society show no relationship to the strength of exercise intentions in older adults (Table 13.4).

Table 13.4   Relationship Between Normative Beliefs and Behavioral Intention to Exercise

	Intention to exercise	
Normative belief	Low	High
Close friends	0.07	1.10[a]
Most members of family	0.36	1.37[a]
Physical educators	1.21	1.90
Physicians	0.43	1.21
Society	1.14	1.10

Note. Beliefs were measured with an arbitrary 7-point scale (-3 to $+3$).
[a]$p < .05$.
Data from Godin and Shephard (1986a).

Primary-care physicians are in a strong position to set subjective norms that encourage active behavior (Mulder, 1981). But in practice it is rare for doctors to have a significant influence on the exercise behavior of their patients. In the early 1980s only a quarter of regular exercisers had been advised to exercise by their physicians (Canada Fitness Survey, 1983; Dishman, Sallis, & Orenstein, 1985). Moreover, such advice had been concentrated on younger adults and had been couched in general terms, with correspondingly little impact on behavior. The President's Council on Physical Fitness and Sports (1973) found that only 3% of adults cited medical advice as their reason for exercising, and none of the subjects seen by Sidney and Shephard (1977) made such a comment. Iverson, Fielding, Crow, and Christenson (1985) reported that doctors offered an exercise prescription to only 3.4% of ambulatory patients. Moreover, 80% of patients had never been given advice to exercise by their doctors (Wechsler, Levine, Idelson, Rohman, & Taylor, 1983; Wyshak, Lamb, Lawrence, & Curran, 1980). Indeed, few physicians regarded regular aerobic exercise as an important matter to discuss with their patients (Valente, Sobal, Muncie, Levine, & Antlitz, 1986; Wechsler et al., 1983), although Riddle (1980) did find an association between jogging behavior and the patient's perception of their physician's beliefs about exercise.

From a public-health standpoint, an important opportunity was missed during this period, as 43% of inactive adults claimed that positive advice from a doctor would have increased their involvement in sport (Perrier Corporation, 1979). The situation now appears to be changing, and Stephens and Craig (1990) found that 56% of those over age 65 were being encouraged to exercise by their doctors. This is fortunate because as people age they increasingly rely on medical advice regarding physical activity (Canada Fitness Survey, 1983).

Godin and Shephard (1990a) noted that the adult population as a whole held a favorable impression of physicians' attitudes toward exercise (Table 13.5). People also had a desire to comply with such beliefs. The exception in the study

Table 13.5   Normative Beliefs Concerning Physician's Expectations in Selected Populations and Motivation to Comply With Physician's Perceived Recommendation

Population	Normative belief	Motivation to comply
Parents (average age 42 years)	1.7 ± 1.5	1.6 ± 1.6
Employees (average age 39 years)	0.9 ± 1.6	0.9 ± 1.5
Disabled (average age 31 years)	−1.5 ± 1.4	−1.2 ± 1.4
Pregnant (average age 26 years)	2.0 ± 1.0	1.1 ± 1.8
Total sample (N = 799)	1.3 ± 1.7	1.1 ± 1.8

Note. Both items were scored on an arbitrary 7-point scale (−3 to +3).
Data from Godin and Shephard (1990b).

was a sample of young adult paraplegics. They perceived that their physicians had a cautious, negative attitude toward their involvement in exercise and they had a corresponding lack of respect for that medical judgment. The sample did not include people beyond retirement age, but it seems likely that some physicians would also show the cautious attitude of "defensive medicine" when advising older patients, whether disabled or not.

Of even greater importance from a public-health standpoint, when physicians advise exercise, they apparently ought to present the case more strongly and specifically, as neither the physician's perceived normative beliefs nor the patient's motivation to comply with such norms was significantly related to the patient's exercise participation (Godin & Shephard, 1986b).

Physical educators, another source of normative social influences that might be expected to promote physical activity, were apparently little more effective than physicians. The influence of family and friends was dominant (as previously suggested by Heinzelmann, 1973, and Oldridge, 1982). It seems likely that with the progressive social isolation of the middle old and very old, positive influences from family and friends diminish progressively. It is also likely that the beliefs or perceived beliefs of such reference groups change with age. The friends of the elderly have themselves become less active, and members of the immediate family may fear that if a parent or an elderly relative is encouraged to engage in vigorous activity, such activity will precipitate serious injury, leading to a dependency that would be disastrous for the next of kin. Stephens and Craig (1990) found that the positive influence of a spouse decreased from 62% in men and 64% in women aged 20 to 24 years to 54% and 41%, respectively, in those over age 65. Likewise, encouragement from friends decreased from 55% in men and 53% in women at 20 to 24 years to 47% in both men and women over age 65. On the other hand, Godin and Shephard (1986a) found no interactions of age or sex with either normative beliefs or the motivation to comply with them in their sample of adults aged 45 to 74 years, although all members of this sample were sufficiently active to volunteer for an exercise class.

The relationship of an independent assessment of subjective norms to the summed product of normative beliefs and the motivation to comply with such norms was weaker than that revealed in the corresponding analysis for attitudes, but it nevertheless remained highly significant ($r = .35$, $p < .001$, Godin & Shephard, 1986a), supporting the use of the Fishbein model in this age group. Social norms had more influence on exercise in the less-educated members of the sample.

Overall Determinants of Exercise Intentions in Older Adults

A multiple regression analysis that tested intentions to exercise against attitudes toward activity, subjective norms, recent exercise behavior, prior experience of sport and physical activity, educational level, and two- and three-way interactions between these variables yielded a cumulative r^2 of .364. The proportion of variance described by the measured factors is of the order anticipated in psychometric analyses: the findings indicate that almost 64% of the variance is attributable either to methodological problems or to other unmeasured variables. Individual terms carrying a significant beta weight included attitude toward exercise (.389) and two-way interactions linking subjective norms with level of education (.207), prior experience of exercise (.141), and sex (.136).

Barriers to Exercise

An exercise intention does not always translate into exercise behavior. Intervening factors include not only obvious physical and psychological barriers to exercise but also motivations to alternative behaviors and role-playing influences (Shephard, 1985).

Godin, Valois, Shephard, and Desharnais (1987) conducted a path analysis of habits, attitudes, subjective norms, intentions, and behavior on a sample of 136 adults ranging in age from 20 to 65 years. Although there was a strong simple correlation between behavioral intention and behavior over the next 3 weeks ($r = .559$), this became statistically insignificant ($r = .073$) when the more sophisticated path analysis allowed for the dominant effect of habit. Nevertheless, intention remained related to exercise behavior over the following 2 months ($r = .581$ in a simple correlation; $r = .412$ in path analysis), perhaps because the influence of occasional barriers became less important over a longer period of observation.

Attitude exerted its influence upon behavior largely through intention, and subjective norms had surprisingly little influence on behavior. The implication for current short-term programs of health promotion seems to be that promoters should emphasize the development of the exercise habit at an early age and focus more attention on strengthening positive attitudes than on developing favorable subjective norms.

There has been extensive discussion of perceived obstacles to exercise in both Canada (Canada Fitness Survey, 1983) and the United States (Dishman et al., 1985). Dishman and his associates stressed the need to diminish or compensate for physical, environmental, and psychological barriers to exercise; to provide knowledge, skills, and reinforcements that encourage physical activity; and to guide the individual in choosing an exercise program of appropriate type and intensity.

The most common barriers adults perceive to regular exercise are "work pressures," "laziness," and "lack of time" (Table 13.6). Likewise, more time is seen as the factor most likely to increase personal participation (Table 13.7). At first inspection, the complaint of lack of time is difficult to reconcile with the 5 to 15 hr per week that most Canadian adults spend watching television (Stephens & Craig, 1990), but the complaint becomes more comprehensible if

Table 13.6   Factors Restricting Participation in Exercise Programs

Obstacle	% currently participating	% not participating
Work pressures	56	39
Laziness	30	26
Lack of facilities	21	13
Lack of time	22	9
Cost	16	10
Injury of illness	17	39

Data from Canada Fitness Survey (1983) for subjects over age 20 years.

Table 13.7   Factors That Would Encourage Personal Participation in Physical Activity

Factor	Percentage of sample citing factor
More time	40
Better facilities	27
Partner	22
Family interest	18
Friend's interest	17
Cheaper facilities	16
Fitness classes	11
Fitness test	9
Organized sports	9
Activities sponsored by employer or union	7
Information on benefits	6
Nothing	20

Data from Canada Fitness Survey (1983).

the time is translated into an equivalent opportunity cost. If we suppose that 2 hr of travel are required to attend a 1-hr organized exercise class and the use of time is valued at an average industrial wage of $15/hr, then the investment of time in travel and participation becomes much greater than the cost of club membership or the purchase of recommended clothing and equipment.

Old age undoubtedly influences the relative importance of many barriers to exercise. Time is more available to the senior citizen. A comparison of findings for those aged 25 to 44 years and those over age 65 indicates that work was a barrier for 63% of younger men and 56% of younger women but for less than 15% of older men and women. Family commitments were a barrier for 35% of younger men and 50% of younger women, but less than 15% of people over age

65 found such commitments a barrier. Other competing interests dropped from 25% and 19% in younger men and women, respectively, to less than 15% in older people. Nevertheless, the minimum time investment needed in order to participate in a group exercise program may increase with retirement. Often older people no longer have access to a convenient work-site class, and they may need to reach alternative facilities by an infrequent bus service or an even less convenient transportation system for the disabled. It is thus fortunate that the interests of the elderly often turn to walking and gardening. There remains a need for health professionals to find ways of incorporating greater amounts of exercise into the normal day of the senior citizen and to find appealing forms of physical activity that do not require long journeys to a distant exercise complex.

Disposable income is generally reduced at retirement, and elderly women make up a large fraction of the poor in most developed societies. Probably because of the shift to low-cost pursuits, cost is seen as less of a barrier for older adults (Stephens & Craig, 1990). Nevertheless, those prescribing exercise should look critically at recommendations that require a large financial investment in membership fees and specialized clothing and equipment.

The social requirements of active leisure—joint participation with other family members, friends, or a partner—are less often available to the elderly. Stephens and Craig (1990) found this was a barrier for 12% of men and 15% of women aged 25 to 44 years but for less than 15% of men and 19% of women over age 65.

Lastly, there are the barriers of illness or injury and the fear that exercise may induce such problems. In the typical scenario, a senior citizen spends 9 to 10 years with some physical disability, which culminates in a final year of almost total dependency. Women live longer than men but also suffer a longer period of dependency (Canada Health Survey, 1982). Illness or injury was seen as a barrier to exercise by 8% of men and 9% of women aged 25 to 44 years but by 19% of men and 34% of women over age 65 (Stephens & Craig, 1990). Illness or physical disability becomes an ever-increasing barrier to participation for many of the very old, and there is consequently a great need for test facilities and programs adapted to the needs of those with various types and degrees of disability. Programs for the disabled should be able to accommodate not only people with various types of locomotor problems but also the growing numbers who have sensory impairments (blindness, deafness, loss of balance) and cognitive loss. Sidney and Shephard (1977) noted the importance the elderly attached to a specific program for seniors, with instructions on how to exercise safely and opportunities for regularly supervised activity. Their observation may be linked to people's age-related fear of injury while exercising (10% of men and women 25-44 years but 15% of men and 21% of women over age 65; Stephens & Craig, 1990).

Motivation to continue in alternative sedentary behavior may be quite strong in the middle-old and very old because medical advisers and other care givers commonly dissuade significant involvement in exercise. Some old people also come to enjoy playing the role of an invalid, and such role-playing militates against effective involvement in a rehabilitation program.

Practical Lessons for Programming

From the foregoing discussion, it is plain that initial motivation and sustained compliance are no easier to achieve as people age. Nevertheless, certain guidelines can be suggested. It is more useful to focus on beliefs than on subjective norms, and appropriate exercise beliefs should be shaped by a simple but sound educational program (Clark, 1985). Given the dominant influence of prior experience, the exercise program should build upon an individual's previous habits, tapping any skills that have been accumulated and using any readily available supplies of specialized clothing and equipment. If new skills are to be learned, detailed instructions must be provided and opportunities allowed for frequent repetition of the required movements (Redford, 1989). Since recent memory is likely to be poor (particularly in the middle old and very old), it is helpful when instructors not only give frequent reminders of the timing of activity sessions but also incorporate as much of the exercise prescription as possible into the normal day (e.g., the walk to the store for a newspaper or to the dining hall for lunch and supper). Potential barriers to action, such as the absence of a suitable companion, a lack of transportation to the exercise site, limited sight or hearing, and cognitive, emotional, or behavioral problems, must be recognized and overcome. Records should be kept of the individual's beliefs about exercise, and feedback about test results should be provided with those beliefs in mind. For instance, if the exerciser's search is for youth, as some of the data suggest, an increment of maximal oxygen intake with training could be presented as a means of reducing biological age.

Above all, exercise must be seen as personally rewarding. A skilled class leader will present participation in such terms: as a means of escape from physical dependency, of earning the respect of significant others, or of gaining a sense of personal fulfillment. For the sake of role modeling, it is often useful to have an older person lead an exercise class. As age increases, lack of ability is increasingly seen as a barrier to participation (less than 10% of men and 18% of women aged 25-44 years but 15% of men and 23% of women over age 65; Stephens & Craig, 1990), and a growing number of men feel ''ill at ease'' in an exercise class (7% of men and 16% of women aged 25-44 years but 15% of men and women over age 65). Failure to meet the unrealistic expectations of a young, very fit class leader can further weaken self-efficacy and motivation among the frail elderly (Sidney & Shephard, 1977).

Impact on Public Health

Regular exercise can add as much as 2 years to the life span of a middle-aged adult, but because of a ''squaring'' of the mortality curve (Fries, 1980), the gain of life expectancy seems reduced to a few months if an individual does not begin to exercise until age 70 or 75 years (Paffenbarger, 1988).

On the other hand, the opportunity for an increase in the quality-adjusted life span remains quite large even in old age. Regular exercise can set back the age when dependencies would otherwise result from a deterioration of physical capacities (aerobic power, muscular strength, and flexibility) by as much as 10 to 20 years. This effect was clearly demonstrated by the results of a retrospective questionnaire that related senior citizens' current dependency to their activity habits at age 50 (Table 13.8).

Finally, there is the potential for vigorous senior citizens to serve as role models. Such people can encourage an active lifestyle not only among their peers but also in younger individuals, for whom the direct economic gains from an increase of physical activity may be much larger (Shephard, 1986). One such role model was Roland Michener, the former governor general of Canada. He would cheerfully jog for a distance of 8 km in his ninth decade of life, and he often embarrassed younger and less fit scientists who were attending health-related meetings in Ottawa by insisting that they accompany him on such expeditions.

Old age is unfortunately marked by a progressive decline in habitual activity. The data suggest that the behavioral model of Fishbein and Ajzen is helpful in clarifying this phenomenon. A review of factors that influence behavioral intentions to exercise among the elderly suggests that attitudes have a larger impact than subjective norms. Short-term health promotion programs should thus focus upon beliefs and attitudes rather than subjective norms. Nevertheless, there is room for health professionals to develop the norm that people should maximize their opportunities for physical activity during retirement. Physicians could play an important role in setting such expectations, as older individuals increasingly seek medical advice before they begin exercising. Habit makes an important contribution to a senior citizen's lifestyle, suggesting that exercise programs for younger people can have a substantial influence upon the exercise behavior of these same individuals as they age. Finally, various external and internal barriers decrease the likelihood that old people will translate an exercise intention into active behavior, so greater effort should be directed to understanding and eliminating such barriers.

Table 13.8   Relationship Between Physical Activity at Age 50 Years and Current Level of Dependency

Level of dependency	Activity score at age 50 years
None	9.28 ± 9.76 ($n = 286$)
Minor disability	8.12 ± 8.94 ($n = 126$)
Severe disability	7.70 ± 9.43 ($n = 173$)
Institutionalized	4.06 ± 6.63 ($n = 25$)

Note. Sample was 674 people aged 65 to 90 years. Units are arbitrary.
Data from Shephard and Montelpare (1988).

References

Canada Fitness Survey. (1983). *Fitness and lifestyle in Canada*. Ottawa, ON: Directorate of Fitness and Amateur Sport.

Canada Health Survey. (1982). Ottawa, ON: Health & Welfare, Canada.

Clark, B.A. (1985). Principles of physical activity programming for the older adult. *Topics in Geriatric Rehabilitation*, **1**, 68-77.

Dishman, R., Sallis, J., & Orenstein, D. (1985). The determinants of physical activity and exercise. *Public Health Reports*, **100**, 158-171.

Fishbein, M., & Ajzen, I. (1975). *Beliefs, attitude, intention and behavior: An introduction to theory and research*. Reading, MA: Addison-Wesley.

Fries, J.F. (1980). Aging, natural death and the compression of morbidity. *New England Journal of Medicine*, **303**, 130-135.

Godin, G., & Shephard, R.J. (1985). Psycho-social predictors of exercise intentions among spouses. *Canadian Journal of Applied Sport Sciences*, **1**, 36-43.

Godin, G., & Shephard, R.J. (1986a). The importance of type of attitude to the study of exercise behavior. *Psychological Reports*, **58**, 991-1000.

Godin, G., & Shephard, R.J. (1986b, June). *Perceived influence of physician and exercise behavior*. Paper presented at the meeting of the Canadian Public Health Association, Vancouver, BC.

Godin, G., & Shephard, R.J. (1986c). Psychosocial factors influencing intentions to exercise in a group of individuals ranging from 45 to 74 years of age. In M. Berridge & G. Ward (Eds.), *International perspectives on adapted physical activity* (pp. 243-249). Champaign, IL: Human Kinetics.

Godin, G., & Shephard, R.J. (1990a). An evaluation of the potential role of the physician in influencing community exercise behavior. *American Journal of Health Promotion*, **4**, 255-259.

Godin, G., & Shephard, R.J. (1990b). Use of attitude-behavior models in exercise promotion. *Sports Medicine*, **10**, 103-121.

Godin, G., Valois, P., & Shephard, R.J. (1986). Perceived physical ability and relation of attitude to behavior. *Perceptual and Motor Skills*, **63**, 1075-1078.

Godin, G., Valois, P., Shephard, R.J., & Desharnais, R. (1987). Prediction of leisure-time exercise behavior: A path analysis (Lisrel V) model. *Journal of Behavioral Medicine*, **10**, 145-158.

Goldberg, G., & Shephard, R.J. (1982). Personality profiles of disabled individuals in relation to physical activity patterns. *Journal of Sports Medicine and Physical Fitness*, **22**, 477-484.

Harris, D.V. (1970). Physical activity history and attitudes of middle-aged men. *Medicine and Science in Sports*, **2**, 203-208.

Heinzelmann, F. (1973). Social and psychological factors that influence the effectiveness of exercise programs. In J.P. Naughton & H.K. Hellerstein (Eds.), *Exercise testing in coronary heart disease* (pp. 275-287). New York: Academic Press.

Iverson, D., Fielding, J., Crow, R., & Christenson, G. (1985). The promotion of physical activity in the United States population: The status of programs in medical, worksite, community and school settings. *Public Health Reports*, **100**, 212-224.

Kenyon, G. (1986). Six scales for assessing attitudes toward physical activity. *Research Quarterly*, **39**, 566-574.

Massie, J., & Shephard, R.J. (1971). Physiological and psychological effects of training. *Medicine and Science in Sports*, **3**, 110-117.

Montoye, H.J. (1975). *Physical activity and health: An epidemiological study of an entire community*. Englewood Cliffs, NJ: Prentice Hall.

Mulder, J.A. (1981). Prescription home exercise therapy for cardiovascular fitness. *Journal of Family Practice*, **13**, 345-348.

Norwegian Confederation of Sports. (1984). *Physical activity in Norway, 1983*. Oslo: Author.

Oldridge, N.B. (1981). Drop-out and potential compliance-improving strategies in exercise rehabilitation. In F.J. Nagle & H.J. Montoye (Eds.), *Exercise in health and disease* (pp. 250-258). Springfield, IL: Charles C Thomas.

Oldridge, N.B. (1982). Compliance and exercise in primary and secondary prevention of coronary heart disease: A review. *Preventive Medicine*, **11**, 56-70.

Paffenbarger, R.S. (1988). Contributions of epidemiology to exercise science and cardiovascular health. *Medicine and Science in Sports and Exercise*, **20**, 426-438.

Perrier Corporation. (1979). *The Perrier Study: Fitness in America*. New York: Author.

President's Council on Physical Fitness and Sports. (1973, May). National Adult Fitness Survey. *Newsletter of Council*, pp. 1-27.

Redford, J.B. (1989). Rehabilitation and the aged. In W. Reichel (Ed.), *Clinical aspects of aging* (3rd ed.) (pp. 177-187). Baltimore: Williams & Wilkins.

Riddle, P. (1980). Attitudes, beliefs, behavioral intentions and behaviors of women and men toward regular jogging. *Research Quarterly*, **51**, 663-674.

Ryckman, R.M., Robbins, M.A., Thornton, B., & Cantrell, P. (1982). Development and validation of a physical self-efficacy scale. *Journal of Personality and Social Psychology*, **42**, 891-900.

Schreyer, R., Lime, D.W., & Williams, D.R. (1984). Characterizing the influence of past experience on recreational behavior. *Journal of Leisure Research*, **16**, 34-50.

Shephard, R.J. (1985). Factors influencing the exercise behavior of patients. *Sports Medicine*, **2**, 348-366.

Shephard, R.J. (1986). *The economic benefits of enhanced fitness*. Champaign, IL: Human Kinetics.

Shephard, R.J. (1987). *Physical activity and aging* (2nd ed.). London: Croom Helm.

Shephard, R.J. (1991). Fitness and aging. In C. Blais (Ed.), *Aging into the twenty-first century* (pp. 22-35). North York, ON: Captus.

Shephard, R.J., & Montelpare, W.M. (1988). Geriatric benefits of exercise as an adult. *Journal of Gerontology (Medical Sciences)*, **43**, M86-M90.

Shephard, R.J., Morgan, P., Finucane, R., & Schimmelfing, L. (1980). Factors influencing recruitment to an occupational fitness program. *Journal of Occupational Medicine*, **22**, 389-398.

Sidney, K.H., Niinimaa, V., & Shephard, R.J. (1983). Attitudes towards exercise and sports: Sex and age differences, and changes with endurance training. *Journal of Sports Sciences*, **1**, 195-210.

Sidney, K.H., & Shephard, R.J. (1977). Attitudes towards health and physical activity in the elderly: Effects of a physical training program. *Medicine and Science in Sports*, **8**, 246-252.

Sofranko, A.J., & Nolan, M.F. (1972). Early life experiences and adult sports participation. *Journal of Leisure Research*, **4**, 6-18.

Sonstroem, R.J., & Walker, M.I. (1973). Relationship of attitudes and locus of control to exercise and physical fitness. *Perceptual and Motor Skills*, **36**, 1031-1034.

Stephens, T., & Craig, C. (1990). *The well-being of Canadians*. Ottawa, ON: Canadian Fitness and Lifestyle Research Institute.

Triandis, H.C. (1977). *Interpersonal behavior*. Pacific Grove, CA: Brooks/Cole.

Valente, C., Sobal, J., Muncie, H., Levine, D., & Antlitz, A. (1986). Health promotion: Physicians' beliefs, attitudes and practices. *American Journal of Preventive Medicine*, **2**, 82-88.

Valois, P., Shephard, R.J., & Godin, G. (1986). Relationship of habit and perceived physical ability to exercise behavior. *Perceptual and Motor Skills*, **62**, 811-817.

Wechsler, H., Levine, S., Idelson, R.K., Rohman, M., & Taylor, J.O. (1983). The physician's role in health promotion: A survey of primary care practitioners. *New England Medical Journal*, **308**, 97-100.

Wyshak, G., Lamb, G.A., Lawrence, R.S., & Curran, W.J. (1980). A profile of the health-promoting behavior of physicians and lawyers. *New England Journal of Medicine*, **303**, 104-107.

Yoesting, D.R., & Burkhead, D.L. (1973). Significance of childhood recreational experience on adult leisure behavior: An explanatory analysis. *Journal of Leisure Research*, **5**, 25-36.

CHAPTER *14*

Physical Activity and Diet in Weight Loss

Denise E. Wilfley
Kelly D. Brownell

Obesity is a major public-health problem. Approximately 27% of women and 24% of men are 20% or more above desirable weight (Kuczmarski, 1992). Conditions related to obesity such as hypertension, diabetes, and cardiovascular disease pose significant threats to health (Bray, 1986; Pi-Sunyer, 1991).

Conventional wisdom suggests that obese people should exercise more, presumably because "it burns calories." It is true that increased activity is beneficial—so much so that the best predictor of long-term maintenance of weight loss is whether a person exercises (Brownell & Wadden, in press). It is unlikely, however, that exercise exerts this powerful effect simply because it burns calories. The mechanisms linking exercise to weight loss are both complex and fascinating. Moreover, the knowledge that exercise is important does not translate into regular activity in most obese people. Improving adherence is a major challenge.

This chapter covers the benefits of physical activity in the obese. We devote particular attention to the mechanisms by which exercise facilitates long-term weight loss, as multiple pathways appear to link exercise to weight change. We explore ways to increase adherence and discuss the importance of tailoring exercise interventions to the special physical and psychosocial needs of obese people. We also examine special issues such as how our culture's preoccupation with shape and weight may perpetuate unhealthy attitudes toward dieting and exercise, how to establish criteria for an individual's "reasonable weight," and when exercise can be psychologically or physically harmful.

Does Exercise Promote Weight Loss?

There has been extensive research to examine the relationship of exercise to weight loss. The results are clear: Regular exercise is a central component of losing weight and is the single best predictor of long-term weight maintenance (King, Taylor, Haskell, & DeBusk, 1988; Pavlou, Krey, & Steffe, 1989; Perri, McAdoo, McAllister, Lauer, & Yancey, 1986). Data indicate a pattern of weight regain when dietary interventions alone are used, whereas diet combined with exercise leads to better maintenance (e.g., Pavlou et al., 1989). Hence, exercise is now recognized as an important predictor of long-term success in weight management (Craighead & Blum, 1989; Epstein, McCurley, Wing, & Valoski, 1990; Hill et al., 1989; Kayman, Bruvold, & Stern, 1990; King, Frey-Hewitt, Dreon, & Wood, 1989; Pavlou et al., 1989; Sikand, Kondo, Foreyt, Jones, & Gotto, 1988).

Correlational studies support this link between exercise and maintenance (Colvin & Olson, 1983; Gormally & Rardin, 1981; Gormally, Rardin, & Black, 1980; Kayman et al., 1990; Marston & Criss, 1984). Kayman et al. (1990) studied formerly obese women who had lost weight and kept it off, comparing them with obese women who had lost weight and regained. Of the maintainers, 90% exercised regularly (minimum of three times a week for more than 30 min), compared with only 34% of the regainers (Figure 14.1).

Experimental studies with random assignment and control groups that compare exercise with no exercise provide the strongest scientific support for the role of exercise in weight control. Several of these studies (Dahlkoetter, Callahan, & Linton, 1979; Duddleston & Bennion, 1970; Harris & Hallbauer, 1973; Hill et al., 1989; Pavlou et al., 1989; Sikand et al., 1988; Stalonas, Johnson, & Christ,

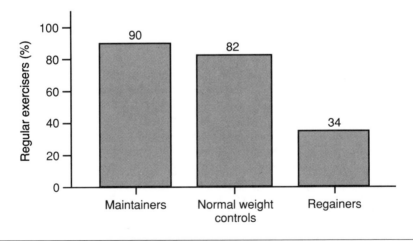

Figure 14.1   Maintenance and relapse after weight loss in women.
Reprinted from Kayman et al. (1990).

1978; van Dale & Saris, 1989) but not all (Belko, Van Loan, Barbieri, & Mayclin, 1987; Lennon, Nagle, Stratman, Shrago, & Dennis, 1985; Phinney, LaGrange, O'Connell, & Danforth, 1988) have found that exercise plus diet leads to greater weight loss than diet alone.

Exercise appears to exert a special influence on weight maintenance. Behavior-modification dietary programs, exercise, and combinations of diet and exercise have about the same short-term effect on weight loss (Grilo, Brownell, & Stunkard, 1993). Therefore, exercise has but a modest effect on initial weight loss, perhaps because dietary compliance is good early in a program and there is little room for additional weight loss.

When the participants in such studies are followed for 1 or 2 years, striking effects of exercise emerge. A study by Pavlou et al. (1989) is noteworthy in this regard. Figure 14.2 displays 8- and 18-month follow-up data from Pavlou et al. (1989). One hundred sixty male members of the Boston Police Department and the Metropolitan District Commission were randomly assigned to one of four 12-week programs (BCDD, or balanced caloric-deficit diet of 1,000 kcal; PSMF, or a ketogenic protein-sparing modified fast; and DPC-70 and DPC-800, two liquid forms of balanced and ketogenic diets) and exercise and nonexercise groups. Note that there is no difference between initial and 18-month follow-up weight for those who did not exercise, regardless of the type of diet used for weight

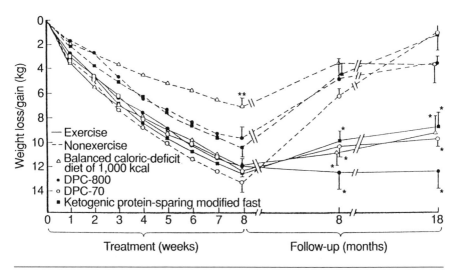

Figure 14.2 Exercise as an adjunct to weight-loss maintenance in moderately obese subjects. Eighteen-month follow-up data confirm the long-term effectiveness of exercise intervention for as short a period as 8 weeks. There is no difference between initial and 18-month follow-up weight for those who did not exercise, regardless of diet used for weight loss. The exercise group, in contrast, maintained weight loss. *Note.* DPC-70 = 420-kcal powdered protein-carbohydrate mix; DPC-800 is an 800-kcal diet provided in powdered form.
Reprinted from Pavlou et al. (1989).

loss. In sharp contrast, the exercise group maintained weight loss. Furthermore, an important predictor of weight maintenance was whether subjects added or stopped exercise during maintenance. As shown in Figure 14.3, participants who ceased exercise at the end of treatment regained weight, whereas those who started exercise at the end of treatment maintained their weight loss at 18-month follow-up.

Exercise facilitates maintenance for those consuming balanced diets (Hill, Newby, Thacker, Sykes, & DiGirolamo, 1988; Pavlou et al., 1989) or extremely low-calorie diets (Pavlou et al., 1989; Sikand et al., 1988). Furthermore, even minimal increases in lifestyle activities (e.g., walking instead of riding, doing errands by walking), which bolster energy expenditure by as little as 200 to 400 kcal per day, result in enhanced maintenance in overweight children (Epstein, Koeske, & Wing, 1984; Epstein, Wing, Koeske, Ossip, & Beck, 1982).

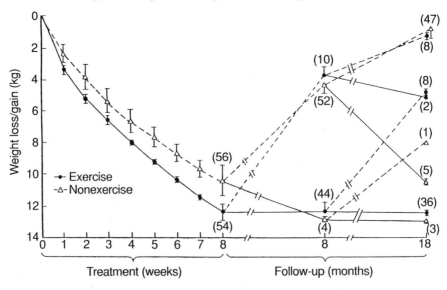

Figure 14.3   The addition or removal of learned exercise appears to be a major contributing factor to weight maintenance. Subjects who ceased exercise regained or demonstrated a strong tendency to return to prestudy weight. Poststudy introduction of exercise (learned but nonsupervised) creates a positive effect. *Note.* Number of subjects is given in parentheses.
Reprinted from Pavlou et al. (1989).

Likely Mechanisms Linking Exercise to Weight Loss

Compelling reasons exist to emphasize physical activity for obese people. Exercise may alter body weight, body composition, appetite, and basal metabolism and can positively affect health status, independent of weight loss. Moreover, exercise can improve psychological functioning, improve self-esteem, and enhance motivation. Therefore, exercise may aid in weight control in many ways (Grilo et al., in press; see Table 14.1).

One can adopt a pragmatic stance with regard to mechanisms and claim that as long as exercise works, defining the precise mechanism is not important. We disagree with this approach and believe that discovery of the mechanism or mechanisms is crucial, not only for scientific reasons but also as a guide in prescribing exercise programs for individuals. For example, if metabolic variables emerge as important, the types and amounts of exercise needed to boost metabolic rate should be prescribed. If psychological mechanisms are more important, consistency, rather than type or amount, may be the central feature of a program. Ultimately, very different programs might be prescribed, depending on the mechanisms linking exercise to weight control.

Exercise Expends Energy

Table 14.2 provides values for caloric expenditure during various physical activities. The chart highlights several important points. First, any activity uses energy, so any increase in activity can promote weight control. Therefore, routine activities such as using stairs and walking are useful ways of expending energy. For example, walking up and down two flights of stairs per day, in place of using an elevator, would account for approximately 6 lb of weight loss per year for an average-weight man (Brownell, Stunkard, & Albaum, 1980). Second, heavier people burn more calories than normal-weight people while doing the same activity because more energy is required to move the extra mass. Nevertheless, many people are dismayed when they learn that even very rigorous physical activities produce relatively small energy deficits (Bjorntorp, 1978). For example, a quarter-pound cheeseburger, a small order of french fries, and a chocolate milkshake from a fast-food restaurant contain about 1,100 kcal. A person must run 11 mi to burn 1,100 kcal.

Table 14.1   Likely Mechanisms Linking Exercise With Success at Weight Control

1. Energy expenditure
2. Minimization of loss of lean body mass
3. Appetite suppression
4. Increased metabolic rate
5. Minimization of effects of weight cycling
6. Reduced risk factors associated with obesity
7. Positive psychological effects

Reprinted from Grilo et al. (1993).

Table 14.2   Calorie Values for 10 Minutes of Activity

	Body weight		
	125	175	250
Personal necessities			
Sleeping	10	14	20
Sitting (watching TV)	10	14	18
Sitting (talking)	15	21	30
Dressing or washing	26	37	53
Standing	12	16	24
Locomotion			
Walking downstairs	56	78	111
Walking upstairs	146	202	288
Walking at 2 mph	29	40	58
Walking at 4 mph	52	72	102
Running at 5.5 mph	90	125	178
Running at 7 mph	118	164	232
Running at 12 mph	164	228	326
Cycling at 5.5 mph	42	58	83
Cycling at 13 mph	89	124	178
Housework			
Making beds	32	46	65
Washing floors	38	53	75
Washing windows	35	48	69
Dusting	22	31	44
Preparing meals	32	46	65
Shoveling snow	65	89	130
Light gardening	30	42	59
Weeding garden	49	68	98
Mowing grass (power)	34	47	67
Mowing grass (manual)	38	52	74
Sedentary occupations			
Sitting (writing)	15	21	30
Light office work	25	34	50
Standing (light activity)	20	28	40
Typing (electric)	19	27	39
Light work			
Assembly line	20	28	40
Auto repair	35	48	69
Carpentry	32	44	64
Bricklaying	28	40	57
Farming chores	32	44	64
House painting	29	40	58

(continued)

Table 14.2   (*continued*)

	Body weight		
	125	175	250
Heavy work			
Using pick & shovel	56	78	110
Chopping wood	60	84	121
Dragging logs	158	220	315
Drilling coal	79	111	159
Recreation			
Badminton	43	65	94
Baseball	39	54	78
Basketball	58	82	117
Bowling (nonstop)	56	78	111
Canoeing at 4 mph	90	128	182
Dancing (moderate)	35	48	69
Dancing (vigorous)	48	66	94
Football	69	96	137
Golfing	33	48	68
Horseback riding	56	78	112
Ping-Pong	32	45	64
Racquetball	75	104	144
Skiing (alpine)	80	112	160
Skiing (water)	60	88	130
Skiing (cross-country)	98	138	194
Squash	75	104	144
Swimming (backstroke)	32	45	64
Swimming (crawl)	40	56	80
Tennis	56	80	115
Volleyball	43	65	94

Reprinted from Brownell (1994).

Weight loss in people who exercise tends to be greater than expected from the direct expenditure of energy (Bray, 1976). Therefore, other physiological or psychological mechanisms are likely to be relevant and must be emphasized in work with overweight individuals.

Exercise May Minimize Loss of Lean Body Mass

As much as 25% of the weight lost through dieting alone may be lean body mass (LBM; McArdle, F.I., Katch, & V.L. Katch, 1991). The loss of LBM decreases when exercise (even low to moderate) is combined with diet (Ballor, McCarthy, &

Wilterdink, 1990). Several studies reveal that regular aerobic exercise, even in the absence of dietary restriction, can produce significant fat loss with minimal loss of lean tissue (Bouchard et al., 1990; Despres, Bouchard, Tremblay, Savard, & Marcotte, 1985; Segal & Pi-Sunyer, 1986). More recently, resistance training has been used to improve the ratio of lean to fat tissue, which may have the added benefit of increasing energy expenditure (Donnelly, N.P. Pronk, Jacobsen, S.J. Pronk, & Jakicic, 1991). Because increasing lean body mass and decreasing body fat may increase metabolic rate (muscle requires more calories than fat does), exercise prescriptions focused on this goal may be especially useful.

Exercise May Suppress Appetite

A number of studies with both humans and animals have examined exercise and appetite (Grilo et al., 1993). A frequent misconception is that increased activity will cause increased food intake and thus provide no net benefit. This regulatory mechanism tends to occur only for certain levels of activity (Grilo et al., 1993).

Human studies suggest that exercise can be effective in regulating appetite. Increasing activity to low or moderate intensity decreases food intake and body weight, but exercise in the more vigorous range leads to increased food intake and stable body weight (Anderson et al., 1991; Epstein, Wing, & Thompson, 1978; Holm, Bjorntorp, & Jagenberg, 1978; Thompson, Jarvie, Lahey, & Cureton, 1982; Woo, Garrow, & Sunyer, 1982). The relationship between physical activity and food intake, however, appears to be affected by gender. Human studies have found compensatory increases in intake among females (Anderson et al., 1991; Woo et al., 1982; Woo & Pi-Sunyer, 1985) but not in males (Anderson et al., 1991).

In sum, exercise is unlikely to increase appetite beyond the level needed to keep body weight stable and often leads to decreased intake. A potential problem exists, however, since people may believe they will be hungrier after they exercise. Dispelling this notion is important.

Exercise May Counter the Metabolic Decline Produced by Dieting

Restriction of caloric intake leads to a rapid reduction in resting metabolic rate (RMR; Barrows & Snook, 1987; Elliot, Goldberg, Kuehl, & Bennett, 1989; McArdle et al., 1991; Mole, Stern, Schultz, Bernauer, & Holcomb, 1989; Ravussin, Burnand, Schutz, & Jequier, 1985; Welle, Amatruda, Forbes, & Lockwood, 1984). Resting energy expenditure may be reduced by 20% or more (Bray, 1976). This decline is noteworthy since RMR accounts for 60% to 70% of total energy expenditure (Bray, 1976; Danforth & Landsberg, 1983; McArdle et al., 1991). Therefore, the body develops ways of conserving energy that may account for the plateau many dieters reach when weight loss slows or stops even though caloric intake remains stable (McArdle et al., 1991).

Exercise may prevent or reduce the decline in the body's metabolic rate produced by dieting (McArdle et al., 1991; Mole et al., 1989; Tremblay, Despres, & Bouchard, 1985; Tremblay et al., 1986). Tremblay and colleagues (1986) found a significant increase in RMR (8% of pretraining values) in obese individuals who engaged in an 11-week training program, despite significant reductions in body weight and body fat. Phinney and colleagues (1988), however, found that when people added physical activity while on extremely low-calorie diets, their metabolic rate was further depressed rather than raised. These conflicting findings underscore the need for more research to define the types and amounts of exercise that have the most beneficial metabolic effects.

Exercise May Minimize the Effects of Weight Cycling

Among the hypothesized but only partly substantiated effects of weight cycling (repeated cycles of weight loss and gain) are increased metabolic efficiency, an increased preference for dietary fat, and altered body composition that favors greater deposition of fat. In addition, weight fluctuation may have serious health consequences (Hamm, Shekelle, & Stamler, 1989; Lissner et al., 1991). Results suggest that exercise may help counteract the metabolic effects of weight cycling to reduce the decline in RMR (van Dale & Saris, 1989), increase weight loss and fat loss (van Dale & Saris, 1989), and prevent increased dietary fat selection (Gerardo-Gettens et al., 1991).

Exercise May Counteract the Health Consequences of Obesity

There is substantial evidence that regular physical activity is associated with good health (Dubbert, 1992; Paffenbarger, Hyde, Wing, & Hsieh, 1986). Recently published epidemiological and experimental studies have revealed that even modest levels of exercise are sufficient for significant health benefits (Blair et al., 1989; DeBusk, Stenestrand, Sheehan, & Haskell, 1990; Leon, Connett, Jacobs, & Rauramaa, 1987).

One study provides convincing evidence that even low levels of activity can have substantial health impact. Blair and colleagues (1989) studied 10,224 men and 3,120 women over an 8-year period. Each person was assigned to a fitness category (based on maximal treadmill testing scores), ranging from very unfit (Fitness Level 1) to very fit (Fitness Level 5). More physically fit individuals had significantly lower mortality rates. Figure 14.4 summarizes these findings. The largest reductions in risk come from moving from very low to moderate levels of exercise, not from being extremely active. This study and others have helped counter the notion that people must exercise vigorously to obtain health benefits (DeBusk et al., 1990; Dubbert, 1992). This fact is particularly important

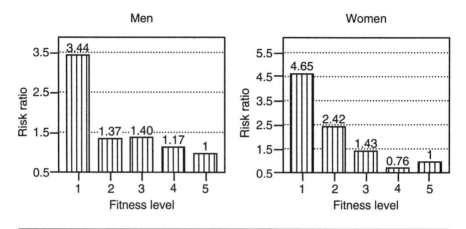

Figure 14.4   The relationship between fitness level and health and projected risk for death.
Note. 1 = very unfit; 5 = very fit.
Reprinted from Brownell (1991b).

for obese people, for whom adherence is greatest in the low- to moderate-intensity range (Epstein, Koeske, & Wing, 1984; Epstein et al., 1990).

Exercise helps offset medical conditions (e.g., high blood pressure, elevated cholesterol, and diabetes) that are prevalent in the obese (Dubbert, 1992). Exercise can provide such benefits independent of weight loss (Bjorntorp, 1992; Bray, 1976; Dubbert, 1992; Powell, Caspersen, Koplan, & Ford, 1989; Wood et al., 1988).

Exercise May Have Positive Psychological Effects

Physical activity improves mood, psychological well-being (especially immediately following exercise), self-concept, and self-esteem (Plante & Rodin, 1990; Rodin & Plante, 1989). In addition, exercise is likely to decrease mild anxiety, depression, and stress. Therefore, exercise may interrupt many of the negative feelings that often precede a dietary lapse (Grilo, Shiffman, & Wing, 1989).

Exercise appears to complement dieting by increasing dietary adherence (Epstein, Koeske, & Wing, 1984; Rodin & Plante, 1989). Rodin and Plante (1989) reported that their weight-control studies suggest that people who do only jumping jacks for 10 min a day three times a week are substantially more successful at weight control than nonexercisers. Similarly, Epstein, Koeske, and Wing (1984) found that diet adherence was related to exercise adherence and that adherence was better in programs with lower caloric expenditure. Therefore, in both studies (Epstein, Koeske, & Wing, 1984; Rodin & Plante, 1989) low caloric expenditure was related to increased dietary adherence and weight loss. Physiological factors (e.g., increased metabolic rate) alone cannot account for this because the type and amount of exercise are so minimal. Rodin and Plante (1989) speculate that such individuals perceive themselves as exercisers who are making positive changes and consequently increase their commitment to restricting food intake.

These results and others suggest that exercise need not be aerobic or of high intensity to engender positive psychological correlates (Doyne et al., 1987; King, Taylor, Haskell, & DeBusk, 1989; Martinsen, Medhus, & Sandvik, 1985; Martinsen, Strand, Paulsson, & Kaggestad, 1989). In fact, high intensity exercise can increase negative mood states such as tension and anxiety (Steptoe & Cox, 1988). Plante and Rodin (1990) conclude that positive psychological benefits may accrue from attempts to get fit as much as from gains attributable to fitness per se. Having the self-image of an exerciser should enhance self-efficacy, which could lead to increased confidence and self-determination. Plante and Rodin (1990) support this hypothesis with the following points:

- Self-efficacy manipulations throughout a 12-week exercise class led to enhanced mood and increased self-concept (Rodin & Plante, 1989).
- King et al. (1989) found that perceived fitness was more closely related to enhanced psychological functioning than was actual fitness (as measured by $\dot{V}O_2$max).
- Doyne et al. (1987) found that anaerobic exercise such as weight lifting may be just as effective in treating depression as aerobic exercise such as running.
- Several studies found that aerobic effects were not necessary for subjects to achieve an antidepressant effect (Martinsen et al., 1985, 1989).

In sum, exercise is an important predictor of success in weight reduction and maintenance and has numerous health and psychological benefits. Regardless of the potential benefits, an exercise program is useful only to the extent that it is followed. In the next section, we address issues that may help or hinder an obese person's ability to comply with an exercise prescription.

Adherence Issues

Although more than 200 studies have been conducted in the past 20 years on various determinants of exercise behavior (Sallis & Hovell, 1990), little systematic investigation has been conducted on obese people. The few articles that do exist are informative, however, and can help in developing programs specific to overweight individuals. The reader is referred to other chapters in this book and to prior reviews for a more general overview of exercise adherence, as they provide a framework from which programs for overweight people can be established (Dishman, 1991; Dubbert, 1992; Grilo et al., 1993; Sallis & Hovell, 1990).

Adherence and the Demographics of Obesity

One reason exercise adherence is a special challenge for the obese is that population groups most prone to obesity are also least likely to exercise. Obesity occurs

groups most prone to obesity are also least likely to exercise. Obesity occurs with especially high prevalence in minority populations (Ernst & Harlan, 1991; Pawson, Martorell, & Mendoza, 1991) and in people of lower socioeconomic status (SES; Sobal & Stunkard, 1989; Van Itallie, 1985). In addition, the incidence of obesity increases with age, particularly in women (Van Itallie, 1985; Williamson, Kahn, Remington, & Anda, 1990). In the case of African-American women aged 45 to 75 years, obesity rates reach as high as 60% (Van Itallie, 1985). Exercise rates for obese people, the elderly, minority groups, and those with low SES are quite low (Caspersen, Christenson, & Pollard, 1986; Sallis & Hovell, 1990).

Obstacles to Exercise for Overweight Individuals

Careful attention to potential physical and psychological barriers to exercise among overweight individuals is critical. Table 14.3 from Grilo et al. (1993) summarizes barriers to exercise.

Physical Burden.   Many overweight people find exercise unpleasant because of their excess weight and poor physical condition. Therefore, weight is a burden to be overcome. Increased activity may be difficult, painful, and fatiguing. The importance of starting overweight people with low- to moderate-intensity programs is clear. Such caution is crucial in order to prevent injuries, enhance exercise self-efficacy, and sustain adherence.

Negative Associations.   Prior negative experiences with exercise can be a major barrier to regular activity. Links between obesity and social rejection are well documented (Allon, 1982; Wadden & Stunkard, 1985). Early negative experiences with peers such as being teased, being picked last for teams, and performing poorly in athletics leave many obese people ashamed of and self-conscious about

Table 14.3   Psychological and Physical Barriers to Exercise in Obese People

Psychological barriers
  Previous negative experiences
    Teased by peers
    Poor performance
    Picked last for teams
    Feeling inadequate
  Lack of confidence
  Lack of knowledge or experience
  Shame of being observed
Physical barriers
  Burden of excess weight
  Low level of fitness

Reprinted from Grilo et al. (1993).

their bodies (Thompson, 1990; Thompson, Fabian, Moulton, Dunn, & Altabe, 1991). Many obese people also manifest disturbances in other areas of life affected by weight such as body image, social interactions, and self-esteem (Wadden & Stunkard, 1985). Hence, the social cost of obesity can be high.

As a result, thoughts of exercise may evoke unpleasant memories, feelings of inadequacy, and shame at the prospect of being observed. It is important for health professionals to help clients identify such feelings and images, to discuss them, and to find ways to make exercise more comfortable and enjoyable. It is helpful to discuss with clients what they would feel comfortable wearing, from shoes to clothing, and to explain where to obtain exercise clothing in large sizes. Health professionals should encourage clients to experiment with different activities until they experience pleasure and satisfaction. This may include exploring opportunities to exercise with other overweight individuals.

Developmental and Gender Issues.   Exercise adoption and maintenance may be enhanced if interventions are tailored to specific life periods, transitions, and developmental milestones (King, 1991). A retired woman with an ill husband will have different developmental and practical concerns than a male middle-aged executive with three children. Table 14.4 presents features and examples of physical-activity programs for several important periods (King, 1991).

It is also important to tailor interventions specifically by gender. For example, many women have not been involved in physical-activity programs. Often women have learned to diet, not exercise, whereas men are frequently taught to exercise solely for competition and thus have difficulty adjusting to lifestyle physical activity.

Adherence Studies

Exercise adherence in obese people has been severely understudied. This is unfortunate because the obese have low exercise participation rates and are at high risk for health problems that can be improved with exercise (Sallis & Hovell, 1990). Gwinup (1975) found that 68% of obese women dropped out of a 1-year program requiring only walking. In a prospective study with a large community sample, Sallis et al. (1986) found that overweight subjects were less likely to adopt exercise than normal-weight subjects.

Intensity.   The literature suggests that a less intense lifestyle, or moderate-intensity activities (those that require less than 60% of maximal capacity, such as walking) may promote better initiation and maintenance than intensive exercise (Dishman, Sallis, & Orenstein, 1985; Dubbert, 1992; Epstein, Koeske, & Wing, 1984; Sallis et al., 1986). Sallis et al. (1986) found that in a large community sample in California, both men and women were more likely to adopt moderate activity than a vigorous fitness regimen. Those taking part in moderate activity showed a dropout rate (25%-35%) roughly half that of

Table 14.4   Features and Examples of Physical-Activity Programs for Several Major Developmental Milestones

Milestone (critical period)	Specific features	Goals and strategies
Adolescence	Rapid physical and emotional changes Increased concern with appearance and weight Need for independence Short-term perspective Increased peer influence	Exercise as part of a program of healthy weight regulation (both sexes) Noncompetitive activities that are fun and varied Emphasis on independence and choice Focus on proximal outcomes (e.g., body image, stress management) Peer involvement and support
Initial work entry	Increased time and scheduling constraints Short-term perspective Employer demands	Choice of activities that are convenient and enjoyable Focus on proximal outcomes Involvement of work site (environmental prompts, incentives) Realistic goal-setting and injury prevention Coeducational noncompetitive activities
Parenting	Increased family demands and time constraints Family-directed focus Postpartum effects on weight and mood	Emphasis on benefits to self and family (e.g., stress management, weight control, well-being) Activities appropriate with children (e.g., walking) Flexible, convenient, personalized regimen Inclusion of activities of daily living Neighborhood involvement and focus Family-based public monitoring and goal setting Availability of child-related services (child care)

(continued)

vigorous exercisers (50%). In addition, moderate activity appears to be more readily maintained over the life span, whereas participation in vigorous activity declines dramatically with age (Sallis et al., 1985). This is especially important in the case of overweight people because obesity increases with age.

Table 14.4   (*continued*)

Milestone (critical period)	Specific features	Goals and strategies
Retirement age	Increased time availability and flexibility	Identification of current and previous enjoyable activities
	Long-term perspective on health, increased health concerns, "readiness"	Matching of activities to current health status
	Care-giving duties, responsibilities (parents, spouse, children or grandchildren)	Emphasis on mild- and moderate-intensity activities, including activities of daily living
		Use of "life path point" information and prompts
		Emphasis on activities engendering independence
		Garnering support of family members and peers
		Availability of necessary services (e.g., caretaking services for significant other)

Reprinted from King (1991).

Epstein and colleagues (Epstein et al., 1982; Epstein, Wing, Koeske, & Valoski, 1985) found that adherence was better among overweight children assigned to low-intensity (lifestyle) regimens than to high-intensity (aerobic exercise) programs. Because lifestyle programs are flexible and easily incorporated into one's daily routine, participants experience fewer barriers (Brownell & Stunkard, 1980; Epstein, Koeske, & Wing, 1984). Moreover, Epstein and colleagues (Epstein et al., 1982, 1985) found that lifestyle exercise was superior to programmed aerobic exercise for long-term weight maintenance (Figures 14.5 and 14.6). Figure 14.5 shows superior maintenance at 17 months (Epstein et al., 1982), and Figure 14.6 extends to 24 months (Epstein et al., 1985). Epstein and colleagues suggest that the long-term superiority of lifestyle exercise over programmed aerobic exercise is related to better long-term adherence.

In sum, recommending lifestyle activity over vigorous programmed exercise is one key to adherence for overweight persons. Adherence may be increased because of the relative ease of incorporating lifestyle exercise into daily life. This in turn may enhance confidence in the ability to perform physical activity (self-efficacy), which may lead to increased adherence. Moderate-intensity activity has many of the health benefits of vigorous exercise (Blair et al., 1989; King, Haskell, Taylor, Kraemer, & DeBusk, 1991; Sallis et al., 1986), with the added benefit of easier maintenance (Dubbert, 1992).

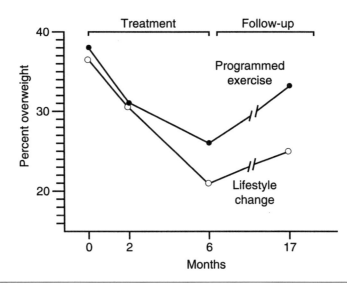

Figure 14.5   Changes in percent overweight for subjects in combined lifestyle and programmed exercise groups during treatment and follow-up.
Reprinted from Epstein et al. (1982).

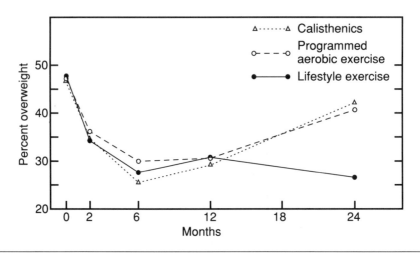

Figure 14.6   Percent overweight for three groups of children at 0, 2, 6, 12, and 24 months follow-up.
Reprinted from Epstein et al. (1985).

Relapse-Prevention Strategies.   Cognitive-behavioral (CBT) programs for exercise adherence that have incorporated components of Marlatt and Gordon's (1985) relapse-prevention model achieve better physical-activity rates at follow-up (Baum, H.B. Clark, & Sandler, 1991; Belisle, Roskies, & Levesque, 1987;

King & Frederiksen, 1984; King, Taylor et al., 1988; Martin et al., 1984). Three components seem particularly useful for increasing adherence:

1. Flexible rather than rigid exercise goals (Martin et al., 1984)
2. Training individuals in specific techniques to cope with missed exercise sessions (King & Frederiksen, 1984)
3. Identifying high-risk situations for relapse and developing coping skills to deal with risk and setbacks (Baum et al., 1991)

Moreover, relapse training resulted in significantly greater weight maintenance than treatment without such training (Baum et al., 1991). Even minimal intervention strategies geared to enhance long-term adherence and weight-loss maintenance are useful (King et al., 1989; Perri et al., 1986).

Stages of Change in Exercise Adoption and Maintenance.   Recently, several researchers have suggested that individuals proceed through specific stages in adopting and maintaining exercise and that each may require different cognitive and behavioral approaches (Dishman, 1991; B.H. Marcus, Rossi, Selby, Niaura, & Abrams, in press; Prochaska, Norcross, Fowler, Follick, & Abrams, in press). The stages of change model proposes that people move through five stages: precontemplation, contemplation, preparation, action, and maintenance (DiClemente et al., 1991).

Dishman (1991) notes that one of this model's potential major contributions is its consideration of individuals' readiness for change. A recent study (B.H. Marcus et al., in press) suggests that exercise programs must accommodate the large percentage of individuals who are not ready to change their exercise habits. Elucidation of client variables such as readiness can facilitate client-treatment matching, thus improving outcome (Fowler, Follick, Abrams, & Rickard-Figueroa, 1985). Client-treatment matching with respect to stages and processes of change in exercise adoption and maintenance is a rapidly growing area, and continued work is needed. The concepts of readiness and matching apply to both exercise and dieting (Brownell & Wadden, in press).

Large-Scale Community and Work Site Interventions.   An excellent review of community-based and work-site interventions was conducted by King (1991). It highlighted the usefulness of programs that consider the needs and characteristics of their target populations. For example, the Community Health Assessment and Promotion Project (Lasco et al., 1989) attempted to alter health behaviors relevant to obesity in approximately 400 people (primarily African-American females). The program was sensitive to the cultural and practical needs of this population (safety, privacy, free transportation, child care) and focused on nutrition and exercise information and the importance of moderate activity such as walking and low-impact aerobics. At the end of 4 months, client participation was over 60%. Another health promotion component might include methods to increase readily available forms of exercise, such as using stairs (Brownell et al., 1980).

Robinson and colleagues (1992) found that adherence to a 6-month endurance-exercise program was improved significantly through the use of incentive-based behavioral management strategies.

Social Support.   All health behaviors, including exercise, are influenced by social context. Attempts to improve weight loss by involving significant others have achieved mixed results, perhaps because of failure to assess the needs and characteristics of the target groups. Wing, M.D. Marcus, Epstein, and Jawad (1991) found a significant interaction between weight-loss treatment (alone versus with spouse support) and gender: Women did better when treated with their spouses, whereas men did better when treated alone. This study demonstrates the need to match support interventions to clients' needs and characteristics. Equivalent studies on social support and exercise adherence in the obese have not been conducted.

Future research is needed to identify the factors that mediate success or failure with spouse, family, or peer interventions for exercise and dietary adherence in the obese. Brownell (1991b) and Brownell and Rodin (1990) provide specific strategies and techniques to aid overweight people in identifying and pursuing the social support they need.

Program Recommendations

Three basic issues confront the clinician:

1. Type of exercise to prescribe
2. Ways to maximize adherence
3. Relapse prevention

Table 14.5, adapted from Grilo et al. (1993), outlines a program for the obese patient. A discussion of its important elements follows.

Avoid a Threshold Mentality

Any activity, even one not normally labeled as exercise, can provide substantial benefit. It is important to avoid the trap of defining physical activity in traditional terms (i.e., 70% of maximal heart rate, three times per week, for at least 15 min). This three-part equation (frequency, intensity, and duration) has been defined as essential for cardiorespiratory conditioning (McArdle et al., 1991). This equation implies an exercise threshold, which suggests that exercise must be performed at specific levels to have any value. Given that any exercise is worthwhile, the threshold mentality can be counterproductive. Instead, we can stress that low to moderate levels of exercise provide many health (Blair et al., 1989), psychological (Rodin &

Table 14.5   Recommendations for Maximizing Exercise Adherence in Obese People

General principles
1. Be sensitive to psychological barriers.
2. Be sensitive to physical barriers.
3. Decrease focus on exercise threshold.
4. Increase focus on enhanced self-efficacy.
5. Emphasize consistency and enjoyment, not amount and type.
6. Begin at a person's fitness level.
7. Encourage people to define routine activities as exercise.
8. Focus on compliance and avoid emphasis on minor metabolic issues (e.g., whether to exercise before or after a meal).
9. Consider lifespan developmental context.
10. Consider sociocultural issues and gender influences.
11. Evaluate social support network.
12. Evaluate stage of change, and intervene accordingly.

Specific interventions
1. Prescription
   a. Provide clear information about importance of activity, including the psychological benefits.
   b. Maximize routine activity. Define daily activities as exercise.
   c. Maximize walking (e.g., walk while doing errands).
   d. Increase use of stairs instead of escalators and elevators.
   e. Incorporate a programmed activity that is enjoyable, fits with lifestyle, and is feasible as client's fitness improves.

2. Behavioral
   a. Introduce self-monitoring, feedback, and goal-setting techniques.
   b. Identify important targets other than weight loss, including physical changes, increased mobility (flexibility, endurance, ease), and reduced heart rate.
   c. Suggest that exercise may help reduce emotional distress when risk for overeating is high.
   d. Stimulus control: Increase exercise cues (e.g., reminders for increasing activity), and decrease competing cues (e.g., do not schedule exercise when it might conflict with work or social obligations).

3. Maintenance and relapse prevention
   a. Use flexible guidelines and goal-setting, but avoid rigid rules.
   b. Identify potential high-risk situations for skipping exercise (e.g., stressful times, busy schedule).
   c. Develop plans to cope with high-risk situations.
   d. Use exercise following dietary lapses to regain a sense of control, mastery, and commitment.
   e. Convey philosophy that a lapse can be used as a signal to re-initiate small amounts of physical activity (e.g., a 2-min walk). Encourage notion that all exercise has a cumulative effect on many domains (e.g., health, mood, sense of mastery).
   f. Use minimal intervention strategies, including phone contacts, that may foster exercise maintenance.

Reprinted from Grilo et al. (1993).

Plante, 1989), and weight-loss benefits (Epstein et al., 1982, 1985). Showing people data from the Blair et al. (1989) study can help make this point clear (see Figure 14.4).

Consistency May Be More Important Than the Type or Amount of Exercise

We believe the most important question to ask about exercise is, "Will I be doing this a year from now?" It is important to help clients choose activities that will be enjoyable in the long run. The focus should be developing a consistent form of activity or set of activities. It is better for a person to play golf twice a week and walk once a week than to run 4 mi a day for a week and then stop entirely.

Provide Thorough Education

It is important to emphasize that even low-intensity exercise leads to enhanced dietary adherence and weight control. Education regarding the physical and psychological benefits of exercise can expand the client's understanding of the potential benefits. Dispelling erroneous notions such as "no pain, no gain" is an essential component. Poor health behaviors can result from inadequate information as well as nonadherence.

Be Sensitive to Obese People's Special Needs

Since the obese have special psychological and physical barriers to exercise, helping them to feel comfortable with exercise and to define even low levels of activity as exercise is an important step toward adherence. Simply conveying understanding and sensitivity can be helpful.

Special Issues

It is important to develop reasonable weight-loss goals and healthy attitudes regarding exercise and diet. We discuss here our culture's preoccupation with shape and weight and how it may perpetuate unhealthy attitudes.

The Role of Exercise in the Search for the Perfect Body

Today's aesthetic ideal is extremely thin and physically fit (Brownell, 1991a; Freedman, 1986; Rodin, 1992). Current standards about ideal body weight and shape, the overstated health benefits of slenderness, and the symbolic connotations of having the ideal body (self-control, success, acceptance) are important factors responsible for the upsurge in dieting and exercise behavior (Brownell, 1991a). Consumers frantically search for information on achieving the perfect body. The amount spent on diet foods, programs, books, and related paraphernalia nearly doubled in the 1980s and is now close to $30 billion (Brownell, 1991a). The drive for thinness has created a burgeoning market for physical-fitness equipment, exercise attire, and health clubs.

Two assumptions fuel this search (Brownell, 1991a). The first is that the body is infinitely malleable, and that with the right diet and exercise program, an individual can achieve the aesthetic ideal. The second assumption is that once the ideal is achieved, the individual will receive considerable rewards, such as interpersonal attraction, career advancement, wealth, and happiness.

Ideal, Healthy, and Reasonable Weight

The body is not infinitely malleable. Genetic factors play a substantial role in limiting our ability to change not only body weight (Stunkard, Foch, Hrubec, 1986; Stunkard, Harris, Pedersen, & McClearn, 1990) but also body shape (Bouchard et al., 1990; Bouchard & Johnson, 1988). Hence, biology may make certain people prone to gain weight or to have specific body shapes and thus may oppose attempts to lose weight (Brownell & Wadden, in press). This creates conflict between cultural pressures and biological realities (Brownell, 1991a).

This mismatch leads to the critical question of how much control people have over weight and shape. It is estimated that current aesthetic ideals (popular models and actresses) have 10% to 15% body fat, compared with 22% to 26% for healthy normal-weight women (Brownell, 1991a; Katch & McArdle, 1988). Miss America contestants work out an average of 14 hr per week, with some approaching 35 hr (Trebbe, 1979). For most people, pursuit of such an ideal is unattainable or unrealistic. Sadly, people who do not meet the ideal are thought to be indulgent, lazy, and lacking in willpower. Yet the amount of exercise and weight loss needed to pursue the ideal is far in excess of what is necessary for healthy living (Katch & McArdle, 1988).

In most weight-loss programs, weight loss to some ideal or goal weight is the desired outcome. Whether or not program staff have developed formal goals, clients have self-imposed goals, which are influenced by visualizations of an aesthetic ideal. The notion of ideal weight may be useful for people who are only mildly overweight (because the ideal is attainable) or for prevention efforts in which excess weight beyond the standard signals the need for intervention. For many people, however, the search for the ideal is an elusive goal and may lead to poor long-term results.

Brownell and Wadden (in press) suggest it is important to think not only of an ideal weight but also of a reasonable weight. Based in part on the weight-maintenance strategies proposed by Brownell and Rodin (1990), Brownell and Wadden (in press) developed questions with which to formulate reasonable weights for clients (Table 14.6). Although these questions are in the formative stage, they may be useful for stimulating clinical work and research on the topic.

Table 14.6   Questions Used as Clinical Criteria to Help Establish a Reasonable Weight for Clients

1. Is there a history of excess weight in your parents or grandparents?
2. What is the lowest weight you have maintained as an adult for at least 1 year?
3. What is the largest size of clothing in which you feel comfortable—at which point you could say ''I look pretty good, considering where I have been''? At what weight would you wear these clothes?
4. Think of a friend or family member (with your age and body frame) who looks normal to you. What does the person weigh?
5. At what weight do you believe you can live with the required changes in eating and exercise?

Note. These questions are based in part on criteria proposed by Brownell and Rodin (1990) and represent clinical impressions. Research-based criteria have not been established. Reprinted from Brownell and Wadden (1992).

They indicate that a reasonable weight would take into account a client's weight history, social circumstances, metabolic profile, and other factors. In some cases, the reasonable and healthy ideals may be the same if an individual can sustain the effort, calorie restriction, and exercise necessary to maintain that weight. On the other hand, the reasonable weight might exceed the ideal weight if biological, psychological, or cultural variables interfere. Nonetheless, any weight loss is likely to be beneficial.

Surprisingly small weight losses can lead to significant improvements in medical conditions (Blackburn & Kanders, 1987; Wassertheil-Smoller et al., 1990). Achieving an important health benefit is one index of successful treatment. Other indexes may include improved mobility or less dependence on others for basic needs. Clients should be encouraged to set weight-loss goals according to several parameters, particularly since a common trap is viewing the achievement of anything but goal weight as failure. Tracking changes in physiological factors such as blood pressure, serum cholesterol, and blood sugar; anthropometric measures (such as skinfold thickness and circumferences); and psychological changes can provide clear evidence of accomplishment to both clients and health professionals. Maintaining such benefits can be a central treatment goal, even if more weight is to be lost.

Exercise Can Be Part of the Solution or Part of the Problem

Although exercise is an important correlate of weight loss, it can become compulsive when performed in pursuit of excessive thinness. An enduring fear of being fat is a hallmark of anorexia nervosa and bulimia nervosa (Fairburn & Cooper, 1984; Garfinkel & Garner, 1982; Striegel-Moore, Silberstein, & Rodin, 1986; Wilson, 1989). Intensive exercise can be a means of weight loss or one of several tactics individuals use to counteract the ingestion of excess calories. One group of researchers investigated the functional role of exercise in 112 women who were regular exercise participants (Davis, Fox, Cowles, Hastings, & Schwass, 1990). Although only a handful were overweight, 77% of these relatively slender and active women wanted to lose weight, and 57% of them were dieting. Another study revealed that 19% of a group of female runners met the diagnostic criteria for bulimia nervosa (Prussin & Harvey, 1991), a much higher prevalence than expected in this group (Pope, Hudson, & Yurgelen-Todd, 1984). Most of the bulimic women cited exercise as their most common compensation tactic for binge episodes. The results did not indicate a particular weight or running profile (i.e., the bulimics were not significantly different from nonbulimics in mileage per week or fastest 10-km race time) but did reveal associated psychological factors (dietary restraint and depression). A survey conducted by *Runner's World* magazine (Brownell, Rodin, & Wilmore, 1988) revealed that among the 4,000 runners who responded, 48% of the females and 21% of the males said they were often, usually, or always "terrified of being fat."

Many studies evaluate whether people diet or exercise, but minimal attention has been given to why they do so. A substantial subset of runners may be motivated by fear of being fat and may indeed be running away from a vision of being fat. Because both diet and exercise can be excessive in some individuals, knowing the exerciser's motivation may help health professionals detect unhealthy exercise and dietary behaviors. For example, Brownell (1991a) suggests that health professionals can ask runners whether they're running from a vision of being fat or toward a vision of being fit. Even the use of fitness as a criterion could create problems, however. Davis et al. (1990) speculate that the pursuit of excessive thinness results from media propaganda implying that one can be physically fit only if one is thin.

Physical activity is a central component of weight loss and the single best predictor of long-term weight maintenance. Even modest levels of exercise are sufficient to offset medical conditions prevalent in the obese. Although most overweight people know they should exercise more, compliance is poor. We suggest several strategies to enhance adherence:

- Being sensitive to the special obstacles overweight people face
- Developing flexible programs that emphasize low to moderate activity
- Using cognitive-behavioral strategies for goal-setting and relapse prevention
- Above all, encouraging overweight people to view any activity as beneficial and to recognize that consistency, not intensity and duration, is the key variable

In short, exercise prescriptions that are interesting, varied, easily accessible, and without negative consequences are more likely to become habitual. The maxim of athletic training, "no pain, no gain," does not apply to a strategy of lifelong regular exercise.

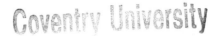

References

Allon, N. (1982). The stigma of overweight in everyday life. In B. Wolman (Ed.), *Psychological aspects of obesity: A handbook* (pp. 130-174). New York: Van Nostrand Reinhold.

Anderson, B., Xu, X., Rebuffe-Scrive, M., Terning, K., Krotkiewski, M., & Bjorntorp, P. (1991). The effects of exercise training on body composition and metabolism in men and women. *International Journal of Obesity*, **15**, 75-81.

Ballor, D.L., McCarthy, J.P., & Wilterdink, E.J. (1990). Exercise intensity does not affect the composition of diet- and exercise-induced body mass loss. *American Journal of Clinical Nutrition*, **51**, 142-146.

Baranowski, T., Bouchard, C., Bar-Or, O., Bricker, T., Heath, G., Kimm, S.Y.S., Malina, R., Obarzanek, E., Pate, R., Strong, W.B., Truman, B., and Washington, S. (1992). Assessment, prevalence, and cardiovascular benefits of physical activity and fitness in youth. *Medicine and Science in Sports and Exercise*, **24**, S240.

Barrows, K., & Snook, J.T. (1987). Effect of a high-protein, very-low-calorie diet on resting metabolism, thyroid hormones, and energy expenditure of obese middle-aged women. *American Journal of Clinical Nutrition*, **45**, 391-398.

Baum, J.G., Clark, H.B., & Sandler, J. (1991). Preventing relapse in obesity through posttreatment maintenance systems: Comparing the relative efficacy of two levels of therapist support. *Journal of Behavioral Medicine*, **14**, 287-302.

Bauman, A., Owen, N., & Rushworth, R.L. (1990). Recent trends and sociodemographic determinants of exercise participation in Australia. *Community Health Studies*, **XIV**, 19-26.

Belisle, M., Roskies, E., & Levesque, M.M. (1987). Improving adherence to physical activity. *Health Psychologist*, **6**, 159-172.

Belko, A.Z., Van Loan, M., Barbieri, T.F., & Mayclin, P. (1987). Diet, exercise, weight loss, and energy expenditure in moderately overweight men. *International Journal of Obesity*, **11**, 93-104.

Berg, M.A., Peltoniemi, J., & Puska, P. (1992). *Health Behaviour Among Finnish Adult Population, Spring, 1991*. National Public Health Institute. Helsinki, Finland: Government Printing Center, Kampin Office.

Bjorntorp, P. (1978). Exercise and obesity. *Psychiatric Clinics of North America*, **1**, 691-696.

Bjorntorp, P. (1992). Physical exercise in the treatment of obesity. In P. Bjorntorp & B.N. Brodoff (Eds.), *Obesity* (pp. 708-711). Philadelphia: Lippincott.

Blackburn, G.L., & Kanders, B.S. (1987). Medical evaluation and treatment of the obese patient with cardiovascular disease. *American Journal of Cardiology*, **60**, 55g-58g.

Blackburn, G., Kanders, B., Brownell, K.D., Wilson, G.T., Adler, J., Stein, L., & Greenberg, I. (1987). The effect of weight cycling on the rate of weight loss in man (Abstract). *International Journal of Obesity*, **11**, 448A.

Blair, S.N., Kohl, H.W., Paffenbarger, R.S., Clark, D.G., Cooper, K.H., & Gibbons, L.W. (1989). Physical fitness and all-cause mortality: A prospective study of healthy men and women. *Journal of the American Medical Association*, **262**, 2395-2401.

Bouchard, C., & Johnson, F.E. (Eds.) (1988). *Fat distribution during growth and later health outcomes*. New York: Liss.

Bouchard, C., Tremblay, A., Despres, J.P., Nadeau, A., Lupien, P.J., Theriault, G., Dussault, J., Moorjani, S., Pinault, S., & Fournier, G. (1990). The response to long-term overfeeding in identical twins. *New England Journal of Medicine*, **322**, 1477-1482.

Bray, G.A. (1976). *The obese patient*. Philadelphia: Saunders.

Bray, G.A. (1986). Effects of obesity on health and happiness. In K.D. Brownell & J.P. Foreyt (Eds.), *Handbook of eating disorders: Physiology, psychology, and treatment of obesity, anorexia, and bulimia* (pp. 3-44). New York: Basic Books.

Brownell, K.D. (1991a). Dieting and the search for the perfect body: Where physiology and culture collide. *Behavior Therapy*, **22**, 1-12.

Brownell, K.D. (1991b). *The LEARN program for weight control*. Dallas: American Health.

Brownell, K.D. (1994). *The LEARN program for weight control*. Dallas: American Health Publishing Company.

Brownell, K.D., & Rodin, J. (1990). *The weight maintenance survival guide*. Dallas: American Health.

Brownell, K.D., Rodin, J., & Wilmore, J.H. (1992). *Eating, body weight, and performance in athletes: Disorders of modern society*. Philadelphia: Lea & Febiger.

Brownell, K.D., & Stunkard, A.J. (1980). Physical activity in the development and control of obesity. In A.J. Stunkard (Ed.), *Obesity* (pp. 300-324). Philadelphia: Saunders.

Brownell, K.D., Stunkard, A.J., & Albaum, J.M. (1980). Evaluation and modification of exercise patterns in the natural environment. *American Journal of Psychiatry*, **137**, 1540-1545.

Brownell, K.D., & Wadden, T.A. (1992). Etiology and treatment of obesity: Towards understanding a serious, prevalent, and refractory disorder. *Journal of Consulting and Clinical Psychology*, **60**, 505-517.

Canada Fitness Survey (1983). *Fitness and aging*. Ottawa: Directorate of Fitness and Amateur Sport.

Caspersen, C.J. (1989). Physical activity epidemiology: Concepts, methods, and applications to exercise science. *Exercise and Sport Sciences Reviews,* **17**, 423-473.

Caspersen, C.J., Christenson, G.M., & Pollard, R.A. (1986). Status of the 1990 physical fitness and exercise objectives—Evidence from NIHS. *Public Health Reporter*, **101**, 587-592.

Caspersen, C.J., & Merrit, R.K. (1992). Trends in physical activity patterns among older adults: The Behavioral Risk Factor Surveillance System, 1986-1990. *Medicine and Science in Sport and Exercise,* **24**, S26.

Caspersen, C.J., Pollard, R.A., & Pratt, S.O. (1988). Scoring physical activity data with special consideration for elderly populations. *Proceedings of the 21st National Meeting of the Public Health Conference on Records and Statistics: Data for an Aging Population.* Washington, DC: July 13–15, 1987, pp. 30-34. DHHS Publication No. (PHS), 88-1214. Washington, DC: U.S. Government Printing Office.

Colvin, R.H., & Olson, S.B. (1983). A descriptive analysis of men and women who have lost significant weight and are highly successful at maintaining the loss. *Addictive Behavior,* **8,** 287-295.

Craighead, L.W., & Blum, M.D. (1989). Supervised exercise in behavioral treatment for moderate obesity. *Behavior Therapy,* **20,** 49-59.

Dahlkoetter, J., Callahan, E.J., & Linton, J. (1979). Obesity and the unbalanced energy equation: Exercise vs. eating habit change. *Journal of Consulting and Clinical Psychology,* **47,** 898-905.

Danforth, E., & Landsberg, L. (1983). Energy expenditure and its regulation. In M.R.C. Greenwood (Ed.), *Obesity* (pp. 103-121). New York: Churchill Livingstone.

Davis, C., Fox, J., Cowles, M., Hastings, P., & Schwass, K. (1990). The functional role of exercise in the development of weight and diet concerns in women. *Journal of Psychosomatic Research,* **34,** 563-574.

DeBusk, R.F., Stenestrand, U., Sheehan, M., & Haskell, W.L. (1990). Training effects of long versus short bouts of exercise in healthy subjects. *American Journal of Cardiology,* **65,** 1010-1013.

Despres, J.P., Bouchard, C., Tremblay, A., Savard, R., & Marcotte, M. (1985). Effects of aerobic training on fat distribution in male subjects. *Medicine and Science in Sports and Exercise,* **17,** 113-118.

DiClemente, C.C., Prochaska, J.O., Fairhurst, S.K., Velicer, W.F., Velasquez, M.M., & Rossi, J.S. (1991). The process of smoking cessation: An analysis of precontemplation, contemplation and preparation stages of change. *Journal of Consulting and Clinical Psychology,* **59,** 295-304.

Dishman, R.K. (1991). Increasing and maintaining exercise and physical activity. *Behavior Therapy,* **22,** 345-378.

Dishman, R.K., Sallis, J.F., & Orenstein, D.R. (1985). The determinants of physical activity and exercise. *Public Health Reporter,* **100,** 158-172.

Donnelly, J.E., Pronk, N.P., Jacobsen, D.J., Pronk, S.J., & Jakicic, J.M. (1991). Effects of a very-low-calorie diet and physical-training regimens on body composition and resting metabolic rate in obese females. *American Journal of Clinical Nutrition,* **54,** 56-61.

Doyne, E.J., Ossip-Klein, D.J., Bowman, E.D., Osborn, K.M., McDougall-Wilson, I.B., & Neimeyer, R.A. (1987). Running versus weight lifting in the treatment of depression. *Journal of Consulting and Clinical Psychology,* **55,** 748-754.

Dubbert, P.M. (1992). Exercise in behavioral medicine. *Journal of Consulting and Clinical Psychology,* **60,** 613.

Duddleston, A.K., & Bennion, M. (1970). Effect of diet and/or exercise on obese college women. Weight loss and serum lipids. *Journal of the American Dietetic Association,* **56,** 126-129.

Ekelund, L.G., Haskell, W.L., Johnson, J.L., Whaley, F.S., Criqui, M.H., and Sheps, D.S. (1988). Physical fitness as a predictor of cardiovascular mortality in asymptomatic North American men: The lipid research clinics mortality follow-up study. *New England Journal of Medicine, 319*, 1379.

Elliot, D.L., Goldberg, L., Kuehl, K.S., & Bennett, W.M. (1989). Sustained depression of resting metabolic rate after massive weight loss. *American Journal of Clinical Nutrition, 49*, 93-96.

Epstein, L.H., Koeske, R., & Wing, R.R. (1984). Adherence to exercise in obese children. *Journal of Cardiac Rehabilitation, 4*, 185-195.

Epstein, L.H., McCurley, J., Wing, R.R., & Valoski, A. (1990). Five-year follow-up of family-based behavioral treatments for childhood obesity. *Journal of Consulting and Clinical Psychology, 58*, 661-664.

Epstein, L.H., Wing, R.R., Koeske, R., Ossip, D.J., & Beck, S. (1982). A comparison of lifestyle change and programmed aerobic exercise on weight and fitness changes in obese children. *Behavior Therapy, 13*, 651-665.

Epstein, L.H., Wing, R.R., Koeske, R., & Valoski, A. (1985). A comparison of lifestyle exercise, aerobic exercise, and calisthenics on weight loss in obese children. *Behavior Therapy, 16*, 345-356.

Epstein, L.H., Wing, R.R., & Thompson, J.K. (1978). The relationship between exercise intensity, caloric intake, and weight. *Addictive Behavior, 3*, 185-190.

Ernst, N.D., & Harlan, W.R. (1991). Obesity and cardiovascular disease in minority populations: Executive summary. Conference highlights, conclusions, and recommendations. *American Journal of Clinical Nutrition, 53*, 1507S-1511S.

Fairburn, C.G., & Cooper, P.J. (1984). The clinical features of bulimia nervosa. *British Journal of Psychiatry, 144*, 238-246.

Fowler, J.L., Follick, M.T., Abrams, D.B., & Rickard-Figueroa, K. (1985). Participant characteristics as predictors of attritition in worksite weight loss. *Addictive Behavior, 10*, 445-448.

Freedman, R. (1986). *Beauty bound*. Lexington, MA: Lexington Books.

Garfinkel, P.E., & Garner, D.M. (1982). *Anorexia nervosa: A multidimensional perspective*. New York: Brunner/Mazel.

Gerardo-Gettens, T., Miller, G.D., Horowitz, B.A., McDonald, R.B., Brownell, K.D., Greenwood, M.R.C., Rodin, J., & Stern, J.S. (1991). Exercise decreases fat selection in female rats during weight cycling. *American Journal of Physiology, 260*, R518-R524.

Godin, G., & Shephard, R.J. (1986). Psychosocial factors influencing intentions to exercise in a group of individuals ranging from 45 to 74 years of age. In M. Berridge and G. Ward (Eds.), International Perspectives on Adapted Physical Activity (pp. 243-249). Champaign, IL: Human Kinetics.

Godin, G., & Shephard, R.J. (1990). An evaluation of the potential role of the physician in influencing community exercise behavior. *American Journal of Health Promotion, 4*, 255-259.

Gormally, J., & Rardin, D. (1981). Weight loss and maintenance changes in diet and exercise for behavioral counseling and nutrition education. *Journal of Consulting and Clinical Psychology, 28*, 295-304.

Gormally, J., Rardin, D., & Black, S. (1980). Correlates of successful response to a behavioral weight control clinic. *Journal of Counseling Psychology*, **27**, 179-191.

Grilo, C.M., Brownell, K.D., & Stunkard, A.J. (1993). The metabolic and psychological importance of exercise in weight control. In A.J. Stunkard & T. Wadden (Eds.), *Obesity: Theory and therapy* (2nd ed.) (pp. 253-273). New York: Raven Press.

Grilo, C.M., Shiffman, S., & Wing, R.R. (1989). Relapse crisis and coping among dieters. *Journal of Consulting and Clinical Psychology*, **57**, 488-495.

Gwinup, G. (1975). Effect of exercise alone on the weight of obese women. *Archives of Internal Medicine*, **13**, 676-680.

Hamm, P., Shekelle, R.B., & Stamler, J. (1989). Large fluctuations in body weight during young adulthood and twenty-five year risk of coronary heart disease in men. *American Journal of Epidemiology*, **129**, 312-318.

Harris, M.B., & Hallbauer, E.S. (1973). Self-directed weight control through eating and exercise. *Behavior Research and Therapy*, **11**, 523-529.

Hill, J.O., Newby, F.D., Thacker, S.V., Sykes, M.N., & DiGirolamo, M. (1988). Influence of food restriction coupled with weight cycling on carcass energy restoration during ad libitum refeeding. *International Journal of Obesity*, **12**, 547-555.

Hill, J.O., Schundlt, D.G., Sbrocco, T., Sharp, T., Pope-Cordel, J., Stetson, B., Kaler, M., & Hime, C. (1989). Evaluation of an alternating-calorie diet with and without exercise in the treatment of obesity. *American Journal of Clinical Nutrition*, **50**, 248-254.

Holm, G., Bjorntorp, P., & Jagenberg, R. (1978). Carbohydrate, lipid, and amino acid metabolism following physical exercise in man. *Journal of Applied Physiology*, **45**, 128-132.

Jacobs, D.R., Jr., Hahn, L.P., Folsom, A.R., Hannan, P.J., Sprafka, J.M., & Burke, G.L. (1991). Time trends in leisure-time physical activity in the upper midwest 1957-1987: University of Minnesota Studies. *Epidemiology*, **2**, 8-15.

Katch, F.I., & McArdle, W.D. (1988). *Nutrition, weight control and exercise* (3rd ed.). Philadelphia: Lea & Febiger.

Kayman, S., Bruvold, W., & Stern, J.S. (1990). Maintenance and relapse after weight loss in women: Behavioral aspects. *American Journal of Clinical Nutrition*, **52**, 800-807.

King, A.C. (1991). Community intervention for promotion of physical activity and fitness. In K.B. Pandolf & J.O. Holloszy (Eds.), *Exercise and sport sciences reviews* (Vol. 19, pp. 211-259). Baltimore: Williams & Wilkins.

King, A.C., & Frederiksen, L.W. (1984). Low-cost strategies for increasing exercise behavior: Relapse preparation training and social support. *Behavior Modification*, **8**, 3-21.

King, A.C., Frey-Hewitt, B., Dreon, D.M., & Wood, P.D. (1989). Diet versus exercise in weight maintenance: The effects of minimal intervention strategies on long-term outcomes in men. *Archives of Internal Medicine*, **149**, 2741-2746.

King, A.C., Haskell, W.L., Taylor, C.B., Kraemer, H.C., & DeBusk, R.F. (1991). Group vs. home-based exercise training in healthy older men and women: A community-based clinical trial. *Journal of the American Medical Association*, **26**, 1535-1542.

King, A.C., Taylor, C.B., Haskell, W.L., & DeBusk, R.F. (1988). Strategies for increasing early adherence to and long-term maintenance of home-based exercise training in healthy middle-aged men and women. *American Journal of Cardiology*, **61**, 628-632.

King, A.C., Taylor, C.B., Haskell, W.B., & DeBusk, R.F. (1989). Influence of regular aerobic exercise on psychological health: A randomized, controlled trial of healthy middle-aged adults. *Health Psychology*, **8**, 305-324.

Kuczmarski, R.J. (1992). Prevalence of overweight and weight gain in the United States. *American Journal of Clinical Nutrition*, **55**, 4955-5025.

Lasco, R.A., Curry, R.H., Dickson, V.J., Powers, J., Menes, S., & Merritt, R.K. (1989). Participation rates, weight loss, and blood pressure changes among obese women in a nutrition-exercise program. *Public Health Reporter*, **104**, 640-646.

Lennon, D., Nagle, F., Stratman, F., Shrago, E., & Dennis, S. (1985). Diet and exercise training effects on resting metabolic rate. *International Journal of Obesity*, **9**, 39-47.

Leon, A.S., Connett, J., Jacobs, D.R., & Rauramaa, R. (1987). Leisure-time physical activity levels and risk of coronary heart disease and death. *Journal of the American Medical Association*, **258**, 2388-2395.

Lissner, L., Odell, P.M., D'Agostino, R.B., Stokes, J., III, Kreger, B.E., Belanger, A.J., & Brownell, K.D. (1991). Variability of body weight and health outcomes in the Framingham population. *New England Journal of Medicine*, **324**, 1839-1844.

Marcus, B.H., Rossi, J.S., Selby, V.C., Niaura, R.S., & Abrams, D.B. (in press). The stages and process of exercise adoption and maintenance. *Health Psychology*.

Marlatt, G.A., & Gordon, J. (Eds.) (1985). *Relapse prevention: Maintenance strategies in the treatment of addictive behaviors*. New York: Guilford.

Martson, A.R., & Criss, J. (1984). Maintenance of successful weight loss: Incidence and prediction. *International Journal of Obesity*, **8**, 435-439.

Martin, J.E., Dubbert, P.M., Katell, A.D., Thompson, J.K., Razynski, J.R., Lake, M., Smith, P.O., Webster, J.S., Sikora, T., & Cohen, R.E. (1984). Behavioral control of exercise in sedentary adults: Studies 1 through 6. *Journal of Consulting and Clinical Psychology*, **52**, 795-811.

Martinsen, E.W., Medhus, A., & Sandvik, L. (1985). Effects of aerobic exercise on depression: A controlled study. *British Medical Journal*, **291**, 109.

Martinsen, E.W., Strand, J., Paulsson, G., & Kaggestad, J. (1989). Physical fitness level in patients with anxiety and depressive disorders. *International Journal of Sports Medicine*, **10**, 58-61.

McArdle, W.D., Katch, F.I., & Katch, V.L. (1991). *Exercise physiology: Energy, nutrition, and human performance*. Philadelphia: Lea & Febiger.

Merritt, R.K., & Caspersen, C.J. (1992). Trends in physical activity patterns among young adults: The Behavioral Risk Factor Surveillance System, 1986-1990. *Medicine and Science in Sport and Exercise, 24,* S26.

Mole, P.A., Stern, J.S., Schultz, C.L., Bernauer, E.M., & Holcomb, B.J. (1989). Exercise reverses depressed metabolic rate produced by severe caloric restriction. *Medicine and Science in Sports and Exercise, 21,* 29-33.

Morris, J.N., Everitt, M.G., Pollard, R., Chave, S.P.W., Semmence, A.M. (1980). Vigorous exercise in leisure-time: Protection against coronary heart disease. *Lancet, 2,* 1207.

Paffenbarger, R.S., Hyde, R.T., Wing, A.L., & Hsieh, C.C. (1986). Physical activity, all-cause mortality, and longevity of college alumni. *New England Journal of Medicine, 314,* 605-613.

Pavlou, K.N., Krey, S., & Steffee, W.P. (1989). Exercise as an adjunct to weight loss and maintenance in moderately obese subjects. *American Journal of Clinical Nutrition, 49,* 1115-1123.

Pawson, I.G., Martorell, R., & Mendoza, F. (1991). Prevalence of overweight and obesity in U.S. Hispanic populations. *American Journal of Clinical Nutrition, 53,* 1522S-1528S.

Perri, M.G., McAdoo, W.G., McAllister, D.A., Lauer, J.B., & Yancey, D.Z. (1986). Enhancing the efficacy of behavior therapy for obesity: Effects of aerobic exercise and a multicomponent maintenance program. *Journal of Consulting and Clinical Psychology, 54,* 670-675.

Phinney, S.D., LaGrange, B.M., O'Connell, M., & Danforth, E. (1988). Effects of aerobic exercise on energy expenditure and nitrogen balance during very low calorie dieting. *Metabolism, 37,* 758-765.

Pi-Sunyer, F.X. (1991). Health implications of obesity. *American Journal of Clinical Nutrition, 53,* 1595S-1603S.

Plante, T.G., & Rodin, J. (1990). Physical fitness and enhanced psychological health. *Current Psychology: Research and Reviews, 9,* 3-24.

Pope, H.G., Jr., Hudson, J.I., & Yurgelen-Todd, D. (1984). Anorexia nervosa and bulimia among 300 women shoppers. *American Journal of Psychiatry, 141,* 292-294.

Powell, K.E., Caspersen, C.J., Koplan, J.P., & Ford, E.S. (1989). Physical activity and chronic disease. *American Journal of Clinical Nutrition, 49,* 999-1006.

Prochaska, J.O., Norcross, J.C., Fowler, J., Follick, M., & Abrams, D.B. (in press). Attendance and outcome in a work site weight control program: Processes and stages of change as process and predictor variables. *Addictive Behaviors.*

Prussin, R.A., & Harvey, P.D. (1991). Depression, dietary restraint, and binge eating in female runners. *Addictive Behaviors, 16,* 295-301.

Ravussin, E., Burnand, B., Schutz, Y., & Jequier, E. (1985). Energy expenditure before and during energy restriction in obese patients. *American Journal of Clinical Nutrition, 41,* 753-759.

Robinson, J.I., Rogers, M.A., Carlson, J.J., Mavis, B.E., Stachnik, T., Stoffelmayr, B., Sprague, H.A., McGrew, C.R., & Van Huss, W.D. (1992). Effects of a

6-month incentive-based exercise program on adherence and work capacity. *Medicine and Science in Sports and Exercise*, **24**, 85-93.

Rodin, J. (1992). *Body traps*. New York: Morrow.

Rodin, J., & Plante, T.G. (1989). The psychological effects of exercise. In R.S. Williams & A. Wallace (Eds.), *Biological effects of physical activity* (pp. 127-137). Champaign, IL: Human Kinetics.

Sallis, J.F., Haskell, W.L., Fortmann, S.P., Vranizun, K.M., Taylor, C.B., & Solomon, D.S. (1986). Predictors of adoption and maintenance of physical activity in a community sample. *Preventive Medicine*, **15**, 331-341.

Sallis, J.F., Haskell, W.L., Wood, P.D., Fortmann, S.P., Rogers, T., Blair, S.N., & Paffenbarger, R.S. (1985). Physical activity assessment methodology in the Five-City Project. *American Journal of Epidemiology*, **121**, 91-106.

Sallis, J.F., & Hovell, M.F. (1990). Determinants of exercise behavior. In K.B. Pandolf & J.O. Holloszy (Eds.), *Exercise and sport sciences reviews* (Vol. 18, pp. 307-336). Baltimore: Williams & Wilkins.

Salonen, J.T., Puska, P., and Tuomilehto, J. (1982). Physical activity and risk of myocardial infarction, cerebral stroke, and death: A longitudinal study in eastern Finland. *American Journal of Epidemiology,* **115**, 526-537.

Segal, K.R., & Pi-Sunyer, F.X. (1986). Exercise, resting metabolic rate, and thermogenesis. *Diabetes Metabolism Review*, **2**, 19.

Shephard, R.J., & Montelpare, W.M. (1988). Geriatric benefits of exercise as an adult. *Journal of Gerontology (Medical Sciences),* **43**, M86-M90.

Sikand, G., Kondo, A., Foreyt, J.P., Jones, P.H., & Gotto, A.M. (1988). Two-year follow-up of patients treated with a very-low-calorie-diet and exercise training. *Journal of the American Dietetic Association*, **88**, 487-488.

Sobal, J., & Stunkard, A.J. (1989). Socioeconomic status and obesity: A review of the literature. *Psychological Bulletin*, **105**, 260-275.

Stalonas, P.M., Johnson, W.G., & Christ, M. (1978). Behavior modification for obesity: The evaluation of exercise, contingency management, and program adherence. *Journal of Consulting and Clinical Psychology*, **46**, 463-469.

Stephens, T., & Craig, C.L. (1989). Fitness and activity measurement in the 1981 Canada Fitness Survey. In: Drury T., ed., National Center for Health Statistics. *Assessing Physical Fitness and Physical Activity in Population-Based Surveys*. DHHS Publication No. (PHS) 89-1253. Hyattsville, MD: Public Health Service.

Stephens, T., & Craig, C.L. (1990). *The Well-Being of Canadians: Highlights of the 1988 Campbell's Survey*. Ottawa, Canada: Canadian Fitness and Lifestyle Research Institute.

Steptoe, A., & Cox, S. (1988). Acute effects of aerobic exercise on mood. *Health Psychology*, **7**, 329-340.

Striegel-Moore, R.H., Silberstein, L.R., & Rodin, J. (1986). Toward an understanding of risk factors for bulimia. *American Psychologist*, **41**, 246-263.

Stunkard, A.J., Foch, T.T., & Hrubec, Z. (1986). A twin study of human obesity. *Journal of the American Medical Association*, **256**, 51-54.

Stunkard, A.J., Harris, J.R., Pedersen, N.L., & McClearn, G.E. (1990). The body mass index of twins who have been reared apart. *New England Journal of Medicine*, **322**, 1483-1487.

Thompson, J.K. (1990). *Body image disturbance: Assessment and treatment.* Elmsford, NY: Pergamon Press.

Thompson, J.K., Fabian, L.J., Moulton, D.O., Dunn, M.E., & Altabe, M.N. (1991). Development and validation of the physical appearance related teasing scale. *Journal of the Personality Assessment*, **56**, 513-521.

Thompson, J.K., Jarvie, G.J., Lahey, B.B., & Cureton, K.J. (1982). Exercise and obesity: Etiology, physiology, and intervention. *Psychological Bulletin*, **91**, 55-79.

Trebbe, A. (1979, September 15). Ideal is body beautiful and clean cut. *USA Today*, pp. 1-2.

Tremblay, A., Despres, J.P., & Bouchard, C. (1985). The effects of exercise-training on energy balance and adipose tissue morphology and metabolism. *Sports Medicine*, **2**, 223-233.

Tremblay, A., Fontaine, E., Poehlman, E.T., Mitchell, D., Perron, L., & Bouchard, C. (1986). The effect of exercise-training on resting metabolic rate in lean and moderately obese individuals. *International Journal of Obesity*, **10**, 511-517.

Uitenbroek, D.G., & McQueen, D.V. (1992). Leisure-time physical activity in Scotland: Trends 1987-1991 and the effect of question wording. *Sozial und Praventivmedizin*, **37**, 113-117.

Valois, P., Shephard, R.J., & Godin, G. (1986). Relationship of habit and perceived physical ability to exercise behavior. *Perceptual and Motor Skills*, **62**, 811-817.

van Dale, D., & Saris, W.H.M. (1989). Repetitive weight loss and weight regain: Effects on weight reduction, resting metabolic rate, and lipolytic activity before and after exercise and/or diet treatment. *American Journal of Clinical Nutrition*, **49**, 409-416.

Van Itallie, T.B. (1985). Health implications of overweight and obesity in the United States. *Annals of Internal Medicine*, **103**, 983-988.

Verbrugge, L.M., & Wirger, D.L. (1987). Sex differentials in health and mortality. *Women and Health*, **12**, 103-145.

Wadden, T.A., & Stunkard, A.J. (1985). Social and psychological consequences of obesity. *Annals of Internal Medicine*, **103**, 1062-1067.

Wassertheil-Smoller, S.W., Blaufox, M.D., Oberman, A., Langford, H.G., Davis, B.R., & Wylie-Rosett, J. (1990). *The TAIM Study: Adequate weight loss alone combined with drug therapy in the treatment of mild hypertension.* Paper presented at the American Heart Association Conference on Cardiovascular Disease Epidemiology, San Diego.

Welle, S.L., Amatruda, J.M., Forbes, G.B., & Lockwood, D.H. (1984). Resting metabolic rates of obese women after rapid weight loss. *Journal of Endocrinology and Metabolism*, **59**, 41-44.

Williamson, D.F., Kahn, H.S., Remington, P.L., & Anda, R.F. (1990). The 10-year incidence of overweight and major weight gain in U.S. adults. *Archives of Internal Medicine*, **150**, 665-672.

Wilson, G.T. (1989). Bulimia nervosa: Models, assessment, and treatment. *Current Opinion in Psychiatry*, **2**, 790-794.

Wing, R.R., Marcus, M.D., Epstein, L.H., & Jawad, A. (1991). A "family-based" approach to the treatment of obese Type II diabetic patients. *Journal of Consulting and Clinical Psychology*, **59**, 156-162.

Woo, R., Garrow, J.S., & Pi-Sunyer, F.X. (1982). Effect of exercise on spontaneous calorie intake in obesity. *American Journal of Clinical Nutrition*, **36**, 470-477.

Woo, R., Pi-Sunyer, F.X. (1985). Effect of increased physical activity on voluntary intake in lean women. *Metabolism*, **34**, 836-841.

Wood, P.D., Stefanick, M.L., Dreon, D.M., Frey-Hewitt, B., Garay, S.C., Williams, P.T., Superko, H.R., Fortmann, S.P., Albers, J.J., Vranizan, K.M., Ellsworth, N.M., Terry, R.B., & Haskell, W.L. (1988). Changes in plasma lipids and lipoproteins in overweight men during weight loss through dieting as compared with exercise. *New England Journal of Medicine*, **319**, 1173-1179.

This chapter was supported in part by a grant from the Jenny Craig Foundation for the Fellowship Program of the Yale Center for Eating and Weight Disorders.

Index